AF752218

ENDOCRINOLOGY RESEARCH AND CLINICAL DEVELOPMENTS

NEUROENDOCRINOLOGY RESEARCH DEVELOPMENTS

ENDOCRINOLOGY RESEARCH AND CLINICAL DEVELOPMENTS

Additional books in this series can be found on Nova's website at:

https://www.novapublishers.com/catalog/index.php?cPath=23_29&series
p=Endocrinology+Research+and+Clinical+Developments

Additional e-books in this series can be found on Nova's website at:

https://www.novapublishers.com/catalog/index.php?cPath=23_29&series
pe=Endocrinology+Research+and+Clinical+Developments

ENDOCRINOLOGY RESEARCH AND CLINICAL DEVELOPMENTS

NEUROENDOCRINOLOGY RESEARCH DEVELOPMENTS

NEJC S. PENKAVA
AND
LOGAN R. HAIGHT
EDITORS

Nova Science Publishers, Inc.

New York

Copyright © 2010 by Nova Science Publishers, Inc.

All rights reserved. No part of this book may be reproduced, stored in a retrieval system or transmitted in any form or by any means: electronic, electrostatic, magnetic, tape, mechanical photocopying, recording or otherwise without the written permission of the Publisher.

For permission to use material from this book please contact us:
Telephone 631-231-7269; Fax 631-231-8175
Web Site: http://www.novapublishers.com

NOTICE TO THE READER

The Publisher has taken reasonable care in the preparation of this book, but makes no expressed or implied warranty of any kind and assumes no responsibility for any errors or omissions. No liability is assumed for incidental or consequential damages in connection with or arising out of information contained in this book. The Publisher shall not be liable for any special, consequential, or exemplary damages resulting, in whole or in part, from the readers' use of, or reliance upon, this material. Any parts of this book based on government reports are so indicated and copyright is claimed for those parts to the extent applicable to compilations of such works.

Independent verification should be sought for any data, advice or recommendations contained in this book. In addition, no responsibility is assumed by the publisher for any injury and/or damage to persons or property arising from any methods, products, instructions, ideas or otherwise contained in this publication.

This publication is designed to provide accurate and authoritative information with regard to the subject matter covered herein. It is sold with the clear understanding that the Publisher is not engaged in rendering legal or any other professional services. If legal or any other expert assistance is required, the services of a competent person should be sought. FROM A DECLARATION OF PARTICIPANTS JOINTLY ADOPTED BY A COMMITTEE OF THE AMERICAN BAR ASSOCIATION AND A COMMITTEE OF PUBLISHERS.

LIBRARY OF CONGRESS CATALOGING-IN-PUBLICATION DATA

Neuroendocrinology research developments / editors, Nejc S. Penkava and Logan R. Haight.
p. ; cm.
Includes bibliographical references and index.
ISBN 978-1-60876-983-4 (hardcover)
1. Neuroendocrinology. I. Penkava, Nejc S. II. Haight, Logan R.
[DNLM: 1. Neurosecretory Systems--physiology. 2. Neuroendocrinology. 3. Stress, Physiological--physiology. WL 102 N494536 2009]
QP356.4.N4838 2009
612.8072--dc22

2009054172

Published by Nova Science Publishers, Inc. † New York

Contents

PREFACE

Neuroendocrinology is the study of the interactions between the nervous system and the endocrine system. The concept arose from the recognition that the secretion of hormones from the pituitary gland is closely controlled by the brain, especially by the hypothalamus. This new book presents the latest research in the field from around the world.

Chapter 1- Arginine vasotocin (AVT) and corticotropin-releasing hormone (CRH) are two regulators of glucocorticoid levels and stress responses in birds. The author have found that CRH administered intracerebroventricularly (icv) appears to be a more potent stimulator of the hypothalamic-pituitary-adrenal (HPA) axis of chickens compared to equimolar amounts of AVT as determined by increased plasma corticosterone (CORT). Although the basal concentration of CORT was lower in males than in females, the former responded to icv administered peptides with a more pronounced increase of CORT levels than the latter. Peripheral administration of AVT (0.25 nmol/kg, iv) to 5-week old male broiler chicks resulted in a modest but significant increase of plasma CORT while CRH was less efficient. The combined iv administration of both peptides in the same doses caused a significantly greater increase of CORT than would be expected by a simple additive effect. The underlying mechanism was investigated by expressing CRH receptor type 1 (CRHR1) and vasotocin VT2 receptors in a mammalian cell line. Using FRET analysis, both receptors were found to form heterodimers in the presence of CRH and AVT. Heterodimerization was accompanied by a significant augmentation of cAMP production compared to administration of CRH alone. The fourth transmembrane domain TM4 of the VT2R provides an important interface for effective receptor dimerization. It is concluded that the relative efficacy of CRH and AVT in stimulating the HPA axis is site-specific and their interaction at the pituitary receptor level may critically contribute to the endocrine output of the HPA system.

Chapter 2- The gastrointestinal system is essential in the control of energy metabolism, not only because it is the site of nutrient absorption, but also because a variety of gastrointestinal hormones and neuropeptides integrate peripheral and central regulation of food intake and body weight. Among these hormones, ghrelin is the only currently identified orexigenic hormone in the circulation. Three major forms of ghrelin have been identified: acyl ghrelin, des-acyl ghrelin and obestatin. Acyl ghrelin is the only one capable of binding and activating the ghrelin receptor. Blocking the action of acyl ghrelin by receptor antagonist, neutralizing antibodies or Spiegelmer RNA has been reported to affect food intake and body weight in preclinical models. However, the long-term use of these approaches is offset by potential increases in circulating ghrelin due to the feed-back regulation. Defining novel pathways to inhibit the production of acyl ghrelin is appealing for the pharmaceutical intervention of obesity and would shift therapeutic focus to gastric targets.

Ghrelin producing cells comprise approximately one quarter of gastric endocrine cells. The secretion of ghrelin is tightly coupled to the fasting or fed state. While it is presumed that precise control in the production and secretion of ghrelin is critical for the maintenance of energy balance, the molecular mechanisms by which ghrelin producing cells modulate transcription and translation of ghrelin to match overall energy status are unknown. Their studies demonstrate that mammalian target of rapamycin (mTOR) is present in the gastric ghrelin cells and its activity is altered during fasting and obesity. In addition, there exists a reciprocal relationship between gastric mTOR signaling and the expression and secretion of ghrelin during changes in energy status. Both *in vivo* and *in vitro* data support the concept that gastric mTOR activity is reciprocally linked to the production of ghrelin and ghrelin O-acyl transferase (GOAT), the enzyme mediating the octanoylation of ghrelin. Consistent with the increase of circulating ghrelin, inhibition of the gastric mTOR activity stimulates food intake. This orexigenic effect of gastric mTOR inhibition can be blocked by antagonist of ghrelin receptor.

In summary, their studies suggest that gastric ghrelin cells may recognize energy status at the organism level. The mTOR signaling may serve as a unique fuel sensor in gastric ghrelin cells, whose activity is linked to the regulation of energy intake through ghrelin.

The gastrointestinal tract, an interface between the body and the external environment, is a highly specialized organ system that allows living individual to consume food in discrete meals as well as a very diverse array of food stuffs to meet nutrient needs [1]. The gastrointestinal system is essential in the control of energy metabolism, not only because it is the site of nutrient absorption, but also because it is the largest endocrine organ in the body and also an important source of gastrointestinal hormones and neuropeptides such as ghrelin, peptide YY (PYY), pancreatic polypeptide (PP), glucagon-like peptide-1 (GLP-1), oxyntomodulin (OXM) and cholecystokinin (CCK). These peptide hormones have been demonstrated to potently influence the food intake and energy metabolism by acting on the hypothalamus and brainstem, the ingestion and energy metabolism center in the central nervous system [2]. Among these hormones, ghrelin is the only currently identified orexigenic hormone in the circulation. Since its discovery in year 1999 [3], ghrelin has been the focus of the search for an efficient intervention of obesity. Much of the effort has been focused on the intervention of the effect of ghrelin at the receptor level. Although the ghrelin antagonism has been documented to be effective in the inhibition of food intake and reduction of body weight, its long-term efficacy may be guarded because of its potential to increase the production of ghrelin [4]. Their recent study has identified an important intracellular mechanism involving mTOR signaling on the regulation of ghrelin production, providing a novel insight into the development of an alternative therapeutic strategy to treat obesity by direct intervention of gastric ghrelin [5]. Here the author summarize the recent advance on ghrelin with focus on the regulation of ghrelin production by gastric fuel sensing mechanism.

Chapter 3- Dogs (*Canis familiaris*) are believed to be one of the oldest domesticated animals (Serpell, 1995), and undoubtedly, they have naturally adapted to humans and established a niche for themselves in modern human society. Considering the numerous other animals inhabiting the planet, the affinity between humans and dogs can be considered special. Recent comparative cognitive studies, involving the comparison of dogs with wolves (*Canis lupus*) or other species, have suggested that this adaptation of dogs to humans is because of dogs' superior social skills and cognitive ability. For example, when dogs and their owners were subjected to the Strange Situation Test, which was developed to examine the attachment patterns of human infants separated from or reunited with their mothers, dogs behaved differently toward their owners as compared to strangers (Topál, Miklósi, Csányi, & Dóka, 1998). However, the behavior of hand-reared wolves did not differ between their owners and strangers (Topál, Gácsi, Miklósi, Virányi, Kubinyi, & Csányi, 2005). These findings lead us assume that dogs can recognize the difference between their owners and strangers and exhibit specific responses to their owners. In contrast, at least under the conditions of the study, wolves cannot distinguish their owners from strangers or respond differently even if they do recognize their owners. Moreover, dogs can select an object indicated to them with using human signals, such as finger pointing or gazing (Hare, Brown, Williamson, & Tomasello, 2002; Virányi, Gácsi, Kubinyi, Topál, Belényi, Ujfalussy & Miklósi, 2008). Several studies have reported that unlike dogs, wolves cannot respond to human gestures (Hare, Brown, Williamson, & Tomasello, 2002; Virányi, Gácsi, Kubinyi, Topál, Belényi, Ujfalussy & Miklósi, 2008), although the results of these studies remain controversial (Udell, Dorey & Wynne, 2008). It was also reported that when both dogs and socialized wolves that had been trained to perform a simple manipulation task were presented with an insoluble version of the same task, the dogs gazed at the presenting human, while the socialized wolves did not (Miklósi, Kubinyi, Topál, Gácsi, Virányi, & Csányi, 2003). All these studies indicate that dogs have the ability to acquire a high level of social skills and cognitive ability such as pointing or gazing. Such abilities help dogs engage in nonverbal communicative interactions with humans, and this may be a reason for why dogs but not wolves adapted to human society, although these animals appear similar.

How have dogs acquired this high level of social skills and cognitive ability? The answer to this question has been suggested by an interesting study on the domestication of the fox (*Vulpes vulpes*), a wild canine. This study conducted in Russia succeeded in domesticating foxes by selecting particular characteristics—lack of fear of or aggression toward humans—as the main index. Interestingly, the domesticated foxes could respond to human gestures just as dogs could, whereas non-selected foxes could not (Hare, Plyusnina, Ignacio, Schepina, Stepika, Wrangham, & Trut, 2005). Hare and Tomasello (2005) proposed the hypothesis that specialized social skills and cognitive ability appeared in dogs after the central nervous system of this animal, which mediates fear and aggression, evolved during the process of domestication. The serotonergic neural system, which is related to aggressive behavior or anxiety, was reportedly changed in domesticated foxes compared to non-selected foxes (Popova, Voitenko, Kulikov, & Avgustinovich, 1991). Furthermore, the basal plasma levels of both adrenocorticotrophic hormone and glucocorticoid and the glucocorticoid response to stress were found to be lower in domesticated foxes than non-selected ones; in other words, a decrease in the activity of the hypothalamus-pituitary-adrenal (HPA) axis was also found (Oskina, 1996). Hare and Tomasello (2005) assumed that this attenuation of HPA axis activity might contribute to the inhibition of the fear response or aggressive behavior toward humans. Although the mechanism by which dogs exhibit superior social skills remains largely unknown, the series of experiments on domesticated foxes have provided one possible explanation: the changes of the central nervous system mediating the fear response and aggression or regulating the activity of the HPA axis are involved in the mechanism.

Chapter 4- Pheochromocytomas are neuroendocrine tumors that may be either sporadic or manifestation of a familial cancer syndromes and are derived from neural-crest. In the present study oncogenes — *k-ras* and *c-myc* were investigated in sporadic human pheochromocytomas in order to identify their involvement. The aim of their investigation was to identify new molecular targets of neuroendocrine carcinogenesis.

Pheochromocytoma samples were tested for activating point mutations of *k-ras* and to the levels of k-Ras and c-Myc protein expression by immunohistochemistry.

The results of their analysis showed that point mutations of *k-ras* were frequent changes, namely 88.9% of pheochromocytomas harbored activating *k-ras* mutations in codon 12. The k-Ras and c-Myc proteins were up regulated in the pheochromocytomas the author investigated. Sixty-one point five percent of samples had moderate upregulation of k-Ras, while strong expression of k-Ras proteins was not observed in any of their pheochromocytoma case. Increased levels of Myc protein were detected in 92.3% of cases. Strong upregulation was observed in 6 pheochromocytoma samples and also in the investigated lymph node metastasis (53.8%). Five out of 10 samples with activating *k-ras* mutation had upregulated levels of both k-Ras and c-Myc.

Their findings on upregulation of *k-ras* and *c-myc* oncogenes expression in pheochromocytoma samples may indicate their collaborative involvement in tumorigenesis and may contribute to better understanding of pheochromocytoma molecular profile.

Keywords: pheochromocytoma, oncogenes, k-ras, c-myc, signal transduction pathways

Chapter 5- Mammalian sex determination is dependent on a proper function of small gene on the smallest chromosome – Sry. Sry triggers the development of tesis in the male, and subsequently, hormonal secretions by the fetal testis are responsible for the proper development of male sexual organs, while in female, sexual development takes place in the absence of any hormonal exposure. Similar mechanisms of hormonal sex differentiation have been proposed for the development of sex differences in the mammalian brain with one important difference. While testosterone (and its derivative dihydrotestosterone) is the main steroid hormone responsible for the proper development of secondary sexual organs, brain sexual differentiation (at least in rodents) towards male depends on the conversion of testosterone to estradiol by cytochrome P450 aromatase, expressed locally in the brain. However, several studies in recent years have suggested that not all sex differences in the brain are dependent on the exposure to sex steroid hormones. Probably still the most compelling evidence came from birds, more specifically from gynandromorphic zebra finch, described by Arnold and co-workers in 2003. This bird, half male, half female, is showing characteristics of one sex on one side of the body and characteristics of the other sex on the other side of the body. And this does not go only for a plumage, but also for the expression of genes in the brain, where expression of female specific transcripts was detected only in the female half of the brain and expression of male specific transcripts in the male part of the brain. In this case, such differences in gene expression certainly cannot be explained by the action of hormones, as hormones are transported by blood and cannot reach only half of the brain. Therefore, there must be other causes for brain sexual differentiation (and perhaps other organ systems) beside sex steroid hormones. To study hormone independent sex differences in mammals, two mice models have been recently developed. Four core genotype (FCG) mice are mice with manipulated Sry gene where genetic sex is not the same as gonadal sex (XY females, XX males). Another valuable model is SF-1 knockout mice, in which gonads regress very early during development, before gonads start to secrete steroid hormones. These mice are therefore never exposed to any endogenous sex steroids and therefore represent a unique model to study sex differences that must develop due to differences in sex chromosome complements.

In the present review, recent results obtained by studies using mostly these two mice models, will be described along with other evidence for sex differences in the brain that develop in the absence of hormone exposure.

Chapter 6- The Hypothalamic-Pituitary-Adrenal (HPA) axis and the locus caeruleus / norepinephrine-sympathetic nervous system (LC/NE-SNS), are involved in the pathophysiology of Posttraumatic Stress Disorder (PTSD), a clustering of symptoms that develop after exposure to traumatic life events. However, diverse biological patterns of disease have been reported and this can be attributed mainly on comorbidity, biological vulverability (genetic and transgenerational effects) and previous stress history and the developmental stage of the individual.

In pediatric PTSD, elevated peripheral cortisol concentrations are noted in the majority of studies, while low cortisol is the most frequent finding in adult studies. Furthermore, in contrast to adult studies, initially elevated evening cortisol in the aftermath of a traumatic event, was predictive of later PTSD development in children. Longitudinal data on pediatric and adolescent PTSD biology have shown that progressive divergence of cortisol and noradrenaline concentrations over time may be responsible for PTSD maintenance and may explain the discrepancies between the child and adult PTSD phenotypes.

Psychobiological abnormalities, through chronically disturbed HPA and LC/NE-SNS activity, in vulnerable periods of development may have irreversible effects on behavioral maturation and may affect specific vulnerable brain areas, altering CNS development, increasing both the biological risk for psychopathology as well as the cardiometabolic risk in later life.

Chapter 7- It is well established that response to stress is one of the fundamental reactions of highly developed organisms. In spite of the fact that more than 70 years have passed since Selye began to study this phenomenon, even now many issues in this particular area of scientific research remain unclear. Therefore there is a good reason to discuss some basic questions which seem important for the future perspectives.

During the last half century new methodologies have allowed scientists to obtain much new data about different aspects of stress reaction. However inadequate expansion of the meaning of the term "stress" has made the concept of stress a bit ambiguous. For that reason it is important to study the fine mechanisms of the interconnections between features of stress at the levels of the genome, the single cell, the organism (neuroendocrine reactions and other "classic" effects) and the population level. Meanwhile, it seems that the current value of some prospective research areas has been underestimated. This applies particularly to the studies of stress that influences genomic integrity in somatic and germ cells of animals.

In this paper I endeavor to mark some prospective research areas connecting the physiology, neuroendocrinology and genetics to study common mechanisms of stress reaction more effectively and try to better interpret its evolutionary significance.

Chapter 8- Corticotrophin-releasing hormone (CRH) and urocortin (UCN) are well-known peptides whose functions, in mammals, include different aspects of stress-response, such as the activation of the hypothalamus-hypophysis-adrenal gland axis and the reduction of the appetite, respectively. Expecially in vertebrates, numerous sequences are now available for CRH, UCN and their paralogs that are collectively dubbed as CRH-family members. Together with a better understanding of their functions, the increased availability of CRH-family member sequences allowed sequence comparison and the consequent flourishing of evolutive hypotheses. Even if problems and conundrums still persist about the origin and the diversification of the CRH-family components, there is growing evidence that this family of peptides, the related receptors and their binding proteins evolved before the split of deuterostomian and protostomian lineages. In invertebrates, CRH-like molecules have been isolated and described mainly in insects whereas no sequence information have so far been derived from other models, such as molluscs or annelids. In insects, the molecules considered as the most probable paralogs of vertebrate CRH-family members are usually ascribed to the group of diuretic hormones. However, in numerous invertebrate taxa, morphological, functional and molecular data indicate the presence of CRH and/or UCN orthologs in circulating and immune-related cell types, that the author refer to as immunocytes. Here the author review the evidence connecting the presence of invertebrate CRH- and UCN-like peptides to the immune and neuroendocrine system, suggesting that their involvement with the stress response is probably one of their most primitive characteristic, despite the different anatomical scenario within which the stress response occurs in divergent metazoan taxa.

Chapter 9- An under- or over-nutritional intrauterine environment and over-nutrition in early postnatal period is associated with long-term metabolic consequences, including obesity, insulin resistance, and type 2 diabetes in adulthood. At least in rodents, leptin surge in neonatal pups may be involved in mediating this programming. Fetal under-nutrition results in reduced or premature leptin surge and maternal obesity induces exaggerated or premature leptin surge. Administration of leptin to neonatal pups to induce premature or supraphysiologicalleptin surge may cause hypothalamic programming that brings about metabolic abnormality in adulthood. Although there are many problems to be clarified, neonatal leptin surge may be involved in establishing hypothalamic neuronal system that controls food intake and energy expenditure.

Chapter 10- Steroids produced in the periphery have long been of interest to reproductive biologists. The emergence of neuroendocrinology as a dominant subfield of behavioral studies appeared to demote steroids to a lesser status than the exciting neuropeptides that clearly interacted with many regions of the brain. Seminal findings in recent years, however, have propelled the study of steroids back onto center stage. In this chapter the author identify the seminal findings and describe why they are revolutionary. These new findings have demonstrated steroids have the capacity to modify the structure and function of brain regions both related to and unrelated to reproduction. The consequences on behavior are likely to be profound. This chapter focuses on one steroid, testosterone, because it occupies a strategic position in the metabolic cascade of the sex steroids. It is a position that can influence the actions of androgens and estrogens, as well as the adrenal precursors of testosterone and the recently identified neurosteroids, on the brain and behavior. The author believe future research will reveal testosterone to have behavioral effects extending well beyond those related to reproduction. Still, the massive literature on testosterone – sociosexual behavior provides a solid background on which to begin that work.

Chapter 11- A significant literature exists on the role of psychosocial factors in cancer initiation and progression, and effects of psychosocial interventions on eventual survival, but research investigating the effects of psychosocial interventions on psychoneuroendocrine and psychoneuroimmune outcomes in cancer patients is rare. There is some evidence that stress-reduction interventions may affect cortisol secretion profiles and aspects of cellular immunity, but the clinical significance of any observed effects is not known. Questions that require additional investigation concern: 1) the significance of various endocrine and immune outcome measures for predicting disease outcome in cancer patients (i.e. disease recurrence and/or survival); 2) the optimal timing of psychosocial interventions to affect biological outcomes (i.e. pre- or post-surgery, chemotherapy); 3) the type and stage of cancers that are potentially most responsive to psychosocial interventions (e.g. early vs. late stage, tumour type), and; 4) consideration of other factors that may be mediating any biological changes seen as a result of psychosocial interventions (i.e. health behaviours). The research in these areas will be reviewed and fruitful directions for future research outlined.

In: Neuroendocrinology Research Developments
Editor: N. S. Penkava and L.R. Haight, pp. 1-33
ISBN: 978-1-60876-983-4
© 2010 Nova Science Publishers, Inc.

Chapter 1

MOLECULAR PROCESSES UNDERLYING NEUROENDOCRINE REGULATION OF STRESS RESPONSES IN AN AVIAN SPECIES

Alexander Jurkevich[1*], Marina V. Mikhailova[2], Farrah N. Madison[1], Lawrence E. Cornett[2] and Wayne J. Kuenzel[1]
[1]Center of Excellence for Poultry Science, University of Arkansas, Fayetteville, AR U.S.A.
[2]Department of Physiology and Biophysics, University of Arkansas for Medical Sciences, Little Rock, AR U.S.A.

ABSTRACT

Arginine vasotocin (AVT) and corticotropin-releasing hormone (CRH) are two regulators of glucocorticoid levels and stress responses in birds. The author have found that CRH administered intracerebroventricularly (icv) appears to be a more potent stimulator of the hypothalamic-pituitary-adrenal (HPA) axis of chickens compared to equimolar amounts of AVT as determined by increased plasma corticosterone (CORT). Although the basal concentration of CORT was lower in males than in females, the former responded to icv administered peptides with a more pronounced increase of CORT levels than the latter. Peripheral administration of AVT (0.25 nmol/kg, iv) to 5-week old male broiler chicks resulted in a modest but significant increase of plasma CORT while CRH was less efficient. The combined iv administration of both peptides in the same doses caused a significantly greater increase of CORT than would be expected by a simple additive effect. The underlying mechanism was investigated by expressing CRH receptor type 1 (CRHR1) and vasotocin VT2 receptors in a mammalian cell line. Using FRET analysis, both receptors were found to form heterodimers in the presence of CRH and AVT. Heterodimerization was accompanied by a significant augmentation of cAMP production compared to administration of CRH alone. The fourth transmembrane domain TM4 of the VT2R provides an important interface for effective receptor dimerization. It is concluded that the relative efficacy of CRH and AVT in stimulating

* Corresponding author: Phone: 479-575-4571, Email: ajurkev@uark.edu

the HPA axis is site-specific and their interaction at the pituitary receptor level may critically contribute to the endocrine output of the HPA system.

INTRODUCTION

Stress is an organismal response to environmental cues. Stress affects numerous processes from regulation of gene transcription to disease resistance and behavioral strategies. In general, it is not a stimulus itself that triggers a stress response, but rather uncommon physical parameters, time of occurrence or semantic value of this stimulus. Single stress episodes can be beneficial because they ensure robustness of an organism. However, repetitive or chronic stresses have potentially detrimental effects on reproduction and health due to continuing exposure to elevated concentrations of endogenous glucocorticoids.

The goal of this chapter is to examine recent advances in understanding the roles of two key regulators of stress response in birds, corticotropine-releasing hormone and arginine vasotocin, acting in the brain and pituitary gland, and to determine molecular mechanisms of their cooperative effects. Mechanistic studies on the neuroendocrine control of stress responses in avian species are scarce. Importance of such studies lies in the fact that birds occupy very diverse ecological habitats where they are exposed to environmental stresses including pollution, climate change and changes in ecosystems. In poultry farming, understanding molecular underpinnings of stress could eventually result in developing husbandry practices that ensure appropriate animal welfare.

1. The Hypothalamic-Pituitary-Adrenal Axis and Neuroendocrine Control of Stress Responses in Birds

Living organisms have developed behavioral and physiological mechanisms to maintain homeostasis in response to environmental challenges. A set of anatomical structures, interconnected by signaling molecules into a neuroendocrine network termed the hypothalamic-pituitary-adrenal (HPA) axis that regulates responses to stress, plays a fundamental role in homeostatic control in all vertebrates (Figure 1). The HPA axis is an important component of the physiological stress response. Hypothalamic hormones corticotropin-releasing hormone (CRH), arginine vasotocin (AVT) and its mammalian ortholog arginine vasopressin (AVP) play a central role in control of the HPA axis. CRH and AVT/AVP are produced in parvocellular neurons of the paraventricular nucleus (PVN) and released into hypophysial portal capillaries at the level of external zone in the median eminence (ME) stimulating pituitary corticotropes to secrete adrenocorticotropic hormone (ACTH; de Goeij et al., 1991; Engler et al., 1999). ACTH triggers the synthesis and secretion of glucocorticoids (corticosterone in birds and rats) from the adrenal gland (Harvey et al., 1984; Carsia et al., 1986; Aguilera, 1994) (see Figure 1). Glucocorticoids, in turn, inhibit the activity of hypophysiotropic hypothalamic neurons and pituitary corticotropes limiting endocrine response of the HPA axis to profound and lasting stressors. Thus, the HPA axis represents a typical hierarchically organized regulatory system with multiple feedback circuits (Plotsky, 1991; Makino et al., 2002; Palsson, 2006).

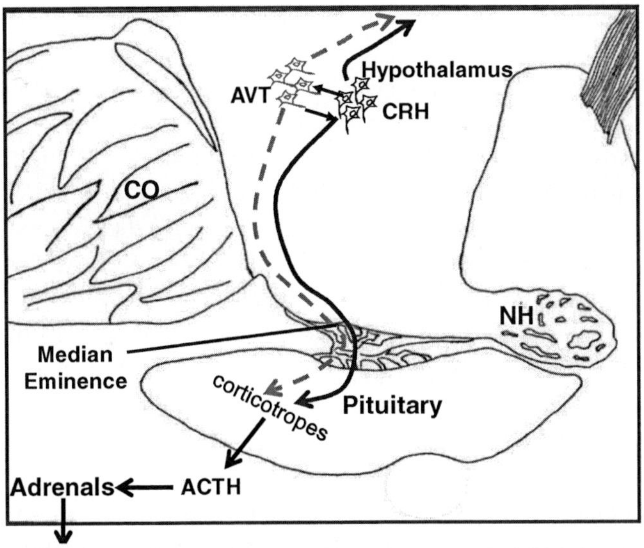

Figure 1. Schematic diagram showing the main components of the hypothalamic-pituitary-adrenal axis in birds. ACTH, adrenocorticotropic hormone; AVT, arginine vasotocin-producing neurons; CO, optic chiasma; CRH, corticotropin-releasing hormone-producing neurons; NH – the neurohypophysis.

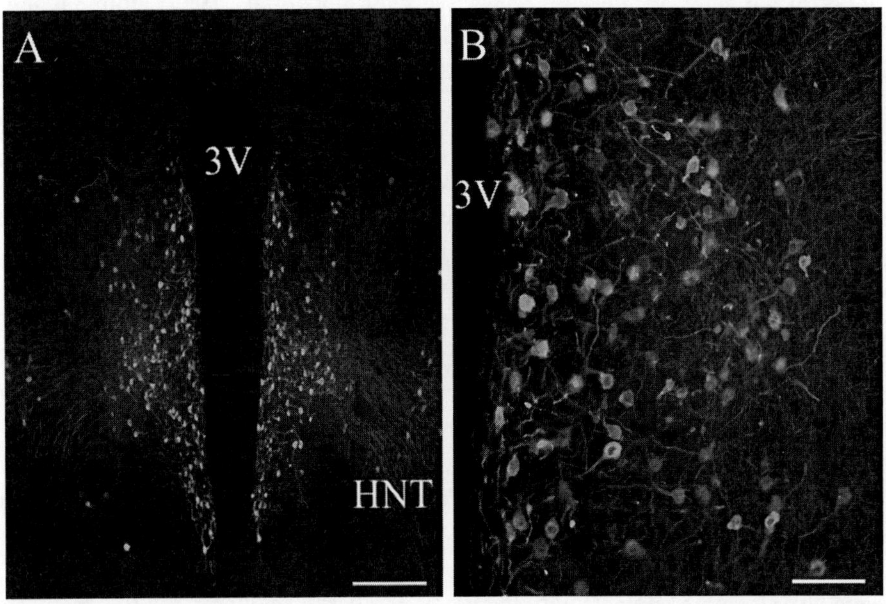

Figure 2. Vasotocin neurons in the hypothalamic paraventricular nucleus of the chicken. A, Low magnification photomicrograph showing magnocellular vasotocinergic neurons and their descending projections forming the hypothalamic-neurohypophyseal tract (HNT). B, High magnification photomicrograph showing a cluster of mostly magnocellular neurons. 3V, the third ventricle. Scale bars, 400 μm (A) and 100 μm (B).

Hypothalamic neurohormones CRH and AVT/AVP belong to two ancient families of peptides – the CRH/urocortin family and the vasotocin/vasopressin/mesotocin/oxytocin family. Both peptide families developed as antagonistic regulators of essential homeostatic mechanisms associated with osmoregulation: the former controlled excretion of body fluids while the latter regulated the retention of water (Acher, 1993; Fekete and Zorrilla, 2007). Their functions related to the control of the HPA axis may be a mechanism that evolved later and is unique to chordates (Chang and Hsu, 2004; Lovejoy and Jahan, 2006). CRH-producing parvocellular neurons have widespread distribution across the brain (Jozsa et al., 1984; Mikami and Yamada, 1984; Ball et al., 1989; Richard et al., 2004) but only those located in the hypothalamic paraventricular nucleus (PVN) and projecting to the external zone of ME stimulate ACTH release from the anterior pituitary (Yoshida, 2008).

In birds and mammals, AVT/AVP is produced in magnocellular and parvocellular neurons of the supraoptic nucleus (SO) and hypothalamic PVN (Figure 2A, B). Parvocellular AVT/AVP-positive neurons are also found in forebrain areas, such as the medial portion of the bed nucleus of stria terminalis (BSTM), medial amygdaloid nucleus and suprachiasmatic nucleus of mammals (De Vries and Miller, 1998) and BSTM of birds (Jurkevich et al., 1997; Aste et al., 1998). It is generally assumed, however, that only AVT/AVP arising from projection of parvocellular hypothalamic neurons to the external zone of the median eminence (ME) reaches pituitary via portal blood vessels and stimulates ACTH release from corticotropes (Mikami and Yamada, 1984; Korf et al., 1988; de Goeij et al., 1991; Engler et al., 1999).

In birds, the ME has distinct anterior and posterior divisions that are linked to almost completely segregated anterior and posterior capillary supplying blood to the cephalic and caudal lobes of the anterior pituitary, respectively (Vitums et al., 1964; Dominic and Singh, 1969). AVT from magnocellular neurons in supraoptic and paraventricular regions is transported along axons passing through the internal zone of the anterior ME and released into the systemic blood stream in the posterior pituitary. It is unlikely that AVT from the systemic circulation has a significant stimulatory effect on ACTH secretion from corticotropes (Engelmann et al., 2004). Moreover, chickens, unlike rats, do not have short portal blood vessels connecting the posterior and anterior pituitary (Neumeier and Lametschwandtner, 1994), and therefore blood enriched with AVT cannot access the anterior pituitary in this manner.

As a matter of interest, studies in mammals provide firm evidence that magnocellular unmyelinated axons passing through the internal zone of ME may release AVP at axonal varicosities called the Herring bodies into portal capillaries supplying the anterior pituitary (Recht et al., 1981; Holmes et al., 1986). This mechanism has yet to be confirmed in birds; however, Herring bodies were noted in the ME of the zebra finch (Oksche et al., 1963) supporting the possibility of magnocellular vasotocinergic control of pituitary functions. In Japanese quail, magnocellular vasotocinergic fibers passing through the internal zone of the anterior ME form collateral branches that cross the external zone of ME and terminate within its palisade layer forming contacts with the portal capillaries (Mikami, 1986). Therefore, there is a possibility that magnocellular neurons in birds may participate in the regulation of the HPA axis.

Magnocellular AVT/AVP neurons located in the PVN (Figure 2) and SO project predominantly through the hypothalamo-neurohypophysial tract (Figure 2A). The tract passes through the internal zone of ME to the posterior pituitary where neurohypophysial hormones are released into the systemic circulation. Studies in mammals, however, demonstrated that projections from about 10% of magnocellular neurons in the SO do not reach the posterior pituitary (Engelmann et al., 2004). In response to stressors magnocellular neurons in the SO and PVN may release AVP from dendrites into the extracellular matrix suggesting paracrine and/or autocrine regulation of local neural circuits via specific vasopressin receptors (Landgraf and Ludwig, 1991; Wotjak et al., 1996; Hurbin et al., 2002). In situ hybridization studies confirmed that the primary source of extracellular AVP in the PVN during exposure to repetitive stress are magnocellular rather than parvocellular neurons (Wotjak et al., 2001). This autocrine regulation limits ACTH secretion and prevents overactivation of the HPA axis during prolonged exposure to stress (Wotjak et al., 2002). Interestingly, CRH neurons in the PVN may execute permissive action on AVP secretion from the SO and on subsequent stimulation of ACTH release (Makara et al., 1982).

Studies in mammals have demonstrated that CRH and AVP may play distinct roles during adaptation to stressful stimuli. While CRH in most mammalian species is considered a primary ACTH secretagogue during acute stress, repeated stress is associated with stimulation of AVP synthesis in parvocellular CRH neurons in the PVN. In rats, acute restraint stress increases the expression of both CRH and AVP genes in parvocellular neurons of the PVN while exposure to repetitive restraint results in a gradual shift to more pronounced stimulation of AVP synthesis (Bartanusz et al., 1993a; Ma et al., 1997; Aubry et al., 1999). In addition, increased AVP co-localization occurs in CRH nerve terminals within external zone of the median eminence (de Goeij et al., 1991; Bartanusz et al., 1993b; Makino et al., 1995; Ma et al., 1997) suggesting augmented release of AVP. An increase in the AVP:CRH secretion ratio may be important for maintaining the secretory capacity of pituitary corticotropes during chronic stress (Aguilera and Rabadan-Diehl, 2000b).

Dual immunofluorescent labeling of coronal brain sections demonstrated that in the PVN of non-stressed chickens CRH and AVT are not co-localized in the same cells (Figure 3A, B). CRH-and AVT-immunoreactive neuronal groups have notably limited overlap. To date, it is unknown whether adaptation to lasting stressors is associated in birds with increased production of AVT by CRH-containing neurons as it occurs in mammals or whether birds have developed different neuroendocrine regulatory strategies.

Activity of parvocellular neurons in the PVN is under control of complex neural pathways including inputs from limbic brain structures – the amygdala and the bed nucleus of stria terminalis (BST; Herman et al., 2005). The medial BST (BSTM) receives highly integrated afferent information and conveys it to the PVN and lateral septum (Montagnese et al., 2008; Abellan and Medina, 2009). Intracerebral release of AVT/AVP within these regions influences a variety of social behaviors and stress responses associated with sociality: confrontation stress, separation stress, and stress due to overpopulation, to name just a few (Delville et al., 1998; Goodson and Evans, 2004; Veenema et al., 2006; Choi et al., 2006). Their studies in chickens have shown that prolonged exposure to stress increased the soma size of parvocellular AVT neurons in the septo-hypothalamic region and decreased temporally the density of their projections to the lateral septum (Jurkevich et al., 1997; Jurkevich et al., 2001). These morphological changes along with findings in mammals (Wotjak et al., 1996) and birds (Goodson and Evans, 2004) suggest the importance of parvocellular neurons in modulating stress-induced responses.

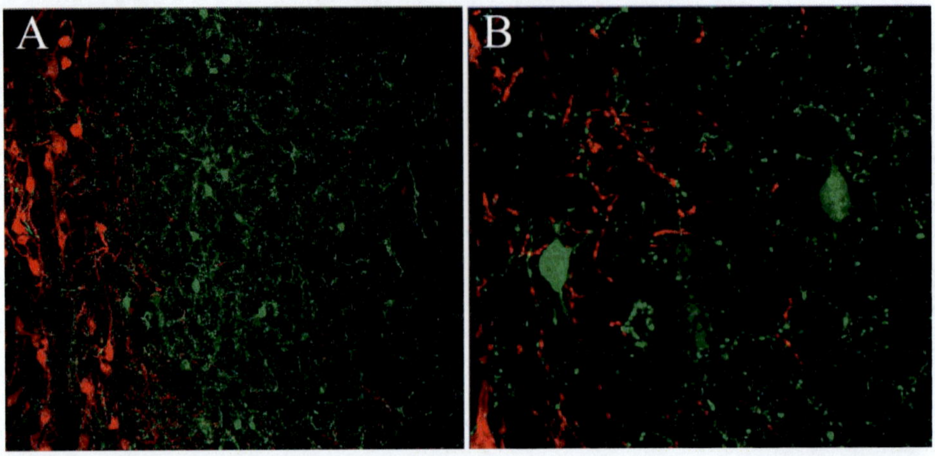

Figure 3. Corticotropin-releasing hormone (CRH) and arginine vasotocin (AVT) in hypothalamic neurons of the chicken. Medium (A) and high magnification (B) photomicrographs of a sagittal brain section immunolabeled for CRH (FITC, green) and AVT (Texas Red, red). Both images are maximum projections of 40 μm-thick stacks of confocal images. Note the differences in CRH and AVT cell sizes. Scale bars, 150 μm (A) and 50 μm (B).

2. The Roles of Corticotropin-Releasing Hormone and Vasotocin in Controlling the Blood Concentration of Corticosterone

Are CRH and AVT equipotent stimulators of the HPA axis? Available data on the relative efficacy of CRH and AVT in stimulating ACTH and glucocorticoid release in birds are conflicting. Higher plasma levels of corticosterone were found in chicks following intracerebroventricular (icv) injections of CRH when compared to chicks received icv injections of AVT (Tachibana et al., 2004). In contrast, intravenously administered AVT was more efficacious than CRH in releasing ACTH and corticosterone in pigeons *Columba livia* (Westerhof et al., 1992; Romero and Wingfield, 2001). Among mammalian species, the relative abilities of AVP and CRH to stimulate ACTH release are variable. In rat and man, CRH is the most potent ACTH secretagogue (Gillies et al., 1982; Brubaker et al., 1982; Vale et al., 1983). In bovine species, AVP and CRH are equipotent in releasing ACTH (Schwartz and Vale, 1988) while AVP is more potent in sheep (Familari et al., 1989; Liu et al., 1990; Kemppainen et al., 1993). In some cases the two hormones when co-administered display synergy in stimulating ACTH release (Gillies et al., 1982; Rivier and Vale, 1983; DeBold et al., 1984).

In order to examine the relative efficacy of CRH and AVT in stimulating the HPA axis of chickens, the author conducted two series of experiments. In the first series, 4 week-old male and female broiler chickens were fitted with unilateral intracerebral cannulas aimed at the lateral ventricle, and with intrajugular catheters. All birds were administerd icv with saline, 10 or 100 pmol of CRH, or 10 or 100 pmol of AVT. Blood samples were taken from the jugular vein remotely via an extended catheter every 15 min for 2 h beginning from the time of peptide injection. Lowest amounts of CRH (10 pmol) were able to increase significantly the levels of corticosterone at 45 and 60 min post-injection in males and at 15, 30 and 105 min post-injection in females when compared to saline injected control groups (Madison et al., 2008). Equimolar amounts of AVT had no significant effect on corticosterone levels in both sexes. The highest amount of CRH (100 pmol) induced a significant increase of corticosterone levels in males and females 15 min post-injection (Figure 4A, B). Corticosterone concentration in plasma continued to rise and remained elevated throughout the 2-h sampling period. In males, plasma levels of corticosterone increased significantly 15 min following administration of 100 pmol AVT and remained elevated during the entire sampling period although this increase was significantly lower than in response to an equimolar amount of CRH (Figure 4A). In females, administration of 100 pmol AVT resulted in increase of plasma corticosterone levels at 30, 45, 90 and 120 min post-injection compared to control females injected with saline (Figure). The results of this study with chickens demonstrated that at the brain level CRH is a more potent stimulant of the HPA axis than AVT. Because primary effects of intracerebroventricularly administered peptides are confined mostly to the brain (see discussion in Madison et al., 2008) their findings could be used to predict the effects of intracerebrally released endogenous CRH and AVT. Once released within the brain, CRH and AVT exert enduring modulatory effects on the pattern of corticosterone secretion. These modulatory effects lasted well beyond the half-life of peptide clearance from cerebrospinal fluid [11-12.4 min (Banks et al., 1987; Martins et al., 1996)] and suggested a likely involvement of secondary mechanisms. One such mechanism could be the presence of ultra short positive feedback loops found in the PVN of rats (Liposits et al., 1985; Imaki et al., 1996). Acting within such a loop, CRH may upregulate its own synthesis and secretion by increasing the expression of CRH and CRH1 type receptor genes (Parkes et al., 1993; Imaki et al., 1996). The presence of similar positive feedback loops controlling AVP release was also confirmed in the lateral septum of rats (Landgraf et al., 1991).

Their results revealed also clear sex differences in basal levels of corticosterone as well as in endocrine responses to centrally administered CRH and AVT. Undisturbed males had significantly lower basal concentration of corticosterone in circulation compared to undisturbed females (Figure 4). Males also responded to icv injections of CRH and AVT with more pronounced release of corticosterone than females. These findings are in agreement with an earlier study showing that adult white leghorn males had significantly higher levels of corticosterone in response to ACTH administration when compared to females (Schmeling and Nockels, 1978). Male broiler chickens exposed to acute stress showed a higher increase in corticosterone levels and benzodiazepine receptors than females (Marin et al., 2002). In general, male chickens have been shown to be more fearful, and therefore they may be more stress-susceptible than females (Banks et al., 1979; Jones, 1987). In seasonal avian breeders differential responsiveness of the HPA axis in males and females could be associated with a specific part of the annual cycle. In spring, free-living male house sparrows responded to capture and restraint stress with higher total corticosterone levels than females (Romero et al., 2006). However during other stages of the annual cycle no sex differences in response to stress were detected. The mechanisms of sex-dependent responsiveness of the avian HPA axis to stressors are poorly understood. One possible explanation could be the presence of sex differences in AVT- and CRH-expressing cells (Jurkevich et al., 1997; Rivalland et al., 2005; Iwasaki-Sekino et al., 2009) or/and distribution of AVT, CRH and glucocorticoid receptors (Koch et al., 2002; Lim et al., 2005).

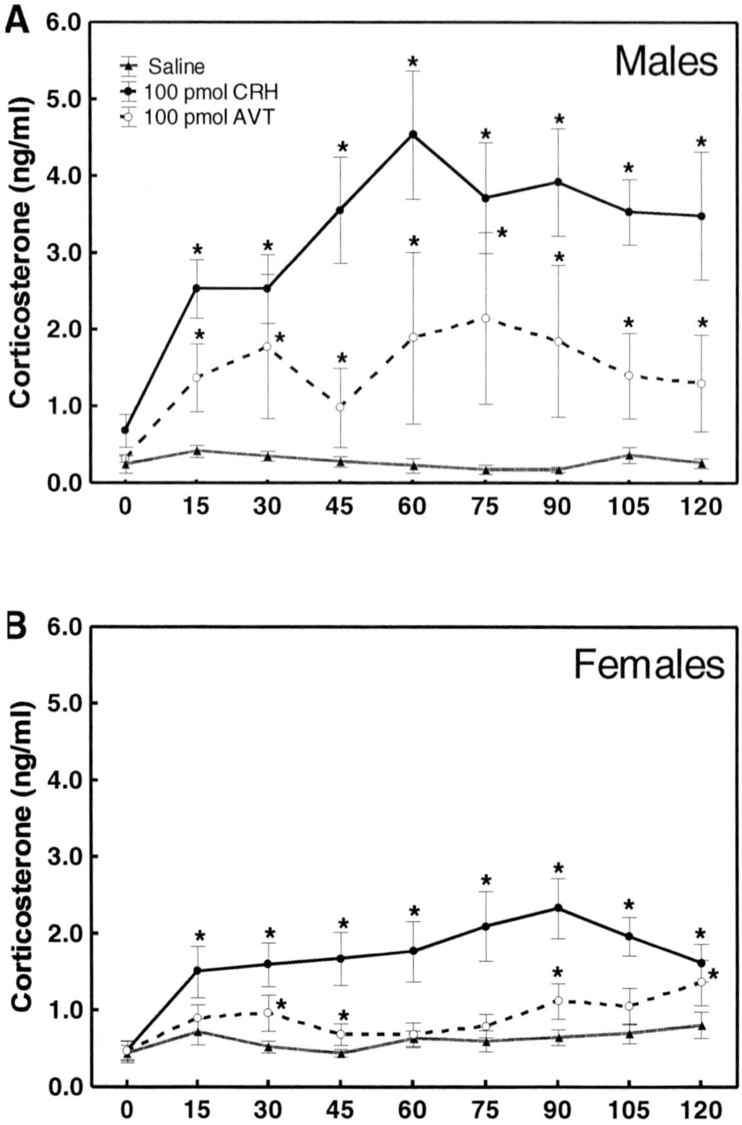

Figure 4. Effects of intracerebroventricular administration of equimolar amounts of CRH and AVT on plasma corticosterone concentration in male (A, n=6/time point) and female (B, n=7/time point) broiler chickens. A zero time point corresponds to the blood sample taken before hormone administration. Data are presented as means ± standard error of means (SEM). An asterisk above the value indicates significant differences ($p<0.05$) between hormone-treated birds and controls for that time point. **Reprinted from General and Comparative Endocrinology, 155(5), Madison et al., "Sex differences in** plasma corticosterone release in undisturbed chickens (*Gallus gallus*) in response to arginine vasotocin and corticosterone releasing hormone", 566-573, *Copyright 2008,* with permission from Elsevier.

In the second series of experiments (Mikhailova et al., 2007) 5 week-old male chickens received peripheral (intravenous, iv) injections of 0.25 nmol/kg AVT or 0.3 nmol/kg CRH. AVT induced a moderate but significant elevation of plasma corticosterone levels while CRH in the nearly equimolar dose was not effective (Figure 5). However when the same doses of

AVT and CRH were given in combination, the concentration corticosterone increased remarkably over the levels induced by each of the peptides alone. Similar synergistic effects of combined administration of AVT/AVP and CRH on ACTH and glucocorticoid release were reported *in vivo* in humans and rats (Rivier and Vale, 1983; DeBold et al., 1984) and *in vitro* (on ACTH release) in a number of various species from fish to mammals (Gillies et al., 1982; Castro et al., 1986; Evans et al., 1988; Familari et al., 1989; Liu et al., 1990; Baker et al., 1996) indicating that cooperative interactions between two hypothalamic peptides have evolved early during phylogeny. These data also suggest that primary synergistic interaction between AVT/AVP and CRH occurs most likely at the level of pituitary corticotropes stimulating subadditive release of ACTH that in turn results in augmented secretion of glucocorticoids from the adrenals. A possible molecular mechanism of this superadditive effect is presented in section 4 of this chapter. Collectively, their results demonstrate that the efficacy of CRH and AVT in stimulating the HPA axis in chickens depends on the site of their action and that concurrent targeting of the pituitary corticotropes by both peptides may result in pronounced superadditive stimulation of the glucocorticoid release.

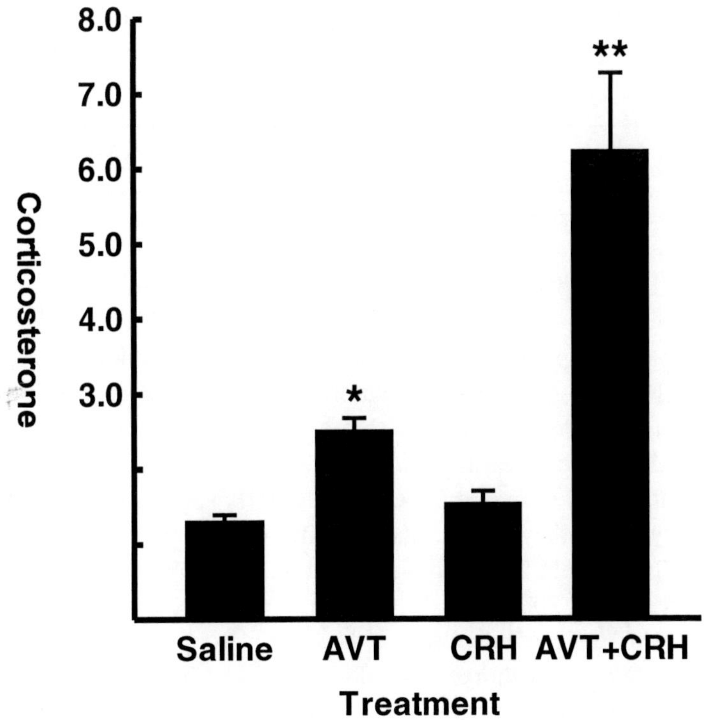

Figure 5. Plasma corticosterone concentration following intravenous administration of CRH and AVT to male chickens (n=6). Corticosterone was measured 30 min after administration of either saline, 0.25 nmol/kg AVT, 0.3 nmol/kg CRH or 0.25 nmol/kg AVT and 0.3 nmol/kg CRH concurrently. Data are presented as means ± SEM. *p<0.05 when compared to the control group, **p<0.01 when compared to the other treatments. Reprinted with permission from Mikhailova et al. "Heterooligomerization between vasotocin and corticotropin-releasing hormone (CRH) receptors augments CRH-stimulated 3',5'-cyclic adenosine monophosphate production", Molecular Endocrinology, 21(9), 2007, 2178-88. *Copyright 2007, The Endocrine Society.*

Table 1. Avian vasotocin receptor isoforms and their functions

Avian AVT receptor isoform	Mammalian AVP/OT receptor homolog	Signal transduction pathway activated	Tissue distribution	Physiological function
VT1	--	Ca^{+2} mobilization	Shell gland, endometrium (birds), brain	Unknown
VT2	V1b	Ca^{+2} mobilization	Corticotropes	ACTH release, social behavior (mammals)
VT3	Oxytocin	Ca^{+2} mobilization	Oviduct (shell gland) myometrium, breast ductal tissue (mammals)	Parturition (mammals), milk ejection (mammals), egg laying (birds)
VT4	V1a	Ca^{+2} mobilization	Vascular smooth muscle, liver, brain	Blood pressure regulation, glucose homeostasis, social behavior (mammals)
--	V2	cAMP production	Kidney collecting ducts (mammals)	Water balance

3. CRH and AVT Receptors Mediating Stress Responses

G protein-coupled receptors for CRH and AVT mediate important signal transduction within the avian HPA axis. Two different isoforms of CRH receptors, termed CRHR1 and CRHR2, have been identified in chickens (Yu et al., 1996; De Groef et al., 2004). Both CRHR1 and CRHR2 are expressed in the main brain parts – tel- and diencephalon, olfactory lobes, cerebellum and brain stem (De Groef et al., 2004). These receptors are also found in the anterior pituitary where they are expressed in different cell types: CRHR1 is expressed in corticotropes (De Groef et al., 2003; Mikhailova et al., 2007) while CRHR2 is expressed in thyrotropes (De Groef et al., 2003).

Receptors for AVT are more diverse. To date, their group has cloned and characterized four isoforms of chicken vasotocin receptors designated as VT1, VT2, VT3 and VT4 (Table 1). The VT1 receptor (VT1R) is expressed in the shell gland and brain (Tan et al., 2000). The VT2R gene is primarily expressed in the pituitary gland (Cornett et al., 2003; Jurkevich et al., 2005). Phylogenetic comparison of the VT2R amino acid sequence with that of other AVP/OT receptor family members has revealed that the VT2R is most closely related to the mammalian vasopressin V1b receptor subtype (Baeyens and Cornett, 2006). The VT3R is a 391 amino acid polypeptide (Gubrij et al., 2005) expressed in the myometrium of the avian shell gland and is likely involved in oviposition (Olson and Hertelendy, 1983; Saito and Koike, 1992). Recently, the expression of the VT3R was found in the brain of a songbird (Leung and Maney, 2009). The screening of the sequenced chicken genome (Hillier et al., 2004) led us to a fourth vasotocin receptor isoform termed the VT4R. The VT4R gene is located on chicken chromosome 1. From phylogenetic analysis, the VT4 receptor has 73% identity with the mammalian V1a receptor and, as its mammalian ortholog, is likely to be expressed in the brain. The brain expression of this receptor was recently confirmed in a songbird (Leung and Maney, 2009).

Out of four AVT receptor isoforms, stress-related functions of the VT2R seem to be the most conspicuous at this time. In chickens, cells containing immunoreactive VT2R were found in the cephalic lobe of the anterior pituitary (Jurkevich et al., 2005). In non-stressed chickens, immunoreactive VT2R is always associated with the plasma membrane (Figure 6A). A series of dual and triple immunofluorescent labeling experiments (Jurkevich et al., 2008) has demonstrated that VT2R is expressed in most corticotropes producing ACTH and α-melanocyte-stimulating hormone (α-MSH) (Figure 7). Some 10% of lactotropes also express the VT2R (Figure 8) (Jurkevich et al., 2008). These findings are in good agreement showing an important role of AVT in regulating endocrine output from corticotropes in birds (Castro et al., 1988; Madison et al., 2008).

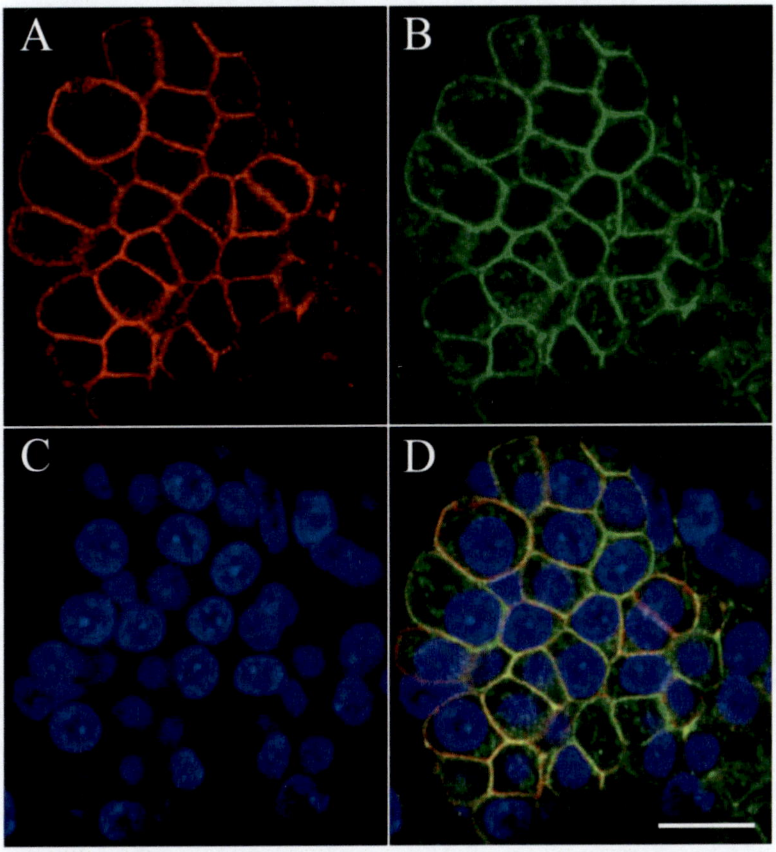

Figure 6. Cells in the cephalic lobe of chicken anterior pituitary gland immunolabeled for vasotocin VT2 receptor (VT2R) and CRH receptor type 1 (CRHR1). Images of 0.8 μm-thick single optical slices taken using a laser scanning confocal microscope. A, Immunofluorescent labeling of VT2R (Rhodamine-Red-X, red). B, Immunofluorescent labeling of CRHR1 (FITC, green). C, Cell nuclei labeled with 4′,6-diamidino-2-phenylindone (DAPI, blue). D, Superimposed images from panels A, B and C to demonstrate colocalization of VT2R and CRHR1 in the plasma membrane. Scale bar, 10 μm.

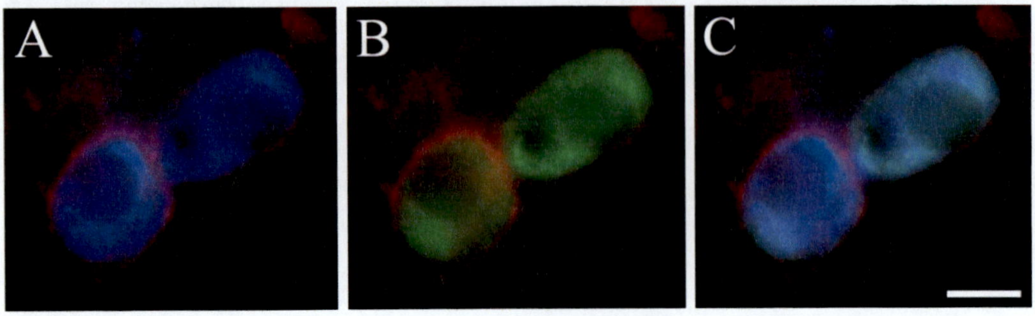

Figure 7. Vasotocin VT2 receptors in pituitary corticotropes of chicken. Triple immunofluorescent labeling using antisera against chicken vasotocin VT2 receptor (VT2R, red), adrenocorticotropic hormone ($ACTH_{1-24}$, blue) and α–melanocyte-stimulating hormone (α-MSH, green). A, Cells labeled for VT2R and ACTH. B, The same cells labeled for VT2R and α-MSH. C, Overlay image of the same cells combining the three color fluorescence images. Scale bar, 5 μm (A-C).

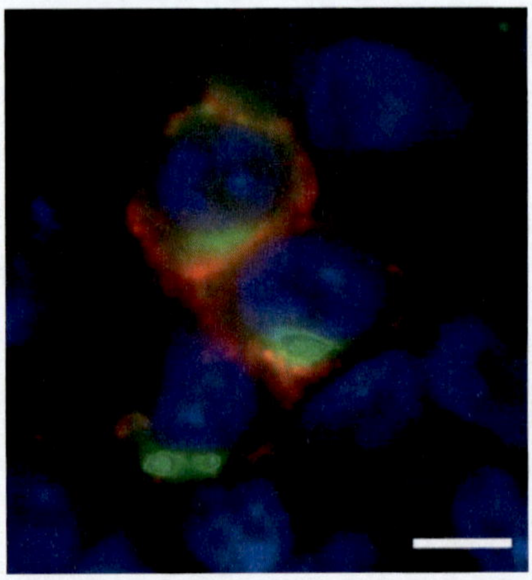

Figure 8. Vasotocin VT2 receptors (VT2R) in pituitary lactotropes of the chicken. Dual immunofluorescent labeling for VT2R (Rhodamine-Red-X, red) and prolactin (FITC, green). Cell nuclei are labeled with DAPI (blue). Scale bar, 5 μm.

In birds the VT2R is considered homologous to the mammalian V1b receptor (Table 1). In mammals, AVP and CRH stimulate secretion of ACTH via V1bR and CRH-R1 receptors, respectively. In contrast to CRH upregulating levels of POMC gene transcripts in the pituitary, AVP has weak or no effect on POMC gene expression (Smith et al., 1993; Aoki et al., 1997); it does, however, influence POMC mRNA stability or processing (Levin et al., 1989). Recent experiments using transgenic mice deficient in either CRHR1 or V1b receptors revealed receptor-specific mechanisms behind hypothalamic control of ACTH release from corticotropes in basal conditions and following stress. Perhaps the most curious finding was that basal levels of ACTH in mice lacking functional CRHR1 or V1b receptors did not differ from their wild-type counterparts (Timpl et al., 1998; Lolait et al., 2007). More detailed analysis revealed a compensatory upregulation of AVP synthesis in the paraventricular nucleus of CRHR1-deficient mice (Muller et al., 2000) while deficiency in V1b receptors did not require upregulation of CRH or oxytocin synthesis in order to maintain basal ACTH levels in undisturbed mice (Lolait et al., 2007). In animals exposed to chronic stress caused by repetitive restraint the presence of functionally intact V1b receptor was necessary for a proper endocrine response of corticotropes. However in an acute stress paradigm the role of V1b receptor was found to be stressor-dependent: V1b receptor was required for a normal HPA axis response to insulin-induced hypoglycemic stress but not to acute restraint (Lolait et al., 2007).

Reactivity of the HPA axis during stress is modulated by the hypothalamic output of CRH and AVP as well as by their interaction with specific receptors on During acute stress, rapid internalization of V1b receptors and subsequent desensitization of the ACTH response to AVP contribute to vasopressinergic mechanisms of plasticity (Hassan and Mason, 2005). In rats, both CRH and AVP receptors are activated during stress, however only changes in pituitary V1b receptor levels correlate with changes in ACTH release (for review see Aguilera, 1994; Aguilera et al., 2004). Importantly, upregulation of V1b receptors in the pituitary during chronic stress is associated with an increase in AVP expression in parvocellular neurons (Aguilera and Rabadan-Diehl, 2000a). More fundamental differences between effects of AVP and CRH on corticotropes occur at the postreceptor level. CRH upregulates levels of POMC gene transcripts while AVP has a weak or no effect on POMC gene expression (Smith et al., 1993; Aoki et al., 1997), but affects POMC mRNA stability or processing (Levin et al., 1989). As mentioned earlier, concurrent action of CRH and AVP/AVT on corticotropes results in synergistic increase of ACTH release. The exact mechanism of this effect is not fully understood. Studies in rats have shown functionally different populations of corticotropes activated solely by CRH, by either CRH or AVP, or by both secretagogues (Jia et al., 1991). It was suggested that synergistic effects may occur only in a latter population of corticotropes (Scott and Dinan, 1998) and likely involve coupling of two intracellular signaling pathways – CRH-activated protein kinase A and AVP-activated protein kinase C (Giguere and Labrie, 1982; Aguilera et al., 1983; Liu et al., 1990).

Robust synergistic effect of CRH and AVT on the HPA axis (see section 3 of this chapter) suggested that both hormones may target the same corticotropes and prompted us to examine whether VT2R and CRH receptors (CRHR) are co-localized in corticotropes. Using dual-labeling immunohistochemistry the author found that VT2R and CRHR are highly co-localized and occur almost solely in the plasma membrane of corticotropes (Figure 7). Abundant co-localization suggested that cooperative effects of CRH and AVT at the level of corticotropes could be an important prerequisite to augment the response of the HPA axis.

As yet, the avian AVT and CRH receptor isoforms involved in the cerebral control of stress responses remain unidentified. In mammals, central vasopressinergic control of the HPA axis is achieved through specific AVP receptors expressed in various brain structures. Out of three known AVP receptor subtypes, the V1a receptor has a major distribution in brain including the olfactory system, basal forebrain, lateral septum, hippocampus, amygdala, SON, PVN and other hypothalamic nuclei, raphe, ventral tegmental area, substantia nigra and nucleus ambiguous (Szot et al., 1994; Ostrowski et al., 1994; Hurbin et al., 2002). Also, the V1a receptor has been shown to be present in rat pituitary gonadotropes (Alonso et al., 1986). Similarly, V1b receptor-expressing and -immunoreactive cells are found in the brain including the olfactory bulbs, basal ganglia, lateral septum, hippocampus, hypothalamus (PVN, SON, suprachiasmatic nucleus) and medial habenula (Vaccari et al., 1998; Hernando et al., 2001). Both V1a and V1b receptor subtypes are co-localized in magnocellular vasopressinergic neurons although the immunohistochemical methods revealed higher staining intensities for the V1a receptor than for the V1b receptor (Hurbin et al., 1998; Hurbin et al., 2002). All neural structures listed above that contained V1a and V1b receptors likewise contain oxytocin (OT) receptors. Additionally, OT receptors occur in the bed nucleus of the stria terminalis, SON, PVN and ventromedial hypothalamic nucleus (Vaccari et al., 1998; Lim et al., 2004). The prevailing distribution of AVP and OT receptors in hypothalamic and limbic areas indicate their roles in behavioral, emotional, endocrine and autonomic components of stress responses (Cullinan et al., 1995). Available results suggest that V1b receptors mediate primarily anxiety- and depression-like components of reaction to stress (Griebel et al., 2003). In contrast, the potential role of central V1a receptors in stress responses is poorly understood. Recent findings revealed important functions of this receptor in neural pathways activating the HPA axis during stress (Wotjak et al., 2002; Ma et al., 2005). A critical role of V1a receptors in socially relevant stress responses has been also demonstrated (Wang et al., 1994; Ebner et al., 1999; Goodson et al., 2006; Ferris et al., 2006).

4. Molecular Interactions between CRH and AVT Receptors

Traditionally, G protein-coupled receptors (GPCR), including receptors for peptide hormones, have been considered to function as monomeric proteins. This concept has been recently challenged by biophysical studies that have demonstrated GPCR oligomerization (reviewed in Park et al., 2004; Milligan, 2009). Increasing evidence suggests that receptor oligomerization may play a role in the modulation of GPCR activity. For example, the formation of heterodimers between type 1 angiotensin II receptors and bradykinin B2 receptors results in increased activation of $G\alpha q$ and $G\alpha i$ proteins (AbdAlla et al., 2000), and dimerization of adenosine A2A and dopamine D3 receptors leads to diminished functional signaling by D3 receptors (Gines et al., 2000). The $GABA_B$, β_2-adrenergic, dopamine and prostaglandin receptors have all been shown to dimerize at some point in their life cycle (Barns, 2006; Milligan, 2009). Functional roles of dimerization include proper packaging, transport, and signal transduction, among others (Maggio et al., 2005), but the specific molecular determinants required for receptor-receptor oligoimerization are still unknown.

Determination of protein-protein interaction is an important step in studying receptor dimerization. Several well developed methods including microscopy, co-immunoprecipitation or co-immunolocalization have being used to determine homo- and heterooligomerization of receptors (Milligan and Bouvier, 2005). However, the protein-protein interaction assays require the use of solvents and detergents for extraction of membrane proteins. As a result of the invasive extraction procedure, the structure of extracted membrane proteins may not represent the actual protein organization in the cell.

The methods based on the use of fluorescent-fused proteins overcome the invasive nature of protein-protein interaction assays. In their laboratory the author use cyan fluorescent protein (CFP) and yellow fluorescent protein (YFP) fused with the chicken CRHR1 and vasotocin VT2 receptors using the pECFP-N1 and pEYFP-N1 vectors respectively. Using confocal microscopy the author found that CRHR1-CFP and VT2R-YFP were expressed on the cell surface in transiently transfected HeLa cells. Upon expression in HeLa cells, the CRHR1-CFP and VT2R-YFP fusion proteins were capable of activating their signal transduction pathways - cyclic AMP production and calcium mobilization, respectively. The VT2R, when expressed in fura-2-loaded HeLa cells, was able to induce a rapid rise of intracellular calcium after the addition of 0.1 μM AVT, similar to the VT2R receptor when expressed in fura-2-loaded COS7 cells in an earlier study (Cornett et al., 2003). Non-transfected fura-2-loaded HeLa cells did not respond to the addition of 0.1 μM AVT (Figure 9). The kinetics of the response was similar for VT2Rs expressed in both cell lines and was consistent with that observed with other Gq-coupled receptors (Ueda et al., 1991; Tanaka et al., 1995).

CRH binding to specific receptors on corticotropes is associated with an increase in intracellular cyclic AMP levels (Perrin et al., 1993; Hillhouse et al., 2002). In non-transfected HeLa cells and cells transfected with the pECFP-N1 expression plasmid, CRH did not increase cyclic AMP production (Figure 10), indicating an absence of CRH receptors in HeLa cells. However, in HeLa cells transfected with CRHR1-CFP, cyclic AMP levels were significantly ($p<0.05$) elevated upon the addition of CRH (Figure 10).

FRET analysis

Fluorescence resonance energy transfer (FRET) analysis is one of the most commonly used non-invasive techniques to study protein-protein interaction. The author used FRET analysis to reveal possible molecular interactions between CRHR1 and VT2 receptors. This method detects the transfer of excitation energy from a donor fluorophore to a nearby acceptor that can occur only over a distance of about 3-7 nm (Marcelli et al., 1998; Periasamy and Day, 1999; Elangovan et al., 2003; Chen et al., 2007). In order to obtain a quantitative measure of FRET efficiency and estimate the distance between donor and acceptor molecules from the same cell, imaging data were processed using PFRET software obtained from the W. K. Keck Center for Cellular Imaging (University of Virginia) (Elangovan et al., 2003). In some instances, dimers can form between two fluorescent protein molecules regardless of the existence of any other dimerization of the proteins fused to these fluorescent proteins (Zacharias et al., 2002). To prevent nonspecific interaction between fluorescent parts of the fluorescent-fused proteins, a single point mutation of Ala^{207} to Lys was performed in the fluorescent parts of the CRHR1-CFP, VT2R-CFP and VT2R-YFP fusion proteins, as well as in the β_2-adrenergic receptor-YFP fusion protein (β_2AR-YFP) which was used as a negative control. The mutated variants of the fusion proteins were expressed in the same cellular compartments as wild-type receptors. FRET analysis of different combinations using mutant and wild-type proteins showed that dimerization of CRHR1 and VT2R occurred between the receptor proteins themselves and not between the fluorescent parts of the fusion proteins. Their results also showed that neither the CRHR1 nor the VT2R were able to dimerize with the β_2-adrenergic receptor. This observation further demonstrated the specificity of the interaction between the CRHR1-CFP and the VT2R-YFP.

Quantitative FRET analysis (Figure 11) demonstrated that CRHR1-CFP and VT2R-YFP formed heterodimers with a computed distance of 5-6 nm between molecules. Based on their calculations, the FRET efficiency was 15-36% which corresponded to possible interaction of the proteins to form oligomers. A low resonance energy transfer signal was obtained in non-transfected HeLa cells. Co-transfection of HeLa cells with CRHR1-CFP and VT2R-YFP resulted in a constitutive resonance energy transfer between the fluorescence donor and acceptor. Addition of either CRH or AVT separately resulted in a small, statistically non-significant, augmentation of FRET efficiency, whereas simultaneous addition of the two neurohormones resulted in a significant ($p<0.05$) increase of FRET efficiency (Figure 12).

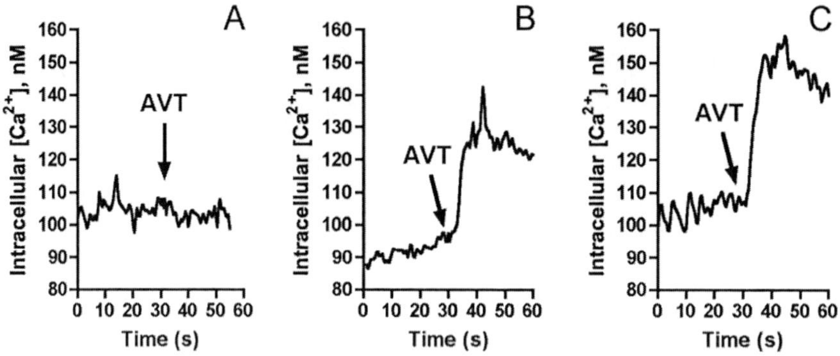

Figure 9. AVT-stimulated calcium mobilization in HeLa cells expressing vasotocin VT2 receptors (VT2R). HeLa cells were either not transfected (control), transfected with pcDNA3/VT2R or pYFP-VT2R, and subsequently treated with 0.1 μM AVT. Changes in fura-2 fluorescence were used to monitor intracellular calcium levels. A, Representative tracing from control HeLa cells that demonstrates unresponsiveness to AVT. B, Representative tracing from HeLa cells that had been transfected with pcDNA3/VT2R 24 hrs prior to fura-2 loading and treatment with AVT. C, Representative tracing from HeLa cells that had been transfected with pYFP-VT2R 24 hrs prior to fura-2 loading and treatment with AVT. Reprinted with permission from Mikhailova et al. "Heterooligomerization between vasotocin and corticotropin-releasing hormone (CRH) receptors augments CRH-stimulated 3',5'-cyclic adenosine monophosphate production", Molecular Endocrinology, 21(9), 2007, 2178-88. *Copyright 2007, The Endocrine Society.*

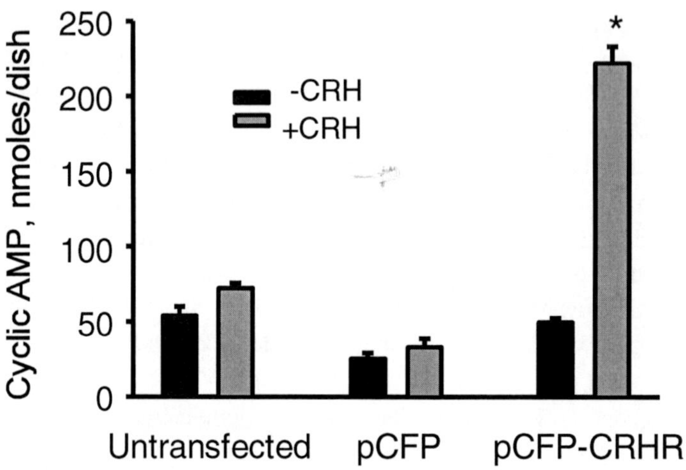

Figure 10. CRH-stimulated cyclic AMP production in HeLa cells expressing CRH receptor 1 (CRHR1). HeLa cells were either not transfected (control), transfected with pCFP, or pCFP-CRHR1, and 24 hours later were treated with 0.1 μM CRH in the presence of 1 mM IBMX, a phosphodiesterase inhibitor. Cells were treated with either vehicle or CRH for 30 min, followed by cell lysis and determination of intracellular cyclic AMP content by enzymeimmunoassay. Values are expressed as the mean ± SEM (n=4). *Significantly ($p<0.001$) different from all other groups. Reprinted with permission from Mikhailova et al. "Heterooligomerization between vasotocin and corticotropin-releasing hormone (CRH) receptors augments CRH-stimulated 3',5'-cyclic adenosine monophosphate production", Molecular Endocrinology, 21(9), 2007, 2178-88. *Copyright 2007, The Endocrine Society.*

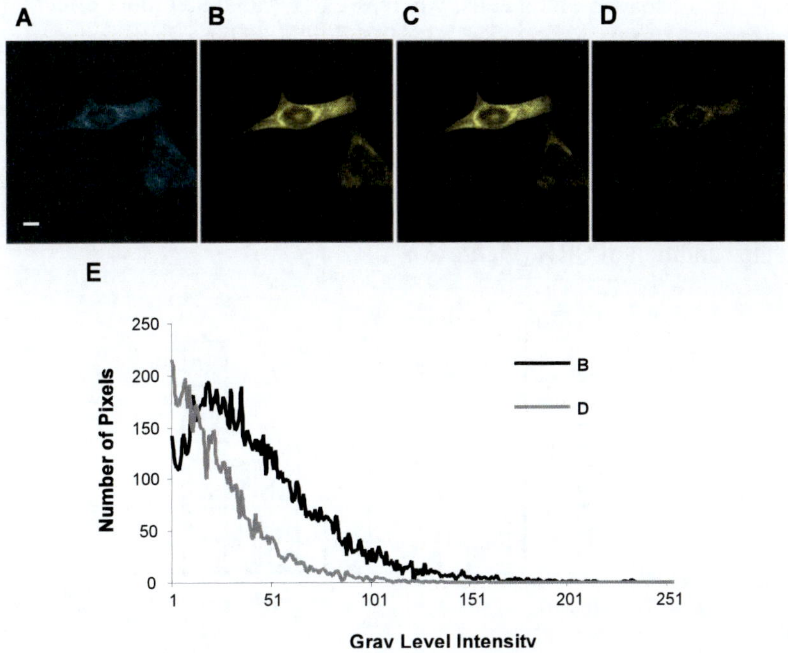

Figure 11. Images illustrating algorithm fluorescence resonance energy transfer (FRET) method. A-D, Laser scanning confocal images of HeLa cells expressing CRHR1 and VT2R. HeLa cells were labeled with CFP (donor, CRHR1) and YFP (acceptor, VT2R). To set the parameters for quantitative FRET, the images of HeLa cells only CRFR1-CFP or VT2R-YFP have been taken with donors and acceptors filter sets (images are not shown). Using a Bio-Rad Radiance 2100 confocal microscope, confocal processed FRET (PFRET) fluorescence signals (non-radiant transfer of energy from CRHR1 donor fluorophore to VT2R acceptor fluorophore) were collected in the same double-labeled cells. Images are representative of 6 experiments. Images collected during: (A) double-labeled donor excitation, donor channel revealing the distribution of CRHR1; (B) double-labeled, donor excitation, acceptor channel; (C) double-labeled acceptor excitation, acceptor channel revealing the distribution of VT2R. (D) PFRET calculated with algorithm methods. E, respective histogram of gray level intensities in images B and D. Scale bar, 20 μM. Reprinted with permission from Mikhailova et al. "Heterooligomerization between vasotocin and corticotropin-releasing hormone (CRH) receptors augments CRH-stimulated 3',5'-cyclic adenosine monophosphate production", Molecular Endocrinology, 21(9), 2007, 2178-88. *Copyright 2007, The Endocrine Society.*

Their results using FRET demonstrate that when transiently expressed in HeLa cells, the avian CRHR1 and VT2R may form heterodimers. The author found that the formation of CRHR1-VT2R heterodimers is augmented in the presence of endogenous ligands for the CRHR1 and VT2R, CRH and AVT, respectively. Neither neurohormone when administered alone was capable of stimulating heterodimer formation. To their knowledge, this is the first demonstration that the CRHR1 and VT2R, normally co-expressed in corticocortropes, can physically interact to form heterodimers.

Molecular signaling in HeLa cells co-expressing CRHR1-CFP and VT2R-YFP.

To obtain functional data on the possible interaction between the neurohormones and/or their respective receptors, CRHR1 and VT2R were transiently co-expressed in HeLa cells and tested for their abilities to mediate stimulation of Ca^{2+} mobilization (Figure 13) and cyclic AMP production (Figure 14). When added alone, AVT but not CRH stimulated Ca^{2+}

mobilization in fura-2-loaded HeLa cells, whereas CRH was much more effective than AVT in stimulating cyclic AMP production. Significantly, in HeLa cells expressing both the CRHR1 and VT2R, cyclic AMP production in the presence of both CRH and AVT was approximately 3-fold higher compared to cyclic AMP levels achieved with CRH administration alone (Figure 14). In contrast, there was no additive or synergistic effect of the two hormones in Ca^{2+} mobilization experiments. The level of calcium mobilization in HeLa cells expressing both the CRHR1 and VT2R obtained with the addition of AVT was not changed with the addition of CRH (Figure13).

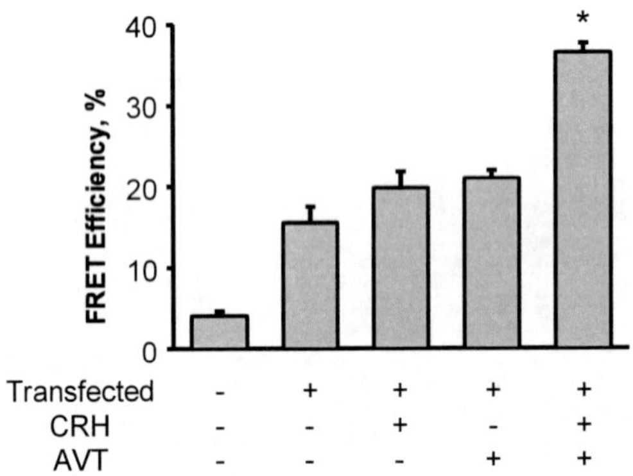

Figure 12. FRET efficiency following treatments with CRH and AVT. HeLa cells were either not transfected or transfected with pCFP-CRHR1 and pYFP-VT2R, and 24 hours later were treated with either vehicle, 0.1 μM CRH, 0.1 μM AVT or with 0.1 μM CRH and 0.1 μM AVT together. FRET measurements were taken 30 min. after hormone addition. Data are the means ± SEM (n=6). *Significantly ($p<0.05$) different from all other groups. Reprinted with permission from Mikhailova et al. "Heterooligomerization between vasotocin and corticotropin-releasing hormone (CRH) receptors augments CRH-stimulated 3',5'-cyclic adenosine monophosphate production", Molecular Endocrinology, 21(9), 2007, 2178-88. *Copyright 2007, The Endocrine Society.*

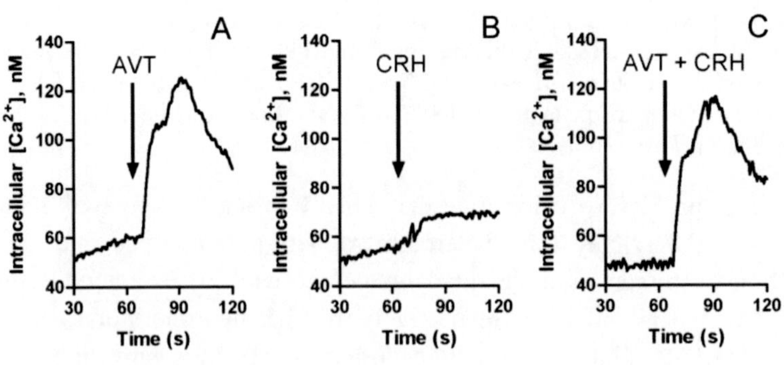

Figure 13. Calcium mobilization in HeLa cells expressing CRHR1-CFP and VT2R-YFP. HeLa cells were transfected with pCFP-CRHR1 and pYFP-VT2R, and 24 hours later treated with either AVT, CRH or AVT and CRH together. Changes in fura-2 fluorescence were used to monitor intracellular calcium levels. A, Transfected HeLa cells were treated with 0.1 μM AVT. B, Transfected HeLa cells were treated with 0.1 μM CRH. C, Transfected HeLa cells were treated with 0.1 μM AVT and 0.1 μM CRH. Reprinted with permission from Mikhailova et al. "Heterooligomerization between vasotocin and corticotropin-releasing hormone (CRH) receptors augments CRH-stimulated 3',5'-cyclic adenosine monophosphate production", Molecular Endocrinology, 21(9), 2007, 2178-88. *Copyright 2007, The Endocrine Society.*

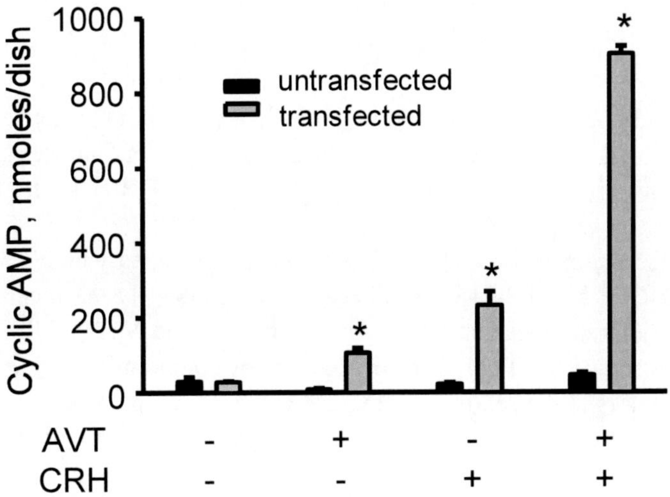

*

Figure 14. Cyclic AMP production in HeLa cells expressing CRHR1-CFP and VT2R-YFP. HeLa cells were either not transfected or transfected with pCFP-CRHR and pYFP-VT2R, and 24 hours later were treated with CRH, AVT or CRH and AVT together in the presence of 1 mM IBMX, a phosphodiesterase inhibitor. Cells were treated with hormones for 30 min, followed by cell lysis and determination of intracellular cyclic AMP content by enzyme immunoassay. Values are expressed as the means ± SEM (n=4). *Significantly ($p<0.001$) different from untransfected cells. Reprinted with **permission from Mikhailova et al. "Heterooligomerization between vasotocin and corticotropin-**releasing hormone (CRH) receptors augments CRH-stimulated 3',5'-cyclic adenosine monophosphate **production", Molecular Endocrinology,** 21(9), 2007, 2178-88. *Copyright 2007, The Endocrine Society.*

Effect of VT2R/β₂AR-YFP/CFP chimera construction on the dimerization of AVT and CRH receptors

Their studies using FRET have shown that CRHR1 and VT2R heterodimerize on the cell membrane of living cells although the exact residues involved remain unknown (Mikhailova et al., 2007). Moreover, it was demonstrated that human V1bR and CRHR1 can form constitutive homo- and heterodimers (Young et al., 2007). An atomic force microscopy analysis of native retinal disc membranes has revealed an organization of molecules of the prototypic GPCR rhodopsin in paracrystalline arrays. Based on these data, the fourth and fifth transmembrane helices (TM4 and TM5) have been inferred to be involved in inter-receptor contact, whereas helices TM1 and TM2, and the intracellular loop connecting helices TM5 and TM6 have been inferred to facilitate the formation of rhodopsin dimer rows. It is not clear, however, whether all GPCRs use these same interfaces or whether some GPCRs use different oligomerization interfaces to achieve functional selectivity. Recent computational and experimental data suggest the involvement of different TM regions in forming the dimerization interface of highly related GPCRs. These findings are also consistent with the possible organization of these receptors into higher-order oligomers, with multiple distinct oligomeric interfaces. As it becomes clearer that oligomeric structures are important for activation (Guo et al., 2005) and have physiological relevance (Ferre et al., 2009), functional models of GPCR dimers/oligomer formation are needed to characterize the structural context of receptor association, and its implication in receptor function.

Of the possible dimer interface sites between GPCRs, computational studies have predicted the TMs, specifically TMs 4-6, to be the probable sites of dimerization (Filizola and Weinstein, 2005). By constructing a chimeric VT2R, with TM4 replaced by 19 amino acids of TM4 form the β_2-adrenergic receptor, and monitoring FRET in the presence of CRH and AVT the author explored the possibility that TM4 of the VT2R participates as one of the possible regions in the formation of the interface of the VT2R-CRHR1 heterodimer (Figure 15).

Following transfection of HeLa cells, VT2/β_2AR-chimera tagged with YFP or CFP, and CRHR1 tagged with CFP or YFP, were localized mainly in the plasma membrane (Figure 16). The observed membrane localization of VT2/β_2AR-YFP and VT2/β_2AR-CFP chimeras implies that the substitution of TM4 from β_2AR did not compromise proper folding and trafficking of the receptors to the cell membrane. The chimeric receptors were able to activate downstream signal transduction pathways and ~~responding~~ to AVT by mobilizing intracellular Ca^{2+}.

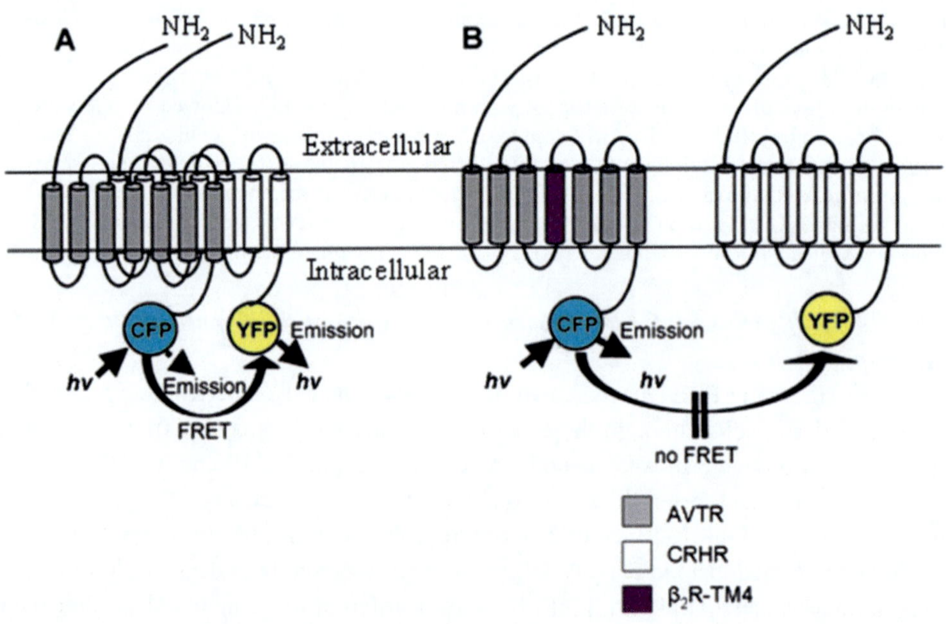

Figure 15. Schematic representation of the interaction between CRHR1 and VT2 receptors.
A, In the presence of CRH and AVT, FRET measurements indicate that the CRHR1 and VT2R are less than 10 nm apart and form heterodimers. B, Repeating the FRET measurements with the CRHR1 and a chimeric VT2R with TM4 substituted with amino acid sequence of TM4 from the β_2-adrenergic receptor (β_2-AR), results in an undetectable FRET signal indicating that the receptors are >10 nm apart. Reprinted with permission from Mikhailova et al. "Transmembrane domain IV of the *Gallus gallus* VT2 vasotocin receptor is essential for forming a heterodimer with the corticotrophin releasing hormone receptor", J Biomedical Optics, 13, 2008, 031208-1-8. *Copyright 2008, The Society of Photo-Optical Instrumentation Engineers.*

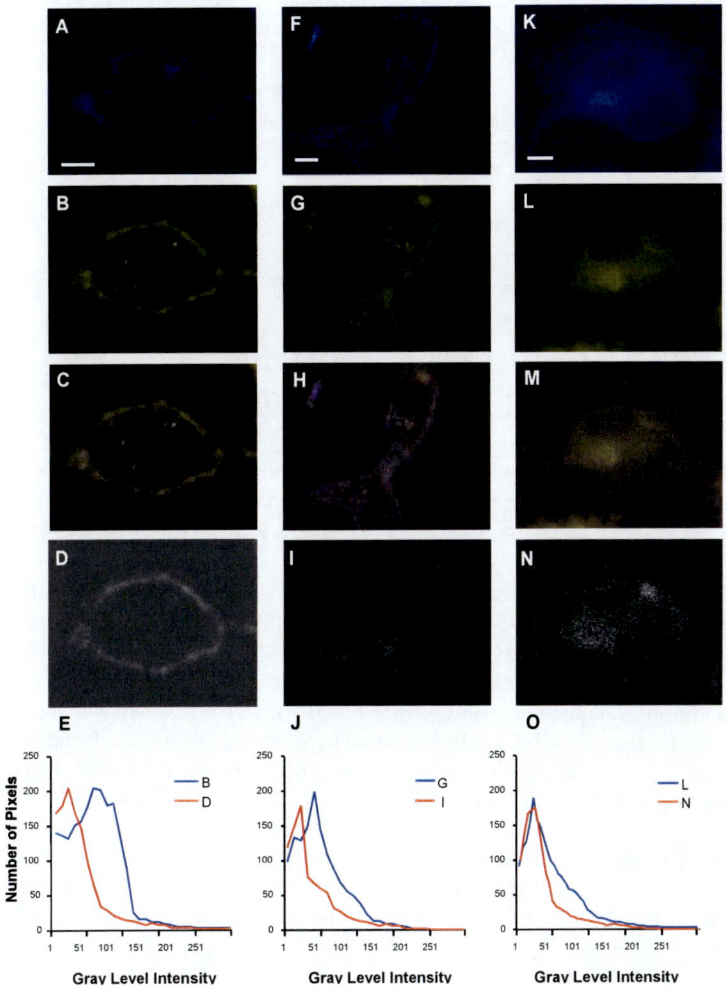

Figure 16. Images for algorithm FRET method. Laser scanning confocal images of HeLa cells coexpressing CRHR1-CFP and VT2R-YFP (A,B,C,D), CRHR1-CFP and VT2R/β_2AR-YFP chimeric receptor (F,G,H,I), and CRHR1-YFP and VT2R/β_2AR-CFP (K, L, M, N). The associated intensity histograms are shown for CRHR1-CFP and VT2R-YFP (E), CRHR1-CFP and VT2R/β_2AR-YFP (J), and CRHR1-YFP and VT2R/β_2AR-CFP (O). HeLa cells were labeled with CFP (donor, CRHR1 or VT2R/β_2AR) and YFP (acceptor, VT2R, VT2R/β_2AR, or CRHR1). To set the parameters for quantitative FRET, the images of HeLa cells expressing only CRHR1-CFP or VT2R/β_2AR-CFP and either VT2R-YFP or VT2R/β_2AR-YFP or CRHR1-YFP were taken with donor and acceptor filter sets (images are not shown). Using confocal microscopy, processed FRET (PFRET) fluorescence signals (non-radiant transfer of energy from CRHR1 or VT2R/β_2AR donor fluorophore to VT2R or VT2R/β_2AR or CRHR1 acceptor fluorophore) were collected in the same double-labeled cells. Images are representative of five experiments.

Images collected during double-labeled donor excitation, donor channel revealing the distribution of CRHR1-CFP (A and F) or VT2R/β_2AR-CFP (K) and; double-labeled, donor excitation, acceptor channel (B, G and L); double-labeled acceptor excitation, acceptor channel revealing the distribution of VT2R-YFP (C), VT2R/β_2AR-YFP (H), or CRHR1-YFP (M). D, I, and N, PFRET calculated with algorithm methods. Scale bar, 20 μm. Reprinted with permission from Mikhailova et al. "Transmembrane domain IV of the *Gallus gallus* VT$_2$ vasotocin receptor is essential for forming a heterodimer with the corticotrophin releasing hormone receptor", J Biomedical Optics, 13, 2008, 031208-1-8. *Copyright 2008, The Society of Photo-Optical Instrumentation Engineers.*

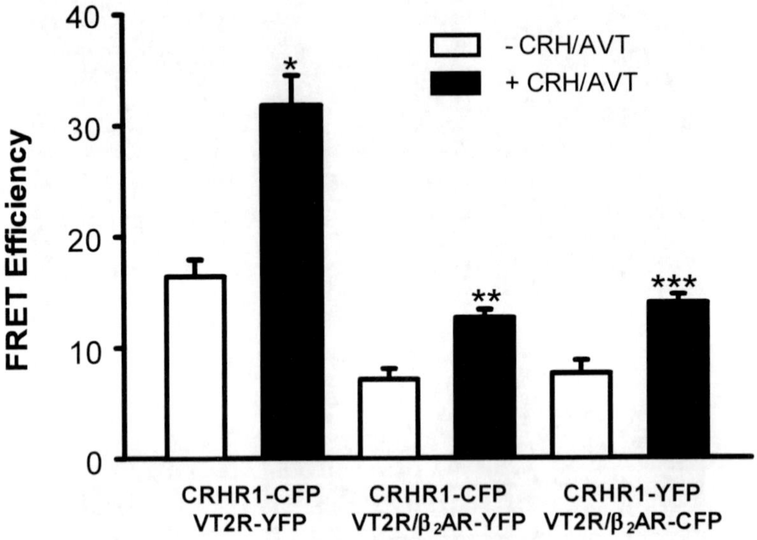

Figure 17. FRET efficiency in HeLa cells expressing CRHR1 and either VT2R or VT2R/ β_2AR following treatment with CRH and AVT. HeLa cells were either transfected with plasmids expressing CRHR1-CFP and VT2R-YFP or CRHR1-CFP and VT2/ β_2AR-YFP, and 24 hours later were treated with either vehicle or 0.1 μM CRH and 0.1 μM AVT together. FRET measurements were taken 30 min. after hormone addition. Data are the means ± SEM (n=5). *FRET efficiency was significantly different ($p<0.011$) than that measured in HeLa cells expressing CRHR1-CFP and VT2R that were not treated with the hormones. **FRET efficiency was significantly different ($p<0.008$) than that measured in HeLa cells expressing CRHR1-CFP and VT2/β_2 AR-YFP that were not treated with the hormones. ***FRET efficiency was significantly different ($p< 0.02$) than that measured in HeLa cells expressing CRHR1-YFP and VT2/β_2 AR-CFP that were not treated with the hormones. Reprinted with permission from Mikhailova et al. "Transmembrane domain IV of the *Gallus gallus* VT_2 vasotocin receptor is essential for forming a heterodimer with the corticotrophin releasing hormone receptor", J Biomedical Optics, 13, 2008, 031208-1-8. *Copyright 2008, The Society of Photo-Optical Instrumentation Engineers.*

Substitution of TM4 from the VT2R with TM4 from the β_2AR affected the interaction between the two receptor proteins (Figure 17). The addition of the CRH and AVT resulted in a significant two-fold FRET increase for both the wild type and VT2R/β_2AR chimera (Figure 17), and confirmed dimerization of the receptors with ligand addition. FRET efficiency was lower with chimeric receptors (15%) compared with the wild receptor (36%), suggesting that the ability of the chimeric VT2R to form herodimers with the CRHR1 in the presence of CRH and AVT was diminished, but not blocked completely. These results suggest that TM4 of VT2R may play a role in the formation of heterodimers between the VT2R and CRHR1. However, their findings do not exclude the possibility that other VT2R regions, notably other transmembrane domains, are involved in the dimerization between the VT2R and CRHR1.

Their findings place the CRHR1 and VT2R in a growing group of G protein-coupled receptors that have been shown, at some point in their life cycle, to form oligomers either as homodimers or as heterodimers with other G protein-coupled receptors (Milligan, 2004; Park et al., 2004; Javitch, 2004; Matsuda et al., 2004). TM4 of the VT2R may play a role in the formation of heterodimers between the VT2R and CRHR1 (Mikhailova et al., 2008). Their results do not exclude the possibility that other VT2R regions, notably other transmembrane domains, are involved in the formation of dimmers between the VT2R and CRHR1. The author believe that the ability of the CRHR1 and VT2R to form heterodimers, especially in the presence of CRH and AVT, may underlie the well-known greater than additive effect and in some cases synergistic effect that is observed in the release of ACTH in the presence of both CRH and AVP in mammalian systems (Leong, 1988; Brooks and Challis, 1989; Arsenijevic et al., 1994), and in the presence of CRH and AVT in at least one non-mammalian vertebrate system (Baker et al., 1996). Their findings indicate that when administered peripherally, simultaneous delivery of CRH and AVT leads to greater circulating corticosterone levels than with administration of either hormone alone. Thus, the domestic chicken can be added to the list of organisms in which CRH and either AVP or AVT have been shown to activate synergistically the hypothalamic-pituitary-adrenal axis.

Conclusion

Although this study focused on the roles of CRH and AVT in the HPA axis, there are several other endogenous regulators that induce ACTH release from the anterior pituitary, including catecholamines, urotensins and cytokines. Regulatory roles of these molecules were beyond the scopes of their study; however, the presence of multiple secretagogues of ACTH and their cross talk, as has been demonstrated for CRH and AVT, suggests a very complex regulatory network importantly contributing to adaptability and survivability of birds in diverse ecological habitats and agricultural settings. Elucidation of these complex interactions could be best achieved by employing the emerging systems biology approach.

Acknowledgments

This work was supported by NSF grants IBN 01111006 and IOS-0842937 and by National Research Initiative Competitive Grant no. 2005-35203-15850 from the USDA Cooperative State Research, Education and Extension Service.

References

AbdAlla, S; Lother, H; Quitterer, U. AT1-receptor heterodimers show enhanced G-protein activation and altered receptor sequestration. *Nature*, 2000 407, 94-98.

Abellan, A; Medina, L. Subdivisions and derivatives of the chicken subpallium based on expression of LIM and other regulatory genes and markers of neuron subpopulations during development. *J Comp Neurol*, 2009, 515, 465-501.

Acher, R. Neurohypophysial peptide systems: Processing machinery, hydroosmotic regulation, adaptation and evolution. *Regul Pept*, 1993, 45, 1-13.

Aguilera, G. Regulation of pituitary ACTH secretion during chronic stress. *Front Neuroendocrinol*, 1994, 15, 321-350.

Aguilera, G; Harwood, JP; Wilson, JX; Morell, J; Brown, JH; Catt, KJ. Mechanisms of action of corticotropin-releasing factor and other regulators of corticotropin release in rat pituitary cells. *J Biol Chem*, 1983, 258, 8039-8045.

Aguilera, G; Nikodemova, M; Wynn, PC; Catt, KJ. Corticotropin releasing hormone receptors: two decades later. *Peptides*, 2004, 25, 319-329.

Aguilera, G; Rabadan-Diehl, C. Regulation of vasopressin V1b receptors in the anterior pituitary gland of the rat. *Exp Physiol*, 2000a, 85 Spec No, 19S-26S.

Aguilera, G; Rabadan-Diehl, C. Vasopressinergic regulation of the hypothalamic-pituitary-adrenal axis: implications for stress adaptation. *Regul Pept*, 2000b, 96, 23-29.

Alonso, G; Szafarczyk, A; Assenmacher, I. Radioautographic evidence that axons from the area of supraoptic nuclei in the rat project to extrahypothalamic brain regions. *Neurosci Lett*, 1986, 66, 251-256.

Aoki, Y; Iwasaki, Y; Katahira, M; Oiso, Y; Saito, H. Regulation of the rat proopiomelanocortin gene expression in AtT-20 cells. I: Effects of the common secretagogues. *Endocrinology*, 1997, 138, 1923-1929.

Arsenijevic, Y; Dubois-Dauphin, M; Tribollet, E; Manning, M; Sawyer, WH; Dreifuss, JJ. Vasopressin-binding sites in the pig pituitary gland: competition by novel vasopressin antagonists suggests the existence of an unusual receptor subtype in the anterior lobe. *J Endocrinol*, 1994, 141, 383-391.

Aste, N; Balthazart, J; Absil, P; Grossmann, R; Mühlbauer, E; Viglietti-Panzica, C; Panzica, GC. Anatomical and neurochemical definition of the nucleus of the stria terminalis in Japanese quail (*Coturnix japonica*). *J Comp Neurol*, 1998, 396, 141-157.

Aubry, JM; Bartanusz, V; Jezova, D; Belin, D; Kiss, JZ. Single stress induces long-lasting elevations in vasopressin mRNA levels in CRF hypophysiotrophic neurones, but repeated stress is required to modify AVP immunoreactivity. *J Neuroendocrinol*, 1999, 11, 377-384.

Baeyens, DA; Cornett, LE. The cloned avian neurohypophysial hormone receptors. *Comp Biochem Physiol B Biochem Mol Biol*, 2006, 143, 12-19.

Baker, BI; Bird, DJ; Buckingham, JC. In the trout, CRH and AVT synergize to stimulate ACTH release. *Regul Pept*, 1996, 67, 207-210.

Ball, GF; Faris, PL; Wingfield, JC. Immunochistochemical localization of corticotropin-releasing factor in selected brain areas of the European starling (*Sturnus vulgaris*) and the song sparrow (*Melospiza melodia*). *Cell Tissue Res*, 1989, 257, 155-161.

Banks, EM; Wood-Gush, DGM; Hughes, BO; Mankovich, NJ. Social rank and priority of access to resources in domestic fowl. *Behav Process*, 1979, 4, 197-209.

Banks, WA; Kastin, AJ; Horvath, A; Michals, EA. Carrier-mediated transport of vasopressin across the blood-brain barrier of the mouse. *J Neurosci Res*, 1987, 18, 326-332.

Barnes, PJ. Receptor heterodimerization: a new level of cross-talk. *J Clin Invest*, 2006 116, 1210-1212.

Bartanusz, V; Aubry, JM; Jezova, D; Baffi, J; Kiss, JZ. Up-regulation of vasopressin mRNA in paraventricular hypophysiotrophic neurons after acute immobilization stress. *Neuroendocrinology*, 1993a, 58, 625-629.

Bartanusz, V; Jezova, D; Bertini, LT; Tilders, FJ; Aubry, JM; Kiss, JZ. Stress-induced increase in vasopressin and corticotropin-releasing factor expression in hypophysiotrophic paraventricular neurons. *Endocrinology*, 1993b 132, 895-902.

Brooks, AN; Challis, JR. Effects of CRF, AVP and opioid peptides on pituitary-adrenal responses in sheep. *Peptides*, 1989, 10, 1291-1293.

Brubaker, PL; Baird, AC; Bennett, HP; Browne, CA; Solomon, S. Corticotropic peptides in the human fetal pituitary. *Endocrinology*, 1982, 111, 1150-1155.

Carsia, RV; Weber, H; Perez, FMJ. Corticotropin-releasing factor stimulates the release of adrenocorticotropin from domestic fowl pituitary cells. *Endocrinology*, 1986, 118, 143-148.

Castro, MG; Estivariz, FE; Iturriza, FC. The regulation of the corticomelanotropic cell activity in Aves--II. Effect of various peptides on the release of ACTH from dispersed, perfused duck pituitary cells. *Comp Biochem Physiol A*, 1986, 83, 71-75.

Castro, MG; Estivariz, FE; Iturriza, FC. The regulation of the corticomelanotropic cell activity in aves. III--Effect of various peptides on the release of MSH from dispersed, perfused duck pituitary cells. Cosecretion of ACTH with MSH. *Comp Biochem Physiol C*, 1988, 91, 389-393.

Chang, CL; Hsu, SY. Ancient evolution of stress-regulating peptides in vertebrates. *Peptides*, 2004, 25, 1681-1688.

Chen, Y; Mauldin, JP; Day, RN; Periasamy, A. Characterization of spectral FRET imaging microscopy for monitoring nuclear protein interactions. *J Microsc*, 2007, 228, 139-152.

Choi, DC; Nguyen, MM; Tamashiro, KL; Ma, LY; Sakai, RR; Herman, JP. Chronic social stress in the visible burrow system modulates stress-related gene expression in the bed nucleus of the stria terminalis. *Physiol Behav*, 2006, 89, 301-310.

Cornett, LE; Kirby, JD; Vizcarra, JA; Ellison, JC; Thrash, J; Mayeux, PR; Crew, MD; Jones, SM; Ali, N; Baeyens, DA. Molecular cloning and functional characterization of a vasotocin receptor subtype expressed in the pituitary gland of the domestic chicken (*Gallus domesticus*): avian homolog of the mammalian V1b-vasopressin receptor. *Regul Pept*, 2003, 110, 231-239.

Cullinan, WE; Herman, JP; Battaglia, DF; Akil, H; Watson, SJ. Pattern and time course of immediate early gene expression in rat brain following acute stress. *Neuroscience*, 1995, 64, 477-505.

De Goeij, DC; Kvetnansky, R; Whitnall, MH; Jezova, D; Berkenbosch, F; Tilders, FJ. Repeated stress-induced activation of corticotropin-releasing factor neurons enhances vasopressin stores and colocalization with corticotropin-releasing factor in the median eminence of rats. *Neuroendocrinology*, 1991, 53, 150-159.

De Groef, B; Goris, N; Arckens, L; Kuhn, ER; Darras, VM. Corticotropin-releasing hormone (CRH)-induced thyrotropin release is directly mediated through CRH receptor type 2 on thyrotropes. *Endocrinology*, 2003, 144, 5537-5544.

De Groef, B; Grommen, SVH; Mertens, I; Schoofs, L; Kuhn, ER; Darras, VM. Cloning and tissue distribution of the chicken type 2 corticotropin-releasing hormone receptor. *Gen Comp Endocrinol*, 2004, 138, 89-95.

De Vries, GJ; Miller, MA. Anatomy and function of extrahypothalamic vasopressin systems in the brain. *Prog Brain Res*, 1998, 119, 3-20.

DeBold, CR; Sheldon, WR; DeCherney, GS; Jackson, RV; Alexander, AN; Vale, W; Rivier, J; Orth, DN. Arginine vasopressin potentiates adrenocorticotropin release induced by ovine corticotropin-releasing factor. *J Clin Invest*, 1984, 73, 533-538.

Delville, Y; Melloni, RH, Jr.; Ferris, CF. Behavioral and neurobiological consequences of social subjugation during puberty in golden hamsters. *J Neurosci*, 1998, 18, 2667-2672.

Dominic, CJ; Singh, RM. Anterior and posterior groups of portal vessels in the avian pituitary. *Gen Comp Endocrinol*, 1969, 13, 22-26.

Ebner, K; Wotjak, CT; Holsboer, F; Landgraf, R; Engelmann, M. Vasopressin released within the septal brain area during swim stress modulates the behavioural stress response in rats. *Eur J Neurosci*, 1999, 11, 997-1002.

Elangovan, M; Wallrabe, H; Chen, Y; Day, RN; Barroso, M; Periasamy, A. Characterization of one- and two-photon excitation fluorescence resonance energy transfer microscopy. *Methods*, 2003, 29, 58-73.

Engelmann, M; Landgraf, R; Wotjak, CT. The hypothalamic-neurohypophysial system regulates the hypothalamic-pituitary-adrenal axis under stress: an old concept revisited. *Front Neuroendocrinol*, 2004, 25, 132-149.

Engler, D; Redei, E; Kola, I. The corticotropin-release inhibitory factor hypothesis: a review of the evidence for the existence of inhibitory as well as stimulatory hypophysiotropic regulation of adrenocorticotropin secretion and biosynthesis. *Endocr Rev*, 1999, 20, 460-500.

Evans, MJ; Brett, JT; McIntosh, RP; McIntosh, JE; McLay, JL; Livesey, JH; Donald, RA. Characteristics of the ACTH response to repeated pulses of corticotrophin-releasing factor and arginine vasopressin *in vitro*. *J Endocrinol*, 1988, 117, 387-395.

Familari, M; Smith, AI; Smith, R; Funder, JW. Arginine vasopressin is a much more potent stimulus to ACTH release from ovine anterior pituitary cells than ovine corticotropin-releasing factor. 1. In vitro studies. *Neuroendocrinology*, 1989, 50, 152-157.

Fekete, EM; Zorrilla, EP. Physiology, pharmacology, and therapeutic relevance of urocortins in mammals: Ancient CRF paralogs. *Front Neuroendocrinol*, 2007, 28, 1-27.

Ferre, S; Baler, R; Bouvier, M; Caron, MG; Devi, LA; Durroux, T; Fuxe, K; George, SR; Javitch, JA; Lohse, MJ; Mackie, K; Milligan, G; Pfleger, KD; Pin, JP; Volkow, ND; Waldhoer, M; Woods, AS; Franco, R. Building a new conceptual framework for receptor heteromers. *Nat Chem Biol*, 2009, 5, 131-134.

Ferris, CF; Lu, SF; Messenger, T; Guillon, CD; Heindel, N; Miller, M; Koppel, G; Robert, BF; Simon, NG. Orally active vasopressin V1a receptor antagonist, SRX251, selectively blocks aggressive behavior. *Pharmacol Biochem Behav*, 2006, 83, 169-174.

Filizola, M; Weinstein, H. The study of G-protein coupled receptor oligomerization with computational modeling and bioinformatics. *FEBS J*, 2005, 272, 2926-2938.

Giguere, V; Labrie, F. Vasopressin potentiates cyclic AMP accumulation and ACTH release induced by corticotropin-releasing factor (CRF) in rat anterior pituitary cells in culture. *Endocrinology*, 1982, 111, 1752-1754.

Gillies, GE; Linton, EA; Lowry, PJ. Corticotropin releasing activity of the new CRF is potentiated several times by vasopressin. *Nature*, 1982, 299, 355-357.

Gines, S; Hillion, J; Torvinen, M; Le, CS; Casado, V; Canela, EI; Rondin, S; Lew, JY; Watson, S; Zoli, M; Agnati, LF; Verniera, P; Lluis, C; Ferre, S; Fuxe, K; Franco, R. Dopamine D1 and adenosine A1 receptors form functionally interacting heteromeric complexes. *Proc Natl Acad Sci U S A*, 2000, 97, 8606-8611.

Goodson, JL; Evans, AK. Neural responses to territorial challenge and nonsocial stress in male song sparrows: segregation, integration, and modulation by a vasopressin V1 antagonist. *Horm Behav*, 2004, 46, 371-381.

Goodson, JL; Evans, AK; Wang, Y. Neuropeptide binding reflects convergent and divergent evolution in species-typical group sizes. *Horm Behav*, 2006, 50, 223-236.

Griebel, G; Simiand, J; Stemmelin, J; Serradeil-Le Gal, C; Steinberg, R. The vasopressin V1b receptor as a therapeutic target in stress-related disorders. *Curr Drug Target CNS Neurol Disord*, 2003, 2, 191-200.

Gubrij, KI; Chaturvedi, CM; Ali, N; Cornett, LE; Kirby, JD; Wilkerson, J; Mikhailova, M; Turner, ML; Baeyens, DA. Molecular cloning of an oxytocin-like receptor expressed in the chicken shell gland. *Comp Biochem Physiol B Biochem Mol Biol*, 2005, 142, 37-45.

Guo, W; Shi, L; Filizola, M; Weinstein, H; Javitch, JA. Crosstalk in G protein-coupled receptors: changes at the transmembrane homodimer interface determine activation. *Proc Natl Acad Sci U S A*, 2005, 102, 17495-17500.

Harvey, S; Phillips, JG; Rees, A; Hall, TR. Stress and adrenal function. *J Exp Zool*, 1984, 232, 633-645.

Hassan, A; Mason, D. Mechanisms of desensitization of the adrenocorticotropin response to arginine vasopressin in ovine anterior pituitary cells. *J Endocrinol*, 2005, 184, 29-40.

Herman, JP; Ostrander, MM; Mueller, NK; Figueiredo, H. Limbic system mechanisms of stress regulation: hypothalamo-pituitary-adrenocortical axis. *Prog Neuropsychopharmacol Biol Psychiatry*, 2005, 29, 1201-1213.

Hernando, F; Schoots, O; Lolait, SJ; Burbach, JP. Immunohistochemical localization of the vasopressin V1b receptor in the rat brain and pituitary gland: anatomical support for its involvement in the central effects of vasopressin. *Endocrinology*, 2001, 142, 1659-1668.

Hillhouse, EW; Randeva, H; Ladds, G; Grammatopoulos, D. Corticotropin-releasing hormone receptors. *Biochem Soc Trans*, 2002, 30, 428-432.

Hillier, LW; Miller, W; Birney, E; Warren, W; Hardison, RC; Ponting, CP; Bork, P; Burt, DW; Groenen, MA; Delany, ME; Dodgson, JB; Chinwalla, AT; Cliften, PF; Clifton, SW; Delehaunty, KD; Fronick, C; Fulton, RS; Graves, TA; Kremitzki, C; Layman, D; Magrini, V; McPherson, JD; Miner, TL; Minx, P; Nash, WE; Nhan, MN; Nelson, JO; Oddy, LG; Pohl, CS; Randall-Maher, J; Smith, SM; Wallis, JW; Yang, SP; Romanov, MN; Rondelli, CM; Paton, B; Smith, J; Morrice, D; Daniels, L; Tempest, HG; Robertson, L; Masabanda, JS; Griffin, DK; Vignal, A; Fillon, V; Jacobbson, L; Kerje, S; Andersson, L; Crooijmans, RP; Aerts, J; van der Poel, JJ; Ellegren, H; Caldwell, RB; Hubbard, SJ; Grafham, DV; Kierzek, AM; McLaren, SR; Overton, IM; Arakawa, H; Beattie, KJ; Bezzubov, Y; Boardman, PE; Bonfield, JK; Croning, MD; Davies, RM; Francis, MD; Humphray, SJ; Scott, CE; Taylor, RG; Tickle, C; Brown, WR; Rogers, J; Buerstedde, JM; Wilson, SA; Stubbs, L; Ovcharenko, I; Gordon, L; Lucas, S; Miller, MM; Inoko, H; Shiina, T; Kaufman, J; Salomonsen, J; Skjoedt, K; Wong, GK; Wang, J; Liu, B; Wang, J; Yu, J; Yang, H; Nefedov, M; Koriabine, M; Dejong, PJ; Goodstadt, L; Webber, C; Dickens, NJ; Letunic, I; Suyama, M; Torrents, D; von, MC; Zdobnov, EM; Makova, K; Nekrutenko, A; Elnitski, L; Eswara, P; King, DC; Yang, S; Tyekucheva, S; Radakrishnan, A; Harris, RS; Chiaromonte, F; Taylor, J; He, J; Rijnkels, M; Griffiths-Jones, S; Ureta-Vidal, A; Hoffman, MM; Severin, J; Searle, SM; Law, AS; Speed, D; Waddington, D; Cheng, Z; Tuzun, E; Eichler, E; Bao, Z; Flicek, P; Shteynberg, DD; Brent, MR; Bye, JM; Huckle, EJ; Chatterji, S; Dewey, C; Pachter, L; Kouranov, A; Mourelatos, Z; Hatzigeorgiou, AG; Paterson, AH; Ivarie, R; Brandstrom, M; Axelsson, E; Backstrom, N; Berlin, S; Webster, MT; Pourquie, O; Reymond, A; Ucla, C; Antonarakis, SE; Long, M; Emerson, JJ; Betran, E; Dupanloup, I; Kaessmann, H; Hinrichs, AS; Bejerano, G; Furey, TS; Harte, RA; Raney, B; Siepel, A; Kent, WJ; Haussler, D; Eyras, E; Castelo, R; Abril, JF; Castellano, S; Camara, F; Parra, G; Guigo,

R; Bourque, G; Tesler, G; Pevzner, PA; Smit, A; Fulton, LA; Mardis, ER; Wilson, RK. Sequence and comparative analysis of the chicken genome provide unique perspectives on vertebrate evolution. *Nature*, 2004, 432, 695-716.

Holmes, MC; Antoni, FA; Aguilera, G; Catt, KJ. Magnocellular axons in passage through the median eminence release vasopressin. *Nature*, 1986, 319, 326-329.

Hurbin, A; Boissin-Agasse, L; Orcel, H; Rabie, A; Joux, N; Desarmenien, MG; Richard, P; Moos, FC. The V1a and V1b, but not V2, vasopressin receptor genes are expressed in the supraoptic nucleus of the rat hypothalamus, and the transcripts are essentially colocalized in the vasopressinergic magnocellular neurons. *Endocrinology*, 1998, 139, 4701-4707.

Hurbin, A; Orcel, H; Alonso, G; Moos, F; Rabie, A. The vasopressin receptors colocalize with vasopressin in the magnocellular neurons of the rat supraoptic nucleus and are modulated by water balance. *Endocrinology*, 2002, 143, 456-466.

Imaki, T; Naruse, M; Harada, S; Chikada, N; Imaki, J; Onodera, H; Demura, H; Vale, W. Corticotropin-releasing factor up-regulates its own receptor mRNA in the paraventricular nucleus of the hypothalamus. *Brain Res Mol Brain Res*, 1996, 38, 166-170.

Iwasaki-Sekino, A; Mano-Otagiri, A; Ohata, H; Yamauchi, N; Shibasaki, T. Gender differences in corticotropin and corticosterone secretion and corticotropin-releasing factor mRNA expression in the paraventricular nucleus of the hypothalamus and the central nucleus of the amygdala in response to footshock stress or psychological stress in rats. *Psychoneuroendocrinology*, 2009, 34, 226-237.

Javitch, JA. The ants go marching two by two: oligomeric structure of G-protein-coupled receptors. *Mol Pharmacol*, 2004, 66, 1077-1082.

Jia, LG; Canny, BJ; Orth, DN; Leong, DA. Distinct classes of corticotropes mediate corticotropin-releasing hormone- and arginine vasopressin-stimulated adrenocorticotropin release. *Endocrinology*, 1991, 128, 197-203.

Jones, RB. Assessment of fear in adult laying hens: correlational analysis of methods and measures. *Br Poult Sci*, 1987, 28, 319-326.

Jozsa, R; Vigh, S; Schally, AV; Mess, B. Localization of corticotropin-releasing factor-containing neurons in the brain of the domestic fowl. An immunohistochemical study. *Cell Tissue Res*, 1984, 236, 245-248.

Jurkevich, A; Barth, SW; Grossmann, R. Sexual dimorphism of arg-vasotocin gene expressing neurons in the telencephalon and dorsal diencephalon of the domestic fowl. An immunocytochemical and *in situ* hybridization study. *Cell Tissue Res*, 1997, 287, 69-77.

Jurkevich, A; Berghman, LR; Cornett, LE; Kuenzel, WJ. Characterization and immunonistochemical vizualization of the vasotocin VT2 receptor in the pituitary of the chicken, *Gallus gallus*. *Gen Comp Endocrinol*, 2005, 143, 82-91.

Jurkevich, A; Berghman, LR; Cornett, LE; Kuenzel, WJ. Immunohistochemical characterization of chicken pituitary cells containing the vasotocin VT2 receptor. *Cell Tissue Res*, 2008, 333, 253-262.

Jurkevich, A; Grossmann, R; Balthazart, J; Viglietti-Panzica, C. Gender-related changes in the avian vasotocin system during ontogeny. *Microsc Res Tech*, 2001, 55, 27-36.

Kemppainen, RJ; Clark, TP; Sartin, JL; Zerbe, CA. Hypothalamic peptide regulation of ACTH secretion from sheep pituitary. *Am J Physiol*, 1993, 265, R840-R845.

Koch, KA; Wingfield, JC; Buntin, JD. Glucocorticoids and parental hyperphagia in ring doves (Streptopelia risoria). *Horm Behav*, 2002, 41, 9-21.

Korf, HW; Panzica, GC; Viglietti-Panzica, C; Oksche, A. Pattern of peptidergic neurons in the avian brain: clusters - local circuitries - projections. *Bas Appl Histochem*, 1988, 32, 55-75.

Landgraf, R; Ludwig, M. Vasopressin release within the supraoptic and paraventricular nuclei of the rat brain: osmotic stimulation via microdialysis. *Brain Res*, 1991, 558, 191-196.

Landgraf, R; Ramirez, AD; Ramirez, VD. The positive feedback action of vasopressin on its own release from rat septal tissue in vitro is receptor-mediated. *Brain Res*, 1991, 545, 137-141.

Leong, DA. A complex mechanism of facilitation in pituitary ACTH cells: recent single-cell studies. *J Exp Biol*, 1988, 139, 151-168.

Leung, CH; Maney, DL. Gene expression of three vasotocin receptor subtypes in the songbird brain. *13th Annual Meeting of the Society for Behavioral Neuroendocrinology*. East Lansing; 2009, Abstract P3.61, 190-191.

Levin, N; Blum, M; Roberts, JL. Modulation of basal and corticotropin-releasing factor-stimulated proopiomelanocortin gene expression by vasopressin in rat anterior pituitary. *Endocrinology*, 1989, 125, 2957-2966.

Lim, MM; Murphy, AZ; Young, LJ. Ventral striatopallidal oxytocin and vasopressin V1a receptors in the monogamous prairie vole (Microtus ochrogaster). *J Comp Neurol*, 2004, 468, 555-570.

Lim, MM; Nair, HP; Young, LJ. Species and sex differences in brain distribution of corticotropin-releasing factor receptor subtypes 1 and 2 in monogamous and promiscuous vole species. *J Comp Neurol*, 2005, 487, 75-92.

Liposits, Z; Paull, WK; Setalo, G; Vigh, S. Evidence for local corticotropin releasing factor (CRF)-immunoreactive neuronal circuits in the paraventricular nucleus of the rat hypothalamus. An electron microscopic immunohistochemical analysis. *Histochemistry*, 1985, 83, 5-16.

Liu, JP; Robinson, PJ; Funder, JW; Engler, D. The biosynthesis and secretion of adrenocorticotropin by the ovine anterior pituitary is predominantly regulated by arginine vasopressin (AVP). Evidence that protein kinase C mediates the action of AVP. *J Biol Chem*, 1990, 265, 14136-14142.

Lolait, SJ; Stewart, LQ; Jessop, DS; Young, WS, III; O'Carroll, AM. The hypothalamic-pituitary-adrenal axis response to stress in mice lacking functional vasopressin V1b receptors. *Endocrinology*, 2007, 148, 849-856.

Lovejoy, DA; Jahan, S. Phylogeny of the corticotropin-releasing factor family of peptides in the metazoa. *Gen Comp Endocrinol*, 2006, 146, 1-8.

Ma, S; Shipston, MJ; Morilak, D; Russell, JA. Reduced hypothalamic vasopressin secretion underlies attenuated adrenocorticotropin stress responses in pregnant rats. *Endocrinology*, 2005, 146, 1626-1637.

Ma, XM; Levy, A; Lightman, SL. Rapid changes in heteronuclear RNA for corticotrophin-releasing hormone and arginine vasopressin in response to acute stress. *J Endocrinol*, 1997, 152, 81-89.

Madison, FN; Jurkevich, A; Kuenzel, WJ. Sex differences in plasma corticosterone release in undisturbed chickens (Gallus gallus) in response to arginine vasotocin and corticotropin releasing hormone. *Gen Comp Endocrinol*, 2008, 155, 566-573.

Maggio, R; Novi, F; Scarselli, M; Corsini, GU. The impact of G-protein-coupled receptor hetero-oligomerization on function and pharmacology. *FEBS J*, 2005, 272, 2939-2946.

Makara, GB; Antoni, FA; Stark, E. Electrical stimulation in the rat of the supraoptic nucleus: failure to alter plasma corticosterone after surgical lesioning of the paraventricular nucleus. *Neurosci Lett*, 1982, 30, 269-273.

Makino, S; Hashimoto, K; Gold, PW. Multiple feedback mechanisms activating corticotropin-releasing hormone system in the brain during stress. *Pharmacol Biochem Behav*, 2002, 73, 147-158.

Makino, S; Smith, MA; Gold, PW. Increased expression of corticotropin-releasing hormone and vasopressin messenger ribonucleic acid (mRNA) in the hypothalamic paraventricular nucleus during repeated stress: association with reduction in glucocorticoid receptor mRNA levels. *Endocrinology*, 1995, 136, 3299-3309.

Marcelli, M; Cunningham, GR; Haidacher, SJ; Padayatty, SJ; Sturgis, L; Kagan, C; Denner, L. Caspase-7 is activated during lovastatin-induced apoptosis of the prostate cancer cell line LNCaP. *Cancer Res*, 1998, 58, 76-83.

Marin, RH; Benavidez, E; Garcia, DA; Satterlee, DG. Sex differences in central benzodiazepine receptor densities and circulating corticosterone release after acute stress in broiler chicks. *Poult Sci*, 2002, 81, 261-264.

Martins, JM; Kastin, AJ; Banks, WA. Unidirectional specific and modulated brain to blood transport of corticotropin-releasing hormone. *Neuroendocrinology*, 1996, 63, 338-348.

Matsuda, M; Imaoka, T; Vomachka, AJ; Gudelsky, GA; Hou, Z; Mistry, M; Bailey, JP; Nieport, KM; Walther, DJ; Bader, M; Horseman, ND. Serotonin regulates mammary gland development via an autocrine-paracrine loop. *Dev Cell*, 2004, 6, 193-203.

Mikami, S. Immunocytochemistry of the avian hypothalamus and adenohypophysis. *Int Rev Cytol*, 1986, 103, 189-248.

Mikami, S; Yamada, S. Immunohistochemistry of the hypothalamic neuropeptides and anterior pituitary cells in the Japanese quail. *J Exp Zool*, 1984, 232, 405-417.

Mikhailova, MV; Blansett, J; Jacobi, SE; Mayeux, PR; Cornett, LE. Transmembrane domain IV of the *Gallus gallus* VT_2 vasotocin receptor is essential for forming a heterodimer with the corticotrophin releasing hormone receptor. *J Biomed Opt*, 2008, 13, 031208.

Mikhailova, MV; Mayeux, PR; Jurkevich, A; Kuenzel, WJ; Madison, FN; Periasamy, A; Chen, Y; Cornett, LE. Heterooligomerization between vasotocin and corticotropin-releasing hormone (CRH) receptors augments CRH-stimulated 3',5'-cyclic adenosine monophosphate production. *Mol Endocrinol*, 2007, 21, 2178-2188.

Milligan, G. G protein-coupled receptor dimerization: function and ligand pharmacology. *Mol Pharmacol*, 2004, 66, 1-7.

Milligan, G. G protein-coupled receptor hetero-dimerization: contribution to pharmacology and function. *Br J Pharmacol*, 2009, 158, 5-14.

Milligan, G; Bouvier, M. Methods to monitor the quaternary structure of G protein-coupled receptors. *FEBS J*, 2005, 272, 2914-2925.

Montagnese, CM; Zachar, G; Balint, E; Csillag, A. Afferent connections of septal nuclei of the domestic chick (Gallus domesticus): A retrograde pathway tracing study. *J Comp Neurol*, 2008, 511, 109-150.

Muller, MB; Landgraf, R; Preil, J; Sillaber, I; Kresse, AE; Keck, ME; Zimmermann, S; Holsboer, F; Wurst, W. Selective activation of the hypothalamic vasopressinergic system in mice deficient for the corticotropin-releasing hormone receptor 1 is dependent on glucocorticoids. *Endocrinology*, 2000, 141, 4262-4269.

Neumeier, C; Lametschwandtner, A. The vascularization of the pituitary gland of the chicken (Gallus domesticus). A scanning electron microscope study of vascular corrosion casts. *Arch Histol Cytol*, 1994, 57, 213-233.

Oksche, A; Farner, DS; Serventy, DL; Wolff, F; Nicholls, CA. The hypothalamo-hypophysial neuro secretory system of the zebra finch, Taeniopygia castanotis. *Cell Tissue Res*, 1963, 58, 846-914.

Olson, DM; Hertelendy, F. Avian shell gland contractility: interaction of PGF_{2a} and arginine vasotocin with Ca^{2+}. *Am J Physiol*, 1983, 244, C150-C157.

Ostrowski, NL; Lolait, SJ; Young, WS, III. Cellular localization of vasopressin V1a receptor messenger ribonucleic acid in adult male rat brain, pineal, and brain vasculature. *Endocrinology*, 1994, 135, 1511-1528.

Palsson B (2006) Systems biology: properties of reconstructed networks. Cambridge: Cambridge University Press.

Park, PS; Filipek, S; Wells, JW; Palczewski, K. Oligomerization of G protein-coupled receptors: past, present, and future. *Biochemistry*, 2004, 43, 15643-15656.

Parkes, D; Rivest, S; Lee, S; Rivier, C; Vale, W. Corticotropin-releasing factor activates c-fos, NGFI-B, and corticotropin-releasing factor gene expression within the paraventricular nucleus of the rat hypothalamus. *Mol Endocrinol*, 1993, 7, 1357-1367.

Periasamy, A; Day, RN. Visualizing protein interactions in living cells using digitized GFP imaging and FRET microscopy. *Methods Cell Biol*, 1999, 58, 293-314.

Perrin, MH; Donaldson, CJ; Chen, R; Lewis, KA; Vale, WW. Cloning and functional expression of a rat brain corticotropin releasing factor (CRF) receptor. *Endocrinology*, 1993, 133, 3058-3061.

Plotsky, PM. Pathways to the secretion of adrenocorticotropin: A view from the portal. *J Neuroendocrinol*, 1991, 3, 1-9.

Recht, LD; Hoffman, DL; Haldar, J; Silverman, AJ; Zimmerman, EA. Vasopressin concentrations in hypophysial portal plasma: insignificant reduction following removal of the posterior pituitary gland. *Neuroendocrinology*, 1981, 33, 88-90.

Richard, S; Martínez-García, F; Lanuza, E; Davies, DC. Distribution of corticotropin-releasing factor-immunoreactive neurons in the central nervous system of the domestic chicken and Japanese quail. *J Comp Neurol*, 2004, 469, 559-580.

Rivalland, ET; Iqbal, J; Clarke, IJ; Turner, AI; Tilbrook, AJ. Co-localization and distribution of corticotrophin-releasing hormone, arginine vasopressin and enkephalin in the paraventricular nucleus of sheep: a sex comparison. *Neuroscience*, 2005, 132, 755-766.

Rivier, C; Vale, W. Interaction of corticotropin-releasing factor and arginine vasopressin on adrenocorticotropin secretion in vivo. *Endocrinology*, 1983, 113, 939-942.

Romero, LM; Cyr, NE; Romero, RC. Corticosterone responses change seasonally in free-living house sparrows (*Passer domesticus*). *Gen Comp Endocrinol*, 2006, 149, 58-65.

Romero, LM; Wingfield, JC. Regulation of the hypothalamic-pituitary-adrenal axis in free-living pigeons. *J Comp Physiol [B]*, 2001, 171, 231-235.

Saito, N; Koike, TI. Alterations in uterine contraction during the oviposition cycle in domestic hens. *Brit Poultry Sci*, 1992, 33, 671-676.

Schmeling, SK; Nockels, CF. Effects of age, sex, and ascorbic acid ingestion on chicken plasma corticosterone levels. *Poultry Sci*, 1978, 57, 527-533.

Schwartz, J; Vale, W. Dissociation of the adrenocorticotropin secretory responses to corticotropin-releasing factor (CRF) and vasopressin or oxytocin by using a specific cytotoxic analog of CRF. *Endocrinology*, 1988, 122, 1695-1700.

Scott, LV; Dinan, TG. Vasopressin and the regulation of hypothalamic-pituitary-adrenal axis function: implications for the pathophysiology of depression. *Life Sci*, 1998, 62, 1985-1998.

Smith, AI; Levin, N; Wallace, CA; Farnworth, P; Blum, M; Roberts, JL. The role of vasopressin on ACTH secretion and biosynthesis in the ovine pituitary gland. *Regul Pept*, 1993, 45, 237-241.

Szot, P; Bale, TL; Dorsa, DM. Distribution of messenger RNA for the vasopressin V_{1a} receptor in the CNS of male and female rats. *Brain Res Mol Brain Res*, 1994, 24, 1-10.

Tachibana, T; Saito, E-S; Saito, S; Tomonaga, S; Denbow, DM; Furuse, M. Comparison of brain arginine-vasotocin and corticotrophin-releasing factor for physiological responses in chicks. *Neurosci Lett*, 2004, 360, 165-169.

Tan, FL; Lolait, SJ; Brownstein, MJ; Saito, N; MacLeod, V; Baeyens, DA; Mayeux, PR; Jones, SM; Cornett, LE. Molecular cloning and functional characterization of a vasotocin receptor subtype that is expressed in the shell gland and brain of the domestic chicken. *Biol Reprod*, 2000, 62, 8-15.

Tanaka, M; Otani, H; Yokode, M; Kita, T. Regulation of apolipoprotein B secretion in hepatocytes from Watanabe heritable hyperlipidemic rabbit, an animal model for familial hypercholesterolemia. *Atherosclerosis*, 1995, 114, 73-82.

Timpl, P; Spanagel, R; Sillaber, I; Kresse, A; Reul, JM; Stalla, GK; Blanquet, V; Steckler, T; Holsboer, F; Wurst, W. Impaired stress response and reduced anxiety in mice lacking a functional corticotropin-releasing hormone receptor 1. *Nat Genet*, 1998, 19, 162-166.

Ueda, N; Mayeux, PR; Walker, PD; Shah, SV. Receptor-mediated increase in cytosolic calcium in LLC-PK1 cells by platelet activating factor and thromboxane A2. *Kidney Int*, 1991, 40, 1075-1081.

Vaccari, C; Lolait, SJ; Ostrowski, NL. Comparative distribution of vasopressin V1b and oxytocin receptor messenger ribonucleic acids in brain. *Endocrinology*, 1998, 139, 5015-5033.

Vale, W; Vaughan, J; Smith, M; Yamamoto, G; Rivier, J; Rivier, C. Effects of synthetic ovine corticotropin-releasing factor, glucocorticoids, catecholamines, neurohypophysial peptides, and other substances on cultured corticotropic cells. *Endocrinology*, 1983, 113, 1121-1131.

Veenema, AH; Blume, A; Niederle, D; Buwalda, B; Neumann, I. Effects of early life stress on adult male aggression and hypothalamic vasopressin and serotonin. *Eur J Neurosci*, 2006, 24, 1711-1720.

Vitums, A; Mikami, S; Oksche, A; Farner, DS. Vascularization of the hypothalamo-hypophysial-complex in the white-crowned sparrow, *Zonotrichia leucophrys gambelii*. *Z Zellforsch Mikrosk Anat*, 1964, 64, 541-569.

Wang, Z; Ferris, CF; De Vries, GJ. Role of septal vasopressin innervation in paternal behavior in prairie voles (*Microtus ochrogaster*). *Proc Natl Acad Sci U S A*, 1994, 91, 400-404.

Westerhof, I; Lumeij, JT; Mol, JA; van den Brom, WE; Rijnberk, A. *In vitro* studies on the effects of ovine corticotrophin-releasing hormone, arginine vasotocin, arginine vasopressin, and haloperidol on adrenocortical function in the racing pigeon (*Columba livia domestica*). *Gen Comp Endocrinol*, 1992, 88, 76-82.

Wotjak, CT; Kubota, M; Liebsch, G; Montkowski, A; Holsboer, F; Neumann, I; Landgraf, R. Release of vasopressin within the rat paraventricular nucleus in response to emotional stress: A novel mechanism of regulating adrenocorticotropic hormone secretion? *J Neurosci*, 1996, 16, 7725-7732.

Wotjak, CT; Ludwig, M; Ebner, K; Russell, JA; Singewald, N; Landgraft, R; Engelmann, M. Vasopressin from hypothalamic magnocellular neurons has opposite actions at the adenohypophysis and in the supraoptic nucleus on ACTH secretion. *Eur J Neurosci*, 2002, 16, 477-485.

Wotjak, CT; Naruo, T; Muraoka, S; Simchen, R; Landgraf, R; Engelmann, M. Forced swimming stimulates the expression of vasopressin and oxytocin in magnocellular neurons of the rat hypothalamic paraventricular nucleus. *Eur J Neurosci*, 2001, 13, 2273-2281.

Yoshida, M. Gene regulation system of vasopressin and corticotropin-releasing hormone. *Gene Regulation and Systems Biology*, 2008, 2, 71-88.

Young, SF; Griffante, C; Aguilera, G. Dimerization between vasopressin v1b and corticotropin releasing hormone type 1 receptors. *Cell Mol Neurobiol*, 2007, 27, 439-461.

Yu, J; Xie, LY; Abou-Samra, AB. Molecular cloning of a type A chicken corticotropin-releasing factor receptor with high affinity for urotensin I. *Endocrinology*, 1996, 137, 192-197.

Zacharias, DA; Violin, JD; Newton, AC; Tsien, RY. Partitioning of lipid-modified monomeric GFPs into membrane microdomains of live cells. *Science*, 2002, 296, 913-916.

In: Neuroendocrinology Research Developments
Editor: N. S. Penkava and L.R. Haight, pp. 35-61

ISBN: 978-1-60876-983-4
© 2010 Nova Science Publishers, Inc.

Chapter 2

GASTRIC FUEL SENSING, GHRELIN PRODUCTION AND FOOD INTAKE

***Geyang Xu*[1]*, Yin Li*[1] *and Weizhen Zhang*[1,2*]**

[1]Department of Physiology and Pathophysiology, Peking University Health Science Center, Beijing 100191, China

[2]Department of Surgery, University of Michigan Medical Center, Ann Arbor, MI 48109-0346, USA

ABSTRACT

The gastrointestinal system is essential in the control of energy metabolism, not only because it is the site of nutrient absorption, but also because a variety of gastrointestinal hormones and neuropeptides integrate peripheral and central regulation of food intake and body weight. Among these hormones, ghrelin is the only currently identified orexigenic hormone in the circulation. Three major forms of ghrelin have been identified: acyl ghrelin, des-acyl ghrelin and obestatin. Acyl ghrelin is the only one capable of binding and activating the ghrelin receptor. Blocking the action of acyl ghrelin by receptor antagonist, neutralizing antibodies or Spiegelmer RNA has been reported to affect food intake and body weight in preclinical models. However, the long-term use of these approaches is offset by potential increases in circulating ghrelin due to the feed-back regulation. Defining novel pathways to inhibit the production of acyl ghrelin is appealing for the pharmaceutical intervention of obesity and would shift therapeutic focus to gastric targets.

Ghrelin producing cells comprise approximately one quarter of gastric endocrine cells. The secretion of ghrelin is tightly coupled to the fasting or fed state. While it is presumed that precise control in the production and secretion of ghrelin is critical for the maintenance of energy balance, the molecular mechanisms by which ghrelin producing cells modulate transcription and translation of ghrelin to match overall energy status are unknown. Their studies demonstrate that mammalian target of rapamycin (mTOR) is present in the gastric ghrelin cells and its activity is altered during fasting and obesity. In addition, there exists a reciprocal relationship between gastric mTOR signaling and the

* Corresponding author: Tel: 734-615-0360; Fax: 734-763-4135; E-mail: weizhenz@umich.edu

expression and secretion of ghrelin during changes in energy status. Both *in vivo* and *in vitro* data support the concept that gastric mTOR activity is reciprocally linked to the production of ghrelin and ghrelin O-acyl transferase (GOAT), the enzyme mediating the octanoylation of ghrelin. Consistent with the increase of circulating ghrelin, inhibition of the gastric mTOR activity stimulates food intake. This orexigenic effect of gastric mTOR inhibition can be blocked by antagonist of ghrelin receptor.

In summary, their studies suggest that gastric ghrelin cells may recognize energy status at the organism level. The mTOR signaling may serve as a unique fuel sensor in gastric ghrelin cells, whose activity is linked to the regulation of energy intake through ghrelin.

The gastrointestinal tract, an interface between the body and the external environment, is a highly specialized organ system that allows living individual to consume food in discrete meals as well as a very diverse array of food stuffs to meet nutrient needs [1]. The gastrointestinal system is essential in the control of energy metabolism, not only because it is the site of nutrient absorption, but also because it is the largest endocrine organ in the body and also an important source of gastrointestinal hormones and neuropeptides such as ghrelin, peptide YY (PYY), pancreatic polypeptide (PP), glucagon-like peptide-1 (GLP-1), oxyntomodulin (OXM) and cholecystokinin (CCK). These peptide hormones have been demonstrated to potently influence the food intake and energy metabolism by acting on the hypothalamus and brainstem, the ingestion and energy metabolism center in the central nervous system [2]. Among these hormones, ghrelin is the only currently identified orexigenic hormone in the circulation. Since its discovery in year 1999 [3], ghrelin has been the focus of the search for an efficient intervention of obesity. Much of the effort has been focused on the intervention of the effect of ghrelin at the receptor level. Although the ghrelin antagonism has been documented to be effective in the inhibition of food intake and reduction of body weight, its long-term efficacy may be guarded because of its potential to increase the production of ghrelin [4]. Their recent study has identified an important intracellular mechanism involving mTOR signaling on the regulation of ghrelin production, providing a novel insight into the development of an alternative therapeutic strategy to treat obesity by direct intervention of gastric ghrelin [5]. Here we summarize the recent advance on ghrelin with focus on the regulation of ghrelin production by gastric fuel sensing mechanism.

1. GHRELIN

The discovery of ghrelin in 1999 is a typical example of reverse pharmacological study. Its receptor was identified and named as the growth hormone secretagogues receptors (GHS-R) in the eighties. A group of small synthetic molecules, named as growth hormone secretagogues, was synthesized and found to stimulate the release of growth hormone from the pituitary. The receptor in response to these agonists was first cloned from the pituitary tissue and named as the growth hormone secretagogue receptor. Sequence analysis identifies this receptor as a member of G-protein-coupled receptor (GPCR) family. Activation of the GHS-R leads to multiple intracellular signaling pathways which includes changes in intracellular calcium, phospholipase C, protein kinase C, and cAMP activated protein kinase A [3,6]. GHS-R is expressed predominantly in the pituitary, hypothalamus and brain cortex, and in multiple peripheral tissues such as the thyroid gland, gastrointestinal organs, pancreas, spleen, myocardium and adrenal gland at much lower expression levels [7]. The endogenous ligand for this orphan GPCR remained unidentified until a group of Japanese scientist discovered in 1999 a unique 28 amino acid peptide in the gastric mucosa, which is potent in binding and activating the GHS-R. Because of its potent stimulation of growth hormone release both *in vivo* and *in vitro*, this endogenous ligand for the GHS-R was names as ghrelin, because 'ghre' is a word root in Proto-Indo-European languages for "grow". Chemical analysis reveals a unique post-translational modification of ghrelin at the Serine 3 residue by octanoylation. No other endogenous peptide has been found to be modified by this mechanism. This octanoylation is critical for ghrelin to bind and activate its receptor GHS-R [3].

1.1. Ghrelin Cell

In all vertebrate species, ghrelin is mainly produced in the stomach. Relative low level of ghrelin can also be found in hypothalamus, pituitary, hippocampus, brain cortex, adrenal gland, intestine, pancreas, and many other tissues [6]. Total gastrectomy [8], a procedure performed in the treatment of gastric cancer or severe gastric ulcers, has been reported to decrease the plasma concentration of ghrelin to ~30–50% of its pre-operation level when measured 30 min after the surgery. This concentration gradually increases to ~70% of the level before the operation. Gastric ghrelin production is therefore proposed to account for ~50–70% of circulating ghrelin. Compensatory production of ghrelin, possibly by the intestines and pancreas, may occur when supply of ghrelin from stomach is limited.

In the stomach, ghrelin-containing cells are more abundant in the fundus than in the pylorus. Four types of endocrine cells have been identified in the oxyntic mucosa: enterochromaffin like (ECL) cells, D cells, enterochromaffin (EC) cells, and X/A-like cells. The relative abundance of these endocrine cells varies between species. In rat oxyntic gland, endocrine cells contain 60–70% of ECL cells, 20% of X/A-like cells, 2–5% of D cells, and 0–2% of EC cells. In human, the corresponding percentages are 30, 20, 22, and 7%. Major products in the granules of these endocrine cells have been identified as histamine and uroguanylin in ECL cells, somatostatin in D cells, and serotonin in EC cells [6]. Ghrelin has been demonstrated to be present in X/A like endocrine cells by *in situ* hybridization at the mRNA level and by immunohistochemical analysis at the protein level. No other peptide hormone has been found to be present in the granule contents of X/A-like cells. Examination by light and electron microscopic immunohistochemistry has revealed the presence of ghrelin in the round, compact, and electron-dense granules compatible with those of X/A-like cells whose hormonal product and physiological functions have not previously been clarified [9]. Ghrelin-immunoreactive cells are also found in the duodenum, jejunum, ileum, and colon. In the intestine, ghrelin concentration gradually decreases from the duodenum to the colon [9].

The pancreas is also a ghrelin-producing organ. Both acyl ghrelin and des-acyl ghrelin are present in the rat pancreatic islets [10]. The cell type producing ghrelin is identified as the islet epsilon (ε) cells instead of α or β cells [11,12]. The pancreatic ghrelin profile changes dramatically during fetal development [13]. Pancreatic ghrelin expressing cells are numerous from mid-gestation to the early postnatal period, comprising 10% of all endocrine cells in the islets, and decrease in number after birth. Both ghrelin mRNA and total ghrelin concentration are abundant in the fetal pancreas, six to seven times greater than in the fetal stomach. Thus the onset of ghrelin expression in pancreatic islets precedes that of gastric ghrelin. Pancreatic ghrelin expression is highest in the prenatal and neonatal periods. In contrast, gastric ghrelin level is low during the prenatal period and increases after birth. Unlike gastric ghrelin, pancreatic ghrelin level is not affected by fasting and re-feeding [13].

1.2. Ghrelin Gene Products

Ghrelin gene spans 5 kb of the genomic DNA on chromosome 3p25–26, consisting of five exons and four introns. The first exon is only 20 bp long, which contributes to part of the 50 un-translated region of ghrelin gene. The putative initiation codon ATG is located at nucleotides 34–36 and is preceded by the consensus initiation sequence, whereas a terminal codon TAG is found 117 codons downstream at position 385–387 [14,15]. Ghrelin gene encodes the 117 amino acid product named as preproghrelin which contains a signal peptide. Ghrelin (i. e., the 28-amino acid GH releasing peptide) is encoded by exons 2 and 3 with the remaining proghrelin peptide sequence contained in exons 4 and 5 [16]. The 5'-upstream regulation region of the ghrelin gene consists of binding sites of several transcriptional factors such as upstream stimulatory factor-1/-2(USF1/2), activator proten-1, CCAAT enhancer binding proteins and cAMP response element binding protein, indicating that these transcription factors may regulate ghrelin expression [16]. A spliced variant without the codon for glutamine in position 14 is produced (pre-pro-des-Gln14-ghrelin mRNA) in rat, mouse and pig [17], while its level is negligible in human [18]. Pre-pro-des-Gln14-ghrelin mRNA is processed in an almost similar manner to preproghrelin, except that this product is devoid of glutamine 14 residue. In addition, a human exon 3-deleted mRNA transcript has been described in breast and prostate cancer [19]. A murine homologue of ghrelin mRNA transcript in which exon 4 is deleted has also been identified in a wide range of murine tissues [14]. It is probable that theses variants, like the pre-pro-des- Gln14-ghrelin mRNA, are products of the ghrelin gene produced by alternative splicing mechanisms.

Full length of ghrelin mRNA encodes preproghrelin, a 117 amino acid peptide. Preproghrelin contains a 23 amino-acid signal peptide and a 94 amino-acid peptide called pro-ghrelin (1–94). Proghrelin includes the 28 amino acid acyl ghrelin (1–28) and a 66 amino acid tail (29–94) named as C-ghrelin [15]. Biochemical studies suggest that proghrelin (1–94) can be cleaved by prohormone convertase 1/3 (PC1/3) in mouse stomach tissue to generate acyl ghrelin *in vivo* [20]. The acyl ghrelin sequence starts from Gly1, which directly follows the signal peptide, and the last two residues of ghrelin are Pro27-Arg28, which correspond to a processing signal for PC1/3. Here, the cleavage most frequently occurs to originate a 28 amino acid peptide, ghrelin (1–28) [20]. Arg28 is occasionally removed from C-terminus of ghrelin (1–28) most likely by a carboxy peptidase B-like enzyme, generating a peptide with 27 amino acids, ghrelin (1–27), which terminates in proline [15]. Although ghrelin (1–27) is present only at a very low level in rat stomach, it is likely 27 and 28 amino acid ghrelin molecules are produced through alternative C-terminal processing of the same ghrelin precursor and that this process may regulate maturation of human ghrelin gene [15]. Both ghrelin (1–28) and ghrelin (1–27) are then subjected to a unique post-translational modification: acylation of the hydroxyl group of Serine 3 residue. This is frequently done with an octanoyl group (C8:0), but modification with decanoyl (C10:0) and decenoyl moieties (C10:1) may also occur [18]. In the human stomach, the des-acyl:acyl ghrelin ratio was found to be about 2:1 [21], but the nonacylated form constitutes >90% of total circulating ghrelin [21], indicating that acyl ghrelin may be de-acylated in the bloodstream. Enzymes responsible for the de-acylation of acyl ghrelin include butyrylcholinesterase and platelet activating factor acetylhydrolase, which are associated with circulating lipids. Other enzymes may also have this capability [22].

The acyltransferase that catalyzes ghrelin octanoylation has been recently identified as ghrelin O-acyltransferase (GOAT) [23], which belongs to a family of membrane-bound O-acyltransferases (MBOATs). GOAT covalently links a medium fatty-acid chain, typically octanoate, to the hydroxyl group of the serine 3 residue of ghrelin. Ingestion of medium-chain fatty acids (MCFAs) or medium-chain triacylglycerols (MCTs) influences the acylation of ghrelin [24]. Nevertheless, it remains to be determined whether ingested MCTs directly modulate the serine 3 residue of ghrelin peptide or indirectly stimulate the acylation of ghrelin through the induction of GOAT. The 66 amino acid tail of wild type proghrelin (29–94) has been proposed to be circulating as a peptide named C-ghrelin [25] or to be processed to smaller peptides, mainly obestatin [26]. Both these products may have physiological relevance. C-ghrelin has been demonstrated to circulate in human plasma at a higher concentration than acyl ghrelin and its level is elevated in heart failure [25]. Peptide consistent in length with the complete C-terminal sequence of proghrelin has been detected in majority of tissues and in circulation in mammals. Its level is responsive to metabolic manipulation in the similar fashion acyl ghrelin (1–28). The tissue distribution of C-ghrelin matches that of ghrelin. The main source of circulating C-ghrelin is likely to be the stomach [21]. A novel peptide derived from the C terminal of proghrelin has been proposed based on comparative genomic analysis. This new peptide is named 'obestatin' because of its potency to suppress the appetite. The structure of obestatin comprises a 23 amino acid sequence derived from proghrelin (53–75) [26]. Obestatin was originally extracted from rat stomach and subsequently shown to be a circulating peptide whose secretion is pulsatile and displays an ultradian rhythmicity similar to ghrelin and growth hormone secretion [27].

1.3. Secretion of Ghrelin

1.3.1. Fluctuation of plasma ghrelin

The clear preprandial rise and postprandial fall in plasma ghrelin level support the contention that ghrelin is an initiation signal for meal consumption. Level of plasma ghrelin increases immediately prior to each meal and falls to baseline within one hour after food intake [28]. The preprandial increase in ghrelin level is observed in human beings who initiate meals voluntarily without any time- and food-related cues. Positive correlation has been demonstrated between plasma ghrelin level and hunger scores [29]. Furthermore, the postprandial suppression of plasma ghrelin level is proportional to the ingested caloric [30]. Inter-meal ghrelin level displays a diurnal rhythm, which rises throughout the day to a zenith at 01:00, then falls overnight to a nadir at 09:00 [28]. The normal, meal-related fluctuations and diurnal rhythm of the ghrelin level are absent after gastric bypass surgery [31]. Plasma ghrelin concentrations in patients with simple obesity [32] and anorexia nervosa [33] are lower and higher, respectively, relative to those of healthy subjects with normal body weight. Among those with type 2 diabetes mellitus, obese patients have lower while lean patients have higher fasting plasma ghrelin concentrations relative to patients with normal body weight. Fasting plasma ghrelin concentration is negatively correlated with body mass index in both non-diabetic and diabetic patients [34]. In summary, ghrelin secretion is up-regulated under conditions of negative energy balance and down-regulated in the setting of positive energy balance.

1.3.2. Regulation of ghrelin secretion by nutrients

Glucose significantly inhibits secretion of ghrelin. Oral infusion of glucose decreases the plasma concentration of total ghrelin within 30 minutes in humans [35] and in rats [36]. It is, however, not clear whether glucose inhibits directly the expression and secretion of gastric ghrelin, or indirectly by an unidentified mechanism. The observation that insulin-induced hypoglycemia up-regulates gastric ghrelin mRNA expression [37] and serum acyl ghrelin level [38] indicates the regulation of ghrelin by glucose may involve multiple mechanisms.

Ingestion of either MCFAs (n-octanoic acid) or MCTs (glyceryltrioctanoate) increases the gastric contents of acyl ghrelin without changing the total ghrelin in mouse [24]. This study suggests that medium-chain fatty acids can be utilized directly for the octanoylation of ghrelin as proposed by the authors. In contrast to this study, infusion of intralipid, a mixture of long-chain triglycerides, decreases plasma total ghrelin in humans [39]. Intraduodenal administration of C12 dodecanoic acid significantly decreases plasma ghrelin, whereas C10 decanoic acid has no effect [40]. Whether the structure of fatty acids will ultimately determine their effect on ghrelin secretion remains to be examined. It is generally accepted that lipid ingestion leads to a smaller decline in ghrelin relative to the administration of glucose.

The effect of amino acids on ghrelin secretion remains controversial. Oral ingestion of a physiological dose of essential amino acids leads to a continuous rise in serum ghrelin level in human [41], while ingestion of proteins has been shown to inhibit ghrelin secretion [42].

1.3.3. Neural control of ghrelin secretion

Autonomic nervous system, especially the parasympathetic nerve, plays an important role in the regulation of ghrelin. In rat and human, ghrelin level rises after administration of muscarinic agonists and falls after delivery of muscarinic antagonists [43,44]. Because gastric mucosa is innervated by the intrinsic enteric nervous system and the extrinsic vagal nervous system derived from the midbrain, it is likely that ghrelin-producing cells are regulated by cholinergic neurons, and this nervous regulation contributes to the pre-prandial reflexive surge of ghrelin. This contention is demonstrated by the observation that vagotomy or blockade of vagus nerve by atropine attenuates the increment of ghrelin induced by fasting [45]. In addition, vagotomy blocks the orexigenic effect of ghrelin. Thus, the efferent fiber of vagus nerve regulates the synthesis of ghrelin, whereas its afferent fiber is critical for ghrelin to exercise its orexigenic effect.

Sympathetic nervous system is also involved in the regulation of ghrelin. Plasma acyl ghrelin concentration is increased by α-adrenergic antagonist and β -adrenergic agonist. It is worth noting that vagotomy inhibits the secretion of gastric ghrelin in the acute phase, while the long term effect of vagotomy is stimulatory, suggesting that ghrelin secretion is modulated by the balance between cholinergic and adrenergic tones that control the enteric nervous system [46].

1.3.4. Hormonal modulation of ghrelin secretion

Insulin

In rat, gastric artery perfusion of insulin significantly inhibits ghrelin release from isolated stomach tissue [47], suggesting a local inhibitory effect of insulin. In addition, insulin may also act on the central nervous system to inhibit ghrelin secretion because intracerebroventricular administration of insulin reduces plasma total ghrelin concentration [48]. Similar observation has been reported in human. Infusion of insulin significantly decreases plasma ghrelin level in patients with euglycemia [49,50]. Fasting plasma acyl ghrelin level is negatively related to insulin concentration [38]. Total ghrelin level is also negatively related to homeostasis model assessment insulin resistance index (HOMA-IR) [51], while it is positively correlated to insulin sensitivity [52]. GLP-1, a potent stimulator for insulin secretion, has been reported to alleviate the pre-prandial rise of ghrelin in human [53]. The inhibitory effect of insulin may underlie the suppression of glucose on ghrelin and the inverse relationship between body weight and ghrelin level. It may also explain the low ghrelin level in patients with type 2 diabetes mellitus. Contradict to this general notion, Toshinai *et al* [37] reported an increment of ghrelin after insulin administration. This may be explained as a result of severe hypoglycemia induced by rapid injection of high dose of insulin. It is worth to note that insulin sensitivity, rather than insulin itself, may play a more important role in the regulation of ghrelin. Whether insulin interacts with growth hormone axis to regulate ghrelin level remains undetermined. Although the insulin-induced hypoglycemia is independent of growth hormone level [54], the negative correlation between insulin and ghrelin has been demonstrated to disappear in patients with growth hormone disorder.

Glucagon

Several observations support the contention that glucagon contributes to the pre-prandial surge of ghrelin. First, glucagon receptor is present in gastric endocrine cells [55]. Second, glucagon concentration increases during fasting. Third, plasma acyl ghrelin concentration rises transiently while des-acyl ghrelin increases persistently after administration of glucagon in rat. Lastly, ghrelin released from the isolated rat stomach is augmented by perfusion of glucagon [47]. The molecular mechanism on how glucagon regulates ghrelin remains to be explored. Previous report suggests that glucagon may directly stimulate the gene transcription of ghrelin [56]. Ghrelin gene promoter has been demonstrated to be up-regulated by glucagon via the mediation of the second messenger cAMP. The physiological regulation of glucagons on ghrelin is complicated by the observation that glucagon suppresses ghrelin secretion [57] via acting on the hypothalamus pituitary axis [58] to stimulate release of growth hormone and glucocorticoids which then inhibit ghrelin secretion.

Growth hormone/insulin-like growth factor-1 (IGF-1)

Growth hormone therapy in growth hormone deficient patients significantly decreases the concentration of plasma acyl ghrelin [59]. Administration of growth hormone in cultured rat gastric tissue inhibits total ghrelin secretion in a time-dependent manner [60]. In rat, growth hormone significantly decreases the gastric ghrelin mRNA and plasma ghrelin level, without changing gastric ghrelin content [61]. These observations support the notion that growth hormone exerts a negative feedback action on ghrelin production and secretion. The concept that IGF-1 may promote ghrelin secretion is supported by following studies. Recombinant human IGF-1 significantly elevates plasma total ghrelin concentration in severely under-nutritioned patients [62]. The IGF-1/IGFBP-3 complex significantly increases ghrelin level in children with low birth weight. IGF-1 may induce ghrelin secretion either directly or indirectly through the reduction of growth hormone [63].

Somatostatin

Somatostatin or its analog octreotide inhibits plasma acyl and total ghrelin levels [64]. On the other hand, an increase in stomach ghrelin mRNA and plasma total ghrelin is detected in somatostatin knockout mice [65]. Since ghrelin increases the level of somatostatin in plasma [66], the inhibitory effect of somatostatin on ghrelin may be considered as a negative feedback modulation.

Leptin

Although some studies report that leptin positively correlates with plasma acyl ghrelin in normal weight woman [67] and up-regulates ghrelin mRNA in mouse stomach [37], it is generally agreed that leptin inhibits the synthesis of ghrelin. Leptin is mainly synthesized and secreted by adipose tissue [68]. Leptin concentration in obese is significantly higher than normal [32]. Reverse relationship has been found between leptin and ghrelin. Gastric ghrelin mRNA increases, whereas leptin mRNA decreases during fasting. Leptin inhibits the transcription of ghrelin and decreases ghrelin release from isolated rat stomach dose-dependently [69]. In contrast to the peripheral effect, central leptin gene therapy decreases plasma leptin level and increases ghrelin level significantly in mice fed with high-fat diet. [70] Thus, peripheral, especially gastric leptin, suppresses ghrelin expression through its receptor in gastric mucosa cells. The effect of leptin on ghrelin secretion is further complicated by its intervention with the body weight, insulin and insulin sensitivity.

Estrogen

Many studies have reported that estrogen up-regulates ghrelin level. Administration of estrogen elevates plasma total ghrelin concentration in female patients with anorexia nervosa [62]. Ghrelin mRNA level rises significantly after estrogen administration in cultured stomach cells [71]. It is likely that the effect of estrogen in the modulation of meal size and growth hormone secretion is partially mediated through ghrelin. Discrepancy in the effect of estrogen on ghrelin secretion, however, exists. Estrogen replacement therapy in post-menopausal women induces plasma total [72] and acyl ghrelin [73]. Plasma acyl ghrelin concentration, numbers of ghrelin expressing cells and ghrelin mRNA level in stomach, increase transiently after ovariectomy in female rats [74]. Reasons for these discrepancy are unclear, but may be attributed to the variation in methods used for estrogen administration such as per oral or transdermal administration, duration of estrogen administration, age and physiological status (such as obesity vs. normal weight, post- or pre-menopausal of experimental subjects), the outcome index measured (total ghrelin or acyl ghrelin), and other experimental methods. The effect of estrogen on ghrelin may explain that plasma ghrelin level in female subjects is higher relative to the male. In human, total ghrelin level is about 3-fold higher in women during the late follicular stage of the cycle than in men [75]. Similarly, ghrelin level is higher in female mice than in male [76].

1.4. Ghrelin and Food Intake

Despite that ghrelin exerts a broad variety of functions ranging from the stimulation of growth hormone release, protection of cardiomyocytes, alteration of inflammatory response, regulation of the gastrointestinal motility and secretion, to modulation of mesenchymal stem cell differentiation, its orexigenic effect is well-documented and receives the most attention [4]. Both peripheral and central administration of acyl ghrelin enhances food intake in mice and rats [77-80]. Daily oral administration of a GHS-R1a antagonist to diet-induced obese mice led to a significant reduction in food intake and body weight due to selective loss of fat mass. Pair-feeding experiments indicate that weight loss is largely a consequence of reduced food intake [81]. Although GHS-R1a antagonist modestly delay gastric emptying at the high dose, delayed gastric emptying does not appear to be a requirement for weight loss because lower doses of GHS-R1a antagonist produce weight loss without affecting the gastric emptying. Reduction in food intake and body weight have also been demonstrated through antagonism of ghrelin by either vaccinating rats with ghrelin immunoconjugate to induce an immune response specific to acyl ghrelin [82] or by a novel type of ghrelin blocking agent named ghrelin RNA Spiegelmer [83]. An RNA Spiegelmer is an oligonucleotide synthesized with unnatural L-enantiomers of ribose in the sugar-phosphate backbone, making them stable *in vivo*. Specific RNA Spiegelmers have been designed to bind specifically and avidly to acyl ghrelin, and thus preventing it from activating the ghrelin receptor *in vitro*. The effect of exogenous ghrelin on neuronal activity in the arcuate nucleus (ARC) has been reported to be efficiently blocked by the RNA Spiegelmer under both *in vitro* and *in vivo* conditions [84]. Infusion of the RNA Spiegelmer to diet-induced obese mice evokes a reduction in food intake, feeding efficiency, fat mass and body weight relative to control groups during the first week of treatment [83,85].

Ghrelin exerts its orexigenic effect via a mechanism involving the central nervous system. Ghrelin fails to stimulate food intake in rats in which the ARC neurons are destroyed [86], suggesting that the hypothalamic ARC is the major target site of ghrelin in the central nervous system. Two groups of neurons have been found in the hypothalamic ARC: an important neural population in which the orexigenic peptides neuropeptide Y (NPY) and agouti-related peptide (AgRP) are present and another population of neurons expressing anorexigenic peptide pro-opiomelanocortin (POMC). Virtually all NPY/AgRP neurons in the ARC contain mRNA for the ghrelin receptor [87]. Intracerebroventricular injection of ghrelin leads to the induction of Fos expression in NPY neurons [88] and an increase in the levels of both NPY and AgRP mRNA in the hypothalamus [89]. The orexigenic effect of ghrelin can be blocked by antagonist of NPY receptor 1 [80], anti-NPY IgG, AgRP inhibitor, or anti-AgRP IgG [4,77]. All of these observations suggest that at least part of the orexigenic effect of ghrelin is mediated by up-regulating the genes encoding these potent appetite stimulating peptides. The finding that ghrelin still stimulates food intake in NPY or AgRP knockout mice, but not in NPY/AgRP double knockout mice, indicates that NPY and AgRP are obligatory mediators for the orexigenic effect of ghrelin [90].

More recently, hypothalamic AMP-activated protein kinase (AMPK) has been shown to involve in the orexigenic effect of ghrelin [91,92]. Administration of ghrelin *in vivo* increases AMPK activity in the hypothalamus. Activation of AMPK may phosphorylate transcription factors of the cAMP responsive element binding protein (CREB) family, which may bind to CRE elements in the NPY promoter to increase its expression and therefore stimulate food intake [93]. In addition, activation of AMPK promotes fatty acid β-oxidation that enables continuous support of the bio-energetic needs for maintaining firing of NPY/AgRP neurons [4,94].

Blocking the action of acyl ghrelin by either receptor antagonist or by neutralizing antibodies or Spiegelmer RNA has been reported to affect food intake and body weight in preclinical models. However, the long-term use of these approaches is offset by potential increases in circulating ghrelin due to the feed-back regulation [4]. So defining novel pathways to inhibit the production of acyl ghrelin is appealing for the pharmaceutical intervention of obesity.

2. Mammalian Target of Rapamycin (mTOR)

Streptomyces hygroscopicus was first isolated from Easter Island, a small triangular-shaped Chilean island located in the South Pacific Ocean, three decades ago. These bacteria secrete a potent anti-fungal macrolide that was named rapamycin. Initially developed as an anti-fungal agent, rapamycin has been widely used as an important immunosuppressive and anti-proliferative medicine. To date, rapamycin (sirolimus as the trade name) has become an FDA (Food and Drug Administration) approved drug used in patients with organ transplantation, in patients with cardiovascular diseases to prevent postangioplastic restenosis, and to treat soft-tissue and bone sarcomas [95].

The mTOR was identified and cloned in the 1990s, shortly after the discovery of two yeast genes, *target of rapamycin 1* and *2* (*TOR1* and *TOR2*) [96], in the budding yeast *Saccharomyces cerevisiae* during a screen for resistance to the immunosuppressant drug rapamycin [97]. Further studies reveal the molecular mechanism of rapamycin inhibition on TOR. Once entering cells, rapamycin binds a small protein receptor called FKBP12 (FK506-binding protein 12 kDa). The rapamycin/FKBP12 complex then specifically binds to TOR and potently interferes with its function, causing cell growth arrest [98]. Extensive genetic studies in yeast have established TOR as an essential molecule in the regulation of cell growth, particularly in response to nutrients. The high degree of conservation among species strongly suggests that TOR is an essential controller of cell growth. The mechanism by which rapamycin inhibits TOR in higher eukaryotes also appears to be conserved [95]. The mammalian TOR, mTOR, is an atypical serine/threonine protein kinase and belongs to the phosphatidylinositol kinase-related kinase (PIKK) family [99]. Its molecular weight is predicted to be 290 kDa [100].

2.1. Structure of mTOR

The mTOR possesses up to 20 tandem HEAT (a protein-protein interaction structure of two tandem anti-parallel α-helices found in huntingtin, elongation factor 3, PR65/A and TOR) repeats at the N-terminal region, followed by an FAT (FRAP, ATM, and TRRAP, all PIKK family members) domain. The kinase domain is located between the FRB (FKBP12/rapamycin binding) domain, which is C-terminal to the FAT domain, and the FATC (FATC-terminus) domain located at the C-terminus of the protein. It is proposed that the HEAT repeats serve to mediate protein-protein interactions, the FRB domain provides a docking site for the FKBP12/rapamycin complex, and the FAT and FATC domains modulate mTOR kinase activity via a mechanism remained to be determined [101]. The binding of rapamycin/FKBP12 to the mTOR FRB domain blocks some of the physiological functions of mTOR [102]. It is still unknown whether rapamycin directly inhibits the intrinsic kinase activity of mTOR. While some scientists believe that the binding prevents mTOR from interacting with its substrates, others have suggested that rapamycin inhibits mTOR autophosphorylation (intrinsic mTOR activity) [101]. Further studies on mTOR phosphorylation are needed to demonstrate that rapamycin does, indeed, contribute to the regulation of mTOR intrinsic kinase activity. The mTOR exists in two different complexes in mammalian cells: mammalian TORC1 (mTORC1) consisting three proteins: raptor (regulatory associated protein of mTOR), mLST8/GβL and mTOR, and mTORC2 consisting mTOR, mLST8 and Rictor. mTORC1 is the only known target of rapamycin[95,100,101].

2.2. Downstream Targets of mTOR

Two proteins: S6K1 (p70 ribosomal protein S6 kinase 1) [103] and 4EBP1 (eIF4E binding protein 1) [104], are the earliest identified and best-studied mTOR downstream effectors. Under basal conditions, S6K1 and 4EBP1 bind to eIF3 (eukaryotic initiation factor 3) and remain inactive. Upon growth stimulations, mTOR binds to eIF3 and phosphorylates S6K1 and 4EBP1 [105]. Phosphorylation of S6K1 releases it from eIF3 and activates its kinase activity. The active S6K1 phosphorylates cellular substrates such as S6 to promote translation and growth [106]. 4EBP1 inhibits cap-dependent mRNA translation via binding to the translation initiator eIF4E (eukaryotic translation initiation factor 4E). Phosphorylation of 4EBP1 by mTOR frees it from eIF4E, relieves its inhibitory effect and stimulates translation initiation [107]. Together, activation of mTOR increases cell growth by promoting protein translation and increasing cell mass. Cells with hyperactive mTOR often gain growth advantage and display a larger size [100].

2.3. Up-Stream Regulators of mTOR

Tuberous sclerosis complex (TSC) is a multi-system disorder characterized by the formation of non-invasive benign tumors in many organs such as brain, lung, skin, heart and kidney [108]. Two independent genes are responsible for TSC disease. *TSC1,* also known as hamartin, encodes a 130-kDa protein with several coiled-coil domains but no known catalytic domains [109]. *TSC2*, also known as tuberin, encodes a 200-kDa protein with a coiled-coil domain and a C-terminal region with homology to the Rap GTPase-activating protein (GAP) [110]. TSC1 and TSC2 form a functional complex that is most stable as a heterodimer [111]. Homozygous inactivation of either TSC1 or TSC2 in mice is lethal to embryos, while heterozygous animals are prone to development of tumors, indicating that both TSC1 and TSC2 function as tumor suppressors [112,113]. In *Drosophila*, inactivation of either *dTSC1* or *dTSC2* increases cell size and cell proliferation while over-expression of both dTSC1 and dTSC2 together decreases cell size, supporting the concept that TSC1 and TSC2 form a functional complex to regulate cell growth [114]. Biochemical studies demonstrate that the TOR pathway is markedly activated in either TSC1 or TSC2 mutant cells [115]. Over-expression of TSC1 and TSC2 suppresses both S6K and 4EBP1 phosphorylation, while transient knock down of TSC2 by RNAi enhances S6K phosphorylation. Furthermore, a rapamycin-resistant S6K mutant is also resistant to inhibition by over-expression of TSC1 and TSC2. These results provide strong evidence that TSC1-TSC2 negatively regulates TOR activity [116].

2.4. mTOR and Energy Metabolism

In addition to its involvement in tumorigenesis, the finding that dys-regulation of mTORC1 in many human metabolic disorders such as obesity and diabetes has boosted an extensive interest in the study of the effect of mTOR on energy metabolism.

2.4.1. mTOR and obesity

Early experiments with rapamycin provide a link between mTOR Complex 1 and adipogenesis. In these studies, rapamycin inhibits both clonal expansion and adipocyte differentiation [117]. Advance studies using gene modified mice have confirmed the role of mTORC1 in the regulation of adipocytes [118]. Defective dTOR signaling leads to loss of fat mass in *Drosophila* [119]. S6K1-deficient mice demonstrate an increase in lipolysis and a reduction in fat mass. S6K1-deficient mice are resistant to diet- and age-induced obesity [120]. Combined disruption of 4E-BP1 and 4E-BP2 in mice renders mice prone to diet-induced obesity. 4E-BP1 and 4E-BP2 double knock out mice demonstrate an increase in the expression of CCAAT/enhancer binding protein δ (C/EBPδ), C/EBPα, and PPARγ. These transcriptional factors are essential in the regulation of adipogenesis and increase in their expression may explain the acceleration in adipogenesis and reduction in energy expenditure observed in these double knock out mice [121]. Moreover, mice with adipose-specific knockout of raptor are lean and resistant to diet-induced obesity, likely because of the increase in mitochondrial uncoupling in white adipose tissue [122]. Taken together, these observations imply that mTORC1 may stimulate adipogenesis, and that elevated mTORC1 activity may contribute to the development of obesity.

2.4.2. mTOR and glucose homeostasis

Given the fact that adipose tissues secrete many hormones that regulate a variety of physiological processes such food intake, energy metabolism and glucose homeostasis, it is not a surprise that mTOR is also involved in the regulation of glucose homeostasis.

Rapamycin has been reported to impair the glucose metabolism by inhibiting the insulin release and increasing insulin resistance [123]. Hyperactive mTORC1 down-regulates IRS1 through the S6K1-dependent negative feedback inhibition. Loss of IRS1 desensitizes the cellular response to insulin, causing insulin resistance which is the fundamental cause of type II diabetes. Thus, dys-regulation of mTORC1 may explain why type-II diabetes is always associated with obesity [124]. Insulin resistance in 4E-BP1 and 4E-BP2 double knock out mice is associated with an increase of ribosomal protein S6 kinase (S6K) activity and an impairment of Akt signaling in muscle, liver, and adipose tissue [121].

2.4.3. Reciprocal relationship between mTOR and nutrients

In mammalian cells, amino acid deprivation causes rapid de-phosphorylation of both 4EBP1 and S6K, while amino acid supplementation stimulates 4E-BP1 and S6K phosphorylation. Rapamycin abolishes these responses, suggesting that mTOR signaling is activated by certain extracellular amino acids [125]. Glucose is another nutrient source that stimulates 4EBP1 and S6K phosphorylation in an mTOR-dependent manner [126]. However, it remains unclear whether glucose itself, glucose metabolites, or glucose-derived products directly stimulate mTOR. It is worth to note that mTOR is more sensitive to amino acids than to glucose. A recent transcriptional profiling of mammalian cells has demonstrated that rapamycin treatment mimics glutamine or leucine starvation more than glucose starvation [127]. Intracellular energy status also affects mTOR signaling. Depletion of ATP levels by the glucose analog 2-deoxyglucose or by the mitochondrial un-coupler rotenone inhibits S6K and 4EBP phosphorylation in an mTOR-dependent manner even in the presence of amino acids. The mTOR has a *K*m of about 1mM for ATP, which is significantly higher than the *K*m for most kinases. These observations suggest that mTOR is an ATP sensor under physiological conditions to regulate translation initiation [128]. However, the intracellular ATP concentration is normally higher than the *K*m for mTOR, implying that a dramatic change of ATP levels within the cells is necessary for altering mTOR kinase activity. Question logically arisen from these observations is whether mTOR serves as the primary physiological ATP sensor or as a result of the activation of its upstream molecules such as AMPK [129]. AMPK, a kinase that is activated by a high AMP/ATP ratio in response to ATP depletion, also modulates S6K activity in an mTOR-dependent manner [129]. AMPK is proposed as a much more sensitive ATP sensor than mTOR because the intracellular AMP concentration is much lower than that of ATP. Thus, a small change in ATP levels could significantly increase the AMP/ATP ratio, suggesting that AMPK may function as a primary physiological sensor of the intracellular energy level to inhibit the mTOR signaling pathway. Further examination demonstrates that AMPK inhibits mTORC1 signaling by phosphorylating TSC2 leading to the enhancement of GAP activity [130]. In summary, mTOR is involved in cellular sensing to extracellular nutrients such as amino acids and glucose.

2.5. mTOR and Food Intake

Down-regulation of the *Drosophila* S6 kinase activity increases food intake, whereas its up-regulation suppresses feeding [131]. In mice, hypothalamus specific expression of dominant-negative S6K increases food intake, while expression of constitutively active S6K inhibits food intake [132]. Studies by Cota *et al* [133] strongly support the notion that hypothalamic mTOR is critical for the regulation of food intake and body weight. Although mTOR and S6K1 are widely expressed in a variety of tissues within the CNS, the phosphorylated form of these two kinases is abundantly localized in the hypothalamus, particularly in the NPY/AgRP and POMC neurons of the ARC. Activity of mTOR pathway in the hypothalamus is tightly linked with energy supply. mTOR activity decreases during fasting and its activity conversely increases during re-feeding. Central administration of leucine, a branch chained amino acid, decreases food intake and body weight by activation of the hypothalamic mTOR signaling. Leptin stimulates hypothalamic mTOR activity, and inhibition of mTOR signaling blunts the anorectic effect of leptin. Furthermore, rapamycin at a dose of 2 mg/kg per week for 16 weeks increases body weight in C57BL/6J mice fed with a high fat diet [134]. All these observations confirm that mTOR is a cellular fuel sensor whose hypothalamic activity is directly tied to the regulation of energy intake.

3. Gastric mTOR Signaling Regulates Ghrelin Production and Food Intake

While extensive studies have examined the hypothalamic fuel sensing mechanisms and its regulation on energy metabolism [135], virtually no attention has been focused on the intracellular fuel sensing mechanism within the gastrointestinal tract. Their recent studies suggest that mTOR signaling pathway regulates fuel sensing in gastric neuroendocrine cells to coordinates the overall energy balance by altering the production of ghrelin [5].

3.1. Expression of mTOR in the Gastric Ghrelin Producing Cells

Immunofluorecent staining of phospho-mTOR (Ser2448) demonstrates strong positive reactivity in cells that are also reactive for ghrelin in the lower 1/3 of the mucosa of the fundus. Almost all ghrelin-positive cells stain positively for phospho-mTOR. Conversely, 28±5% of phospho-mTOR positive gastric mucosal cells are positive for ghrelin. Presence of mTOR in the ghrelin producing cells supports the concept that mTOR may serve as a critical intracellular fuel sensing mechanism in the gastric mucosa. Two experimental findings provide evidence that gastric mTOR is linked with overall energy supply at the organismal level. Gastric mTOR activity is decreased in fasting mice relative to the fed animal. On the other hand, a significant increase in the expression of gastric phospho-mTOR (Ser2448) (pmTOR) and phospho-S6 (Ser235/236) (pS6) is detected in *db/db* obese mice relative to db/m animals, suggesting that gastric mTOR signaling is altered by long-term changes in nutritional status.

3.2. Reciprocal Relationship between Gastric mTOR Signaling and Ghrelin Production

While mTOR signaling is inhibited by fasting, gastric ghrelin mRNA level is significantly increased in fasted mice relative to control animals. Consistent with the change of ghrelin mRNA, gastric preproghrelin level is significantly increased after fasting, as are levels of circulating total ghrelin and acyl ghrelin. These results indicate that gastric mTOR signaling is negatively coordinating with the production of ghrelin during fasting.

In contrast to the starvation, positive energy balance as is the case of obesity up-regulates mTOR signaling and inhibits the production of ghrelin. Decrease in gastric ghrelin mRNA is observed in *db/db* mice relative to the db/m animals. Gastric preproghrelin, plasma total ghrelin and acyl ghrelin levels demonstrate significant decreases in the *db/db* mice compared to db/m mice. It is therefore obvious that there exists a reciprocal relationship between gastric mTOR signaling and ghrelin production.

3.3. Regulation of Ghrelin Production by Gastric mTOR Signaling

If mTOR signaling is linked to the production of ghrelin, then changes in gastric mTOR activity would be expected to alter the production and secretion of ghrelin. Rapamycin, a well-characterized mTOR inhibitor [98], demonstrates a significant effect on the inhibition of gastric phospho-S6 (Ser235/236), a marker of mTOR activity, in C57BL/6J mice. The decrease in gastric mTOR signaling in mice treated with rapamycin is associated with a significant increase in gastric ghrelin mRNA expression, gastric preproghrelin levels, circulating total ghrelin and acyl ghrelin compared with control animals.

Inhibition of gastric mTOR signaling by rapamycin also affects ghrelin expression in obese mice. Intraperitoneal injection of rapamycin significantly inhibits gastric phospho-S6 (Ser235/236) levels in *db/db* mice. The decrement in the gastric mTOR signaling is accompanied by significant increases in gastric ghrelin mRNA levels, tissue preproghrelin content, circulating total ghrelin and acyl ghrelin in *db/db* mice treated with rapamycin. Rapamycin-induced increases in gastric ghrelin mRNA, tissue preproghrelin content, circulating total ghrelin and acyl ghrelin are smaller in obese mice relative to those observed in *db/m* animals.

The fact that atropine demonstrates no effect on rapamycin inhibition of gastric S6 phosphorylation or preproghrelin levels, but abolishes increases in circulating total ghrelin and acyl ghrelin induced by rapamycin indicates that cholinergic innervation of the gastric mucosa is critical in release of mucosal ghrelin into the circulation but not the up-regulation of gastric preproghrelin by rapamycin. Moreover, intraperitoneal administration of L-leucine at a dose of 0. 45 g/kg for six days significantly increases phospho-S6 level, with decreased gastric ghrelin mRNA, gastric preproghrelin content, plasma total ghrelin and acyl ghrelin in C57BL/6J mice compared to controls, which indicates that activation of mTOR signaling in the gastric mucosa would suppress production of ghrelin.

3.4. Regulation of Ghrelin Promoter activity by mTOR

Consistent with *in vivo* studies, rapamycin significantly decreases phosphorylation of mTOR and increases preproghrelin content in 3T3-L1 cells in which ghrelin expression and secretion have been reported [136]. Release of ghrelin into media is dose-dependently regulated by rapamycin. Experiments assaying the activity of the ~3kb human ghrelin promoter (h-ghrelin) demonstrate that mTOR signaling modulates the transcription of the ghrelin gene. Rapamycin significantly increases luciferase activity in HEK 293 cells transfected with ghrelin promoter-luciferase plasmid relative to control, suggesting that down-regulation of mTOR signaling leads to an increase in the activity of ghrelin promoter. Over-expression of mTOR in HEK293 cells decreases ghrelin promoter activity, while over-expression of TSC1 or TSC2, the negative regulators of mTOR signaling, significantly increases ghrelin promoter activity by inhibiting mTOR signaling.

3.5. Regulation of Ghrelin O-acyl Transferase by Gastric mTOR Signaling

The discovery of GOAT in year 2008 extends the therapeutic options for obesity by manipulating the production of acyl ghrelin. Drugs that inhibit GOAT might be able to prevent diet-induced obesity and provide an effective therapy for type-2 diabetes by increasing insulin secretion and enhancing peripheral insulin sensitivity [137]. Changes in gastric mTOR activity have been demonstrated to alter transcription of the GOAT gene, providing an alternative potential approach for designing the therapeutic intervention of obesity.

3.5.1. Reciprocal changes in gastric mTOR signaling and expression of GOAT in fasting and obese mice

Inhibition of gastric mTOR signaling by fasting significantly up-regulates the expression of GOAT transcript relative to fed animals. Experiments using *db/db* obese mice show that long term changes in energy status increase gastric mTOR signaling and results in decrements in GOAT expression relative to control *db/m* mice. This observation suggests a reciprocal relationship between gastric mTOR activity and expression of GOAT mRNA and provides evidence to support the hypothesis that gastric mTOR activity may influence the octanoylation of ghrelin via regulating the expression of GOAT.

3.5.2. Inhibition of gastric mTOR signaling increases GOAT transcription and activation of gastric mTOR signaling attenuates GOAT transcription

Systemic administration of rapamycin at a dose of 1 mg/kg inhibits gastric mTOR activity, while stimulates the expression of GOAT mRNA, an effect which parallels changes in production of both total and acyl ghrelin. In *db/db* obese mice, inhibition of gastric mTOR signaling by rapamycin also results in increments in the transcription of GOAT gene, although increases are less than observed in the db/m control mice. Conversely, up-regulation of gastric mTOR signaling by L-leucine significantly attenuates the expression of GOAT mRNA in the gastric fundus.

3.6. Gastric mTOR Signaling Regulates Food Intake via Ghrelin

Intraperitoneal administration of rapamycin significantly increases food intake relative to the control animals. The orexigenic effect of rapamycin can be blocked by D-Lys-3-GHRP-6, an antagonist for ghrelin receptor. However, antagonism of ghrelin receptor by D-Lys-3-GHRP-6 demonstrates no effect on rapamycin-induced decrease of gastric phospho-S6. Rapamycin-induced increments in gastric ghrelin mRNA and plasma total ghrelin are not affected by administration of D-Lys-3-GHRP6, suggesting that antagonism of the ghrelin receptor does not interfere the effect of rapamycin on the production and secretion of ghrelin. These study provides evidence that rapamycin may act to alter the production of ghrelin to affect the food intake.

4. Conclusion

Obesity, a major health problem in the world [138], is defined as a condition in which energy intake consistently outpaces energy expenditure leading to the accumulation of excess fat to an extent that health is negatively affected. The development of obesity is caused by small but cumulative discrepancies between caloric intake and energy expenditure. Current understanding of the mechanisms underlying the development of obesity is incomplete, and contemporary treatment is often ineffective. Their study [5] suggests that the gastric mucosa is a critical tissue in which fuel sensing mechanism exists to integrate with the hypothalamus to regulate the overall energy balance by alterations in production and secretion of ghrelin. The existence of a fuel-sensing pathway within the gastric mucosa may also provide opportunities for the therapy of obesity.

Acknowledgment

This work was supported by grants from the National Natural Science Foundation of China (30971434, 30871194, 30740096, 30890043, and 30700376), the '985' Program at Peking University (985-2-097-121), the Major National Basic Research Grant of China (No. 2010CB912504).

References

[1] Schneeman, B. O. (2002). Gastrointestinal physiology and functions. *Br J Nutr, 88 Suppl 2*, S159-63.

[2] Hameed, S., Dhillo, W. S. & Bloom, S. R. (2009). Gut hormones and appetite control. *Oral Dis, 15*, 18-26.

[3] Kojima, M., Hosoda, H., Date, Y., Nakazato, M., Matsuo, H. & Kangawa, K. (1999). Ghrelin is a growth-hormone-releasing acylated peptide from stomach. *Nature, 402*, 656-60.

[4] Depoortere, I. (2009). Targeting the ghrelin receptor to regulate food intake. *Regul Pept, 156*, 13-23.

[5] Xu, G., Li, Y., An, W., Li, S., Guan, Y., Wang, N., Tang, C., Wang, X., Zhu, Y., Li, X., Mulholland, M. W. & Zhang, W. (2009). Gastric mammalian target of rapamycin signaling regulates ghrelin production and food intake. *Endocrinology, 150*, 3637-44.

[6] Kojima, M. & Kangawa, K. (2005). Ghrelin: structure and function. *Physiol Rev, 85*, 495-522.

[7] Gnanapavan, S., Kola, B., Bustin, S. A., Morris, D. G., McGee, P., Fairclough, P., Bhattacharya, S., Carpenter, R., Grossman, A. B. & Korbonits, M. (2002). The tissue distribution of the mRNA of ghrelin and subtypes of its receptor, GHS-R, in humans. *J Clin Endocrinol Metab, 87*, 2988.

[8] Jeon, T. Y., Lee, S., Kim, H. H., Kim, Y. J., Son, H. C., Kim, D. H. & Sim, M. S. (2004). Changes in plasma ghrelin concentration immediately after gastrectomy in patients with early gastric cancer. *J Clin Endocrinol Metab, 89*, 5392-6.

[9] Date, Y., Kojima, M., Hosoda, H., Sawaguchi, A., Mondal, M. S., Suganuma, T., Matsukura, S., Kangawa, K. & Nakazato, M. (2000). Ghrelin, a novel growth hormone-releasing acylated peptide, is synthesized in a distinct endocrine cell type in the gastrointestinal tracts of rats and humans. *Endocrinology, 141*, 4255-61.

[10] Date, Y., Nakazato, M., Hashiguchi, S., Dezaki, K., Mondal, M. S., Hosoda, H., Kojima, M., Kangawa, K., Arima, T., Matsuo, H., Yada, T. & Matsukura, S. (2002). Ghrelin is present in pancreatic alpha-cells of humans and rats and stimulates insulin secretion. *Diabetes, 51*, 124-9.

[11] Prado, C. L., Pugh-Bernard, A. E., Elghazi, L., Sosa-Pineda, B. & Sussel, L. (2004). Ghrelin cells replace insulin-producing beta cells in two mouse models of pancreas development. *Proc Natl Acad Sci U S A, 101*, 2924-9.

[12] Wierup, N., Svensson, H., Mulder, H. & Sundler, F. (2002). The ghrelin cell: a novel developmentally regulated islet cell in the human pancreas. *Regul Pept, 107*, 63-9.

[13] Chanoine, J. P. & Wong, A. C. (2004). Ghrelin gene expression is markedly higher in fetal pancreas compared with fetal stomach: effect of maternal fasting. *Endocrinology, 145*, 3813-20.

[14] Jeffery, P. L., Duncan, R. P., Yeh, A. H., Jaskolski, R. A., Hammond, D. S., Herington, A. C. & Chopin, L. K. (2005). Expression of the ghrelin axis in the mouse: an exon 4-deleted mouse proghrelin variant encodes a novel C terminal peptide. *Endocrinology, 146*, 432-40.

[15] Soares, J. B. & Leite-Moreira, A. F. (2008). Ghrelin, des-acyl ghrelin and obestatin: three pieces of the same puzzle. *Peptides, 29*, 1255-70.

[16] Yin, X., Li, Y., Xu, G., An, W. & Zhang, W. (2009). Ghrelin fluctuation, what determines its production? *Acta Biochim Biophys Sin (Shanghai), 41*, 188-97.

[17] Hosoda, H., Kojima, M., Matsuo, H. & Kangawa, K. (2000). Purification and characterization of rat des-Gln14-Ghrelin, a second endogenous ligand for the growth hormone secretagogue receptor. *J Biol Chem, 275*, 21995-2000.

[18] Hosoda, H., Kojima, M., Mizushima, T., Shimizu, S. & Kangawa, K. (2003). Structural divergence of human ghrelin. Identification of multiple ghrelin-derived molecules produced by post-translational processing. *J Biol Chem, 278*, 64-70.

[19] Yeh, A. H., Jeffery, P. L., Duncan, R. P., Herington, A. C. & Chopin, L. K. (2005). Ghrelin and a novel preproghrelin isoform are highly expressed in prostate cancer and

ghrelin activates mitogen-activated protein kinase in prostate cancer. *Clin Cancer Res, 11*, 8295-303.

[20] Zhu, X., Cao, Y., Voogd, K. & Steiner, D. F. (2006). On the processing of proghrelin to ghrelin. *J Biol Chem, 281*, 38867-70.

[21] Bang, A. S., Soule, S. G., Yandle, T. G., Richards, A. M. & Pemberton, C. J. (2007). Characterisation of proghrelin peptides in mammalian tissue and plasma. *J Endocrinol, 192*, 313-23.

[22] De Vriese, C., Gregoire, F., Lema-Kisoka, R., Waelbroeck, M., Robberecht, P. & Delporte, C. (2004). Ghrelin degradation by serum and tissue homogenates: identification of the cleavage sites. *Endocrinology, 145*, 4997-5005.

[23] Yang, J., Brown, M. S., Liang, G., Grishin, N. V. & Goldstein, J. L. (2008). Identification of the acyltransferase that octanoylates ghrelin, an appetite-stimulating peptide hormone. *Cell, 132*, 387-96.

[24] Nishi, Y., Hiejima, H., Hosoda, H., Kaiya, H., Mori, K., Fukue, Y., Yanase, T., Nawata, H., Kangawa, K. & Kojima, M. (2005). Ingested medium-chain fatty acids are directly utilized for the acyl modification of ghrelin. *Endocrinology, 146*, 2255-64.

[25] Pemberton, C., Wimalasena, P., Yandle, T., Soule, S. & Richards, M. (2003). C-terminal pro-ghrelin peptides are present in the human circulation. *Biochem Biophys Res Commun, 310*, 567-73.

[26] Zhang, J. V., Ren, P. G., Avsian-Kretchmer, O., Luo, C. W., Rauch, R., Klein, C. & Hsueh, A. J. (2005). Obestatin, a peptide encoded by the ghrelin gene, opposes ghrelin's effects on food intake. *Science, 310*, 996-9.

[27] Zizzari, P., Longchamps, R., Epelbaum, J. & Bluet-Pajot, M. T. (2007). Obestatin partially affects ghrelin stimulation of food intake and growth hormone secretion in rodents. *Endocrinology, 148*, 1648-53.

[28] Cummings, D. E., Purnell, J. Q., Frayo, R. S., Schmidova, K., Wisse, B. E. & Weigle, D. S. (2001). A preprandial rise in plasma ghrelin levels suggests a role in meal initiation in humans. *Diabetes, 50*, 1714-9.

[29] Cummings, D. E., Frayo, R. S., Marmonier, C., Aubert, R. & Chapelot, D. (2004). Plasma ghrelin levels and hunger scores in humans initiating meals voluntarily without time- and food-related cues. *Am J Physiol Endocrinol Metab, 287*, E297-304.

[30] Erdmann, J., Topsch, R., Lippl, F., Gussmann, P. & Schusdziarra, V. (2004). Postprandial response of plasma ghrelin levels to various test meals in relation to food intake, plasma insulin, and glucose. *J Clin Endocrinol Metab, 89*, 3048-54.

[31] Cummings, D. E., Weigle, D. S., Frayo, R. S., Breen, P. A., Ma, M. K., Dellinger, E. P. & Purnell, J. Q. (2002). Plasma ghrelin levels after diet-induced weight loss or gastric bypass surgery. *N Engl J Med, 346*, 1623-30.

[32] Tschop, M., Weyer, C., Tataranni, P. A., Devanarayan, V., Ravussin, E. & Heiman, M. L. (2001). Circulating ghrelin levels are decreased in human obesity. *Diabetes, 50*, 707-9.

[33] Soriano-Guillen, L., Barrios, V., Campos-Barros, A. & Argente, J. (2004). Ghrelin levels in obesity and anorexia nervosa: effect of weight reduction or recuperation. *J Pediatr, 144*, 36-42.

[34] Erdmann, J., Lippl, F., Wagenpfeil, S. & Schusdziarra, V. (2005). Differential association of basal and postprandial plasma ghrelin with leptin, insulin, and type 2 diabetes. *Diabetes, 54*, 1371-8.

[35] Baldelli, R., Bellone, S., Castellino, N., Petri, A., Rapa, A., Vivenza, D., Bellone, J., Broglio, F., Ghigo, E. & Bona, G. (2006). Oral glucose load inhibits circulating ghrelin levels to the same extent in normal and obese children. *Clin Endocrinol (Oxf), 64*, 255-9.

[36] Guo, Z. F., Ren, A. J., Zheng, X., Qin, Y. W., Cheng, F., Zhang, J., Wu, H., Yuan, W. J. & Zou, L. (2008). Different responses of circulating ghrelin, obestatin levels to fasting, re-feeding and different food compositions, and their local expressions in rats. *Peptides, 29*, 1247-54.

[37] Toshinai, K., Mondal, M. S., Nakazato, M., Date, Y., Murakami, N., Kojima, M., Kangawa, K. & Matsukura, S. (2001). Upregulation of Ghrelin expression in the stomach upon fasting, insulin-induced hypoglycemia, and leptin administration. *Biochem Biophys Res Commun, 281*, 1220-5.

[38] Kim, S. W., Kim, K. W., Shin, C. S., Park do, J., Park, K. S., Cho, B. Y., Lee, H. K. & Kim, S. Y. (2007). Acylated ghrelin secretion is acutely suppressed by oral glucose load or insulin-induced hypoglycemia independently of basal growth hormone secretion in humans. *Horm Res, 67*, 211-9.

[39] Gormsen, L. C., Gjedsted, J., Gjedde, S., Vestergaard, E. T., Christiansen, J. S., Jorgensen, J. O., Nielsen, S. & Moller, N. (2006). Free fatty acids decrease circulating ghrelin concentrations in humans. *Eur J Endocrinol, 154*, 667-73.

[40] Feltrin, K. L., Patterson, M., Ghatei, M. A., Bloom, S. R., Meyer, J. H., Horowitz, M. & Feinle-Bisset, C. (2006). Effect of fatty acid chain length on suppression of ghrelin and stimulation of PYY, GLP-2 and PP secretion in healthy men. *Peptides, 27*, 1638-43.

[41] Groschl, M., Knerr, I., Topf, H. G., Schmid, P., Rascher, W. & Rauh, M. (2003). Endocrine responses to the oral ingestion of a physiological dose of essential amino acids in humans. *J Endocrinol, 179*, 237-44.

[42] Blom, W. A., Lluch, A., Stafleu, A., Vinoy, S., Holst, J. J., Schaafsma, G. & Hendriks, H. F. (2006). Effect of a high-protein breakfast on the postprandial ghrelin response. *Am J Clin Nutr, 83*, 211-20.

[43] Sugino, T., Yamaura, J., Yamagishi, M., Kurose, Y., Kojima, M., Kangawa, K., Hasegawa, Y. & Terashima, Y. (2003). Involvement of cholinergic neurons in the regulation of the ghrelin secretory response to feeding in sheep. *Biochem Biophys Res Commun, 304*, 308-12.

[44] Broglio, F., Gottero, C., Van Koetsveld, P., Prodam, F., Destefanis, S., Benso, A., Gauna, C., Hofland, L., Arvat, E., van der Lely, A. J. & Ghigo, E. (2004). Acetylcholine regulates ghrelin secretion in humans. *J Clin Endocrinol Metab, 89*, 2429-33.

[45] Williams, D. L., Grill, H. J., Cummings, D. E. & Kaplan, J. M. (2003). Vagotomy dissociates short- and long-term controls of circulating ghrelin. *Endocrinology, 144*, 5184-7.

[46] Hosoda, H. & Kangawa, K. (2008). The autonomic nervous system regulates gastric ghrelin secretion in rats. *Regul Pept, 146*, 12-8.

[47] Kamegai, J., Tamura, H., Shimizu, T., Ishii, S., Sugihara, H. & Oikawa, S. (2004). Effects of insulin, leptin, and glucagon on ghrelin secretion from isolated perfused rat stomach. *Regul Pept, 119*, 77-81.

[48] Ueno, M., Carvalheira, J. B., Oliveira, R. L., Velloso, L. A. & Saad, M. J. (2006). Circulating ghrelin concentrations are lowered by intracerebroventricular insulin. *Diabetologia, 49*, 2449-52.

[49] Saad, M. F., Bernaba, B., Hwu, C. M., Jinagouda, S., Fahmi, S., Kogosov, E. & Boyadjian, R. (2002). Insulin regulates plasma ghrelin concentration. *J Clin Endocrinol Metab, 87*, 3997-4000.

[50] Flanagan, D. E., Evans, M. L., Monsod, T. P., Rife, F., Heptulla, R. A., Tamborlane, W. V. & Sherwin, R. S. (2003). The influence of insulin on circulating ghrelin. *Am J Physiol Endocrinol Metab, 284*, E313-6.

[51] Greenman, Y., Golani, N., Gilad, S., Yaron, M., Limor, R. & Stern, N. (2004). Ghrelin secretion is modulated in a nutrient- and gender-specific manner. *Clin Endocrinol (Oxf), 60*, 382-8.

[52] Purnell, J. Q., Weigle, D. S., Breen, P. & Cummings, D. E. (2003). Ghrelin levels correlate with insulin levels, insulin resistance, and high-density lipoprotein cholesterol, but not with gender, menopausal status, or cortisol levels in humans. *J Clin Endocrinol Metab, 88*, 5747-52.

[53] Hagemann, D., Holst, J. J., Gethmann, A., Banasch, M., Schmidt, W. E. & Meier, J. J. (2007). Glucagon-like peptide 1 (GLP-1) suppresses ghrelin levels in humans via increased insulin secretion. *Regul Pept, 143*, 64-8.

[54] Ryber, L., Obrink, K., Houe, N., Frystyk, J. & Jorgensen, J. O. (2006). Serum ghrelin levels are suppressed in hypopituitary patients following insulin-induced hypoglycaemia irrespective of GH status. *Clin Endocrinol (Oxf), 65*, 210-4.

[55] Katayama, T., Shimamoto, S., Oda, H., Nakahara, K., Kangawa, K. & Murakami, N. (2007). Glucagon receptor expression and glucagon stimulation of ghrelin secretion in rat stomach. *Biochem Biophys Res Commun, 357*, 865-70.

[56] Wei, W., Wang, G., Qi, X., Englander, E. W. & Greeley, G. H., Jr. (2005). Characterization and regulation of the rat and human ghrelin promoters. *Endocrinology, 146*, 1611-25.

[57] Arafat, M. A., Otto, B., Rochlitz, H., Tschop, M., Bahr, V., Mohlig, M., Diederich, S., Spranger, J. & Pfeiffer, A. F. (2005). Glucagon inhibits ghrelin secretion in humans. *Eur J Endocrinol, 153*, 397-402.

[58] Arafat, A. M., Perschel, F. H., Otto, B., Weickert, M. O., Rochlitz, H., Schofl, C., Spranger, J., Mohlig, M. & Pfeiffer, A. F. (2006). Glucagon suppression of ghrelin secretion is exerted at hypothalamus-pituitary level. *J Clin Endocrinol Metab, 91*, 3528-33.

[59] Eden Engstrom, B., Burman, P., Holdstock, C. & Karlsson, F. A. (2003). Effects of growth hormone (GH) on ghrelin, leptin, and adiponectin in GH-deficient patients. *J Clin Endocrinol Metab, 88*, 5193-8.

[60] Seoane, L. M., Al-Massadi, O., Barreiro, F., Dieguez, C. & Casanueva, F. F. (2007). Growth hormone and somatostatin directly inhibit gastric ghrelin secretion. An in vitro organ culture system. *J Endocrinol Invest, 30*, RC22-5.

[61] Qi, X., Reed, J., Englander, E. W., Chandrashekar, V., Bartke, A. & Greeley, G. H., Jr. (2003). Evidence that growth hormone exerts a feedback effect on stomach ghrelin production and secretion. *Exp Biol Med (Maywood), 228*, 1028-32.

[62] Grinspoon, S., Miller, K. K., Herzog, D. B., Grieco, K. A. & Klibanski, A. (2004). Effects of estrogen and recombinant human insulin-like growth factor-I on ghrelin secretion in severe undernutrition. *J Clin Endocrinol Metab, 89*, 3988-93.

[63] Iniguez, G., Salazar, T., Roman, R., Avila, A., Gunn, R. D. & Cassorla, F. (2006). Effects of the IGF-I/IGFBP-3 complex on GH and ghrelin nocturnal concentrations in low birth weight children. *Clin Endocrinol (Oxf), 65*, 687-92.

[64] Shimada, M., Date, Y., Mondal, M. S., Toshinai, K., Shimbara, T., Fukunaga, K., Murakami, N., Miyazato, M., Kangawa, K., Yoshimatsu, H., Matsuo, H. & Nakazato, M. (2003). Somatostatin suppresses ghrelin secretion from the rat stomach. *Biochem Biophys Res Commun, 302*, 520-5.

[65] Luque, R. M., Gahete, M. D., Hochgeschwender, U. & Kineman, R. D. (2006). Evidence that endogenous SST inhibits ACTH and ghrelin expression by independent pathways. *Am J Physiol Endocrinol Metab, 291*, E395-403.

[66] Arosio, M., Ronchi, C. L., Gebbia, C., Cappiello, V., Beck-Peccoz, P. & Peracchi, M. (2003). Stimulatory effects of ghrelin on circulating somatostatin and pancreatic polypeptide levels. *J Clin Endocrinol Metab, 88*, 701-4.

[67] Krzyzanowska-Swiniarska, B., Kempa, A., Miazgowski, T. & Pilarska, K. (2007). Serum acylated ghrelin, adiponectin and leptin levels in normal-weight and obese premenopausal women. *Horm Metab Res, 39*, 835-9.

[68] Zhang, Y., Proenca, R., Maffei, M., Barone, M., Leopold, L. & Friedman, J. M. (1994). Positional cloning of the mouse obese gene and its human homologue. *Nature, 372*, 425-32.

[69] Zhao, Z., Sakata, I., Okubo, Y., Koike, K., Kangawa, K. & Sakai, T. (2008). Gastric leptin, but not estrogen and somatostatin, contributes to the elevation of ghrelin mRNA expression level in fasted rats. *J Endocrinol, 196*, 529-38.

[70] Dube, M. G., Beretta, E., Dhillon, H., Ueno, N., Kalra, P. S. & Kalra, S. P. (2002). Central leptin gene therapy blocks high-fat diet-induced weight gain, hyperleptinemia, and hyperinsulinemia: increase in serum ghrelin levels. *Diabetes, 51*, 1729-36.

[71] Sakata, I., Tanaka, T., Yamazaki, M., Tanizaki, T., Zheng, Z. & Sakai, T. (2006). Gastric estrogen directly induces ghrelin expression and production in the rat stomach. *J Endocrinol, 190*, 749-57.

[72] Lambrinoudaki, I. V., Christodoulakos, G. E., Economou, E. V., Vlachou, S. A., Panoulis, C. P., Alexandrou, A. P., Kouskouni, E. E. & Creatsas, G. C. (2008). Circulating leptin and ghrelin are differentially influenced by estrogen/progestin therapy and raloxifene. *Maturitas, 59*, 62-71.

[73] Kellokoski, E., Poykko, S. M., Karjalainen, A. H., Ukkola, O., Heikkinen, J., Kesaniemi, Y. A. & Horkko, S. (2005). Estrogen replacement therapy increases plasma ghrelin levels. *J Clin Endocrinol Metab, 90*, 2954-63.

[74] Matsubara, M., Sakata, I., Wada, R., Yamazaki, M., Inoue, K. & Sakai, T. (2004). Estrogen modulates ghrelin expression in the female rat stomach. *Peptides, 25*, 289-97.

[75] Barkan, A. L., Dimaraki, E. V., Jessup, S. K., Symons, K. V., Ermolenko, M. & Jaffe, C. A. (2003). Ghrelin secretion in humans is sexually dimorphic, suppressed by somatostatin, and not affected by the ambient growth hormone levels. *J Clin Endocrinol Metab, 88*, 2180-4.

[76] Liu, Y. L., Yakar, S., Otero-Corchon, V., Low, M. J. & Liu, J. L. (2002). Ghrelin gene expression is age-dependent and influenced by gender and the level of circulating IGF-I. *Mol Cell Endocrinol, 189*, 97-103.

[77] Nakazato, M., Murakami, N., Date, Y., Kojima, M., Matsuo, H., Kangawa, K. & Matsukura, S. (2001). A role for ghrelin in the central regulation of feeding. *Nature, 409*, 194-8.

[78] Wren, A. M., Small, C. J., Ward, H. L., Murphy, K. G., Dakin, C. L., Taheri, S., Kennedy, A. R., Roberts, G. H., Morgan, D. G., Ghatei, M. A. & Bloom, S. R. (2000). The novel hypothalamic peptide ghrelin stimulates food intake and growth hormone secretion. *Endocrinology, 141*, 4325-8.

[79] Asakawa, A., Inui, A., Kaga, T., Yuzuriha, H., Nagata, T., Ueno, N., Makino, S., Fujimiya, M., Niijima, A., Fujino, M. A. & Kasuga, M. (2001). Ghrelin is an appetite-stimulatory signal from stomach with structural resemblance to motilin. *Gastroenterology, 120*, 337-45.

[80] Shintani, M., Ogawa, Y., Ebihara, K., Aizawa-Abe, M., Miyanaga, F., Takaya, K., Hayashi, T., Inoue, G., Hosoda, K., Kojima, M., Kangawa, K. & Nakao, K. (2001). Ghrelin, an endogenous growth hormone secretagogue, is a novel orexigenic peptide that antagonizes leptin action through the activation of hypothalamic neuropeptide Y/Y1 receptor pathway. *Diabetes, 50*, 227-32.

[81] Asakawa, A., Inui, A., Kaga, T., Katsuura, G., Fujimiya, M., Fujino, M. A. & Kasuga, M. (2003). Antagonism of ghrelin receptor reduces food intake and body weight gain in mice. *Gut, 52*, 947-52.

[82] Carlson, M. J. & Cummings, D. E. (2006). Prospects for an anti-ghrelin vaccine to treat obesity. *Mol Interv, 6*, 249-52.

[83] Helmling, S., Maasch, C., Eulberg, D., Buchner, K., Schroder, W., Lange, C., Vonhoff, S., Wlotzka, B., Tschop, M. H., Rosewicz, S. & Klussmann, S. (2004). Inhibition of ghrelin action in vitro and in vivo by an RNA-Spiegelmer. *Proc Natl Acad Sci U S A, 101*, 13174-9.

[84] Becskei, C., Bilik, K. U., Klussmann, S., Jarosch, F., Lutz, T. A. & Riediger, T. (2008). The anti-ghrelin Spiegelmer NOX-B11-3 blocks ghrelin- but not fasting-induced neuronal activation in the hypothalamic arcuate nucleus. *J Neuroendocrinol, 20*, 85-92.

[85] Shearman, L. P., Wang, S. P., Helmling, S., Stribling, D. S., Mazur, P., Ge, L., Wang, L., Klussmann, S., Macintyre, D. E., Howard, A. D. & Strack, A. M. (2006). Ghrelin neutralization by a ribonucleic acid-SPM ameliorates obesity in diet-induced obese mice. *Endocrinology, 147*, 1517-26.

[86] Tamura, H., Kamegai, J., Shimizu, T., Ishii, S., Sugihara, H. & Oikawa, S. (2002). Ghrelin stimulates GH but not food intake in arcuate nucleus ablated rats. *Endocrinology, 143*, 3268-75.

[87] Willesen, M. G., Kristensen, P. & Romer, J. (1999). Co-localization of growth hormone secretagogue receptor and NPY mRNA in the arcuate nucleus of the rat. *Neuroendocrinology, 70*, 306-16.

[88] Toshinai, K., Date, Y., Murakami, N., Shimada, M., Mondal, M. S., Shimbara, T., Guan, J. L., Wang, Q. P., Funahashi, H., Sakurai, T., Shioda, S., Matsukura, S., Kangawa, K. & Nakazato, M. (2003). Ghrelin-induced food intake is mediated via the orexin pathway. *Endocrinology, 144*, 1506-12.

[89] Kamegai, J., Tamura, H., Shimizu, T., Ishii, S., Sugihara, H. & Wakabayashi, I. (2001). Chronic central infusion of ghrelin increases hypothalamic neuropeptide Y and Agouti-related protein mRNA levels and body weight in rats. *Diabetes, 50*, 2438-43.

[90] Chen, H. Y., Trumbauer, M. E., Chen, A. S., Weingarth, D. T., Adams, J. R., Frazier, E. G., Shen, Z., Marsh, D. J., Feighner, S. D., Guan, X. M., Ye, Z., Nargund, R. P., Smith, R. G., Van der Ploeg, L. H., Howard, A. D., MacNeil, D. J. & Qian, S. (2004). Orexigenic action of peripheral ghrelin is mediated by neuropeptide Y and agouti-related protein. *Endocrinology, 145*, 2607-12.

[91] Lopez, M., Lage, R., Saha, A. K., Perez-Tilve, D., Vazquez, M. J., Varela, L., Sangiao-Alvarellos, S., Tovar, S., Raghay, K., Rodriguez-Cuenca, S., Deoliveira, R. M., Castaneda, T., Datta, R., Dong, J. Z., Culler, M., Sleeman, M. W., Alvarez, C. V., Gallego, R., Lelliott, C. J., Carling, D., Tschop, M. H., Dieguez, C. & Vidal-Puig, A. (2008). Hypothalamic fatty acid metabolism mediates the orexigenic action of ghrelin. *Cell Metab, 7*, 389-99.

[92] Kola, B., Hubina, E., Tucci, S. A., Kirkham, T. C., Garcia, E. A., Mitchell, S. E., Williams, L. M., Hawley, S. A., Hardie, D. G., Grossman, A. B. & Korbonits, M. (2005). Cannabinoids and ghrelin have both central and peripheral metabolic and cardiac effects via AMP-activated protein kinase. *J Biol Chem, 280*, 25196-201.

[93] Thomson, D. M., Herway, S. T., Fillmore, N., Kim, H., Brown, J. D., Barrow, J. R. & Winder, W. W. (2008). AMP-activated protein kinase phosphorylates transcription factors of the CREB family. *J Appl Physiol, 104*, 429-38.

[94] Andrews, Z. B., Liu, Z. W., Walllingford, N., Erion, D. M., Borok, E., Friedman, J. M., Tschop, M. H., Shanabrough, M., Cline, G., Shulman, G. I., Coppola, A., Gao, X. B., Horvath, T. L. & Diano, S. (2008). UCP2 mediates ghrelin's action on NPY/AgRP neurons by lowering free radicals. *Nature, 454*, 846-51.

[95] Yang, Q. & Guan, K. L. (2007). Expanding mTOR signaling. *Cell Res, 17*, 666-81.

[96] Kunz, J., Henriquez, R., Schneider, U., Deuter-Reinhard, M., Movva, N. R. & Hall, M. N. (1993). Target of rapamycin in yeast, TOR2, is an essential phosphatidylinositol kinase homolog required for G1 progression. *Cell, 73*, 585-96.

[97] Heitman, J., Movva, N. R. & Hall, M. N. (1991). Targets for cell cycle arrest by the immunosuppressant rapamycin in yeast. *Science, 253*, 905-9.

[98] Abraham, R. T. & Wiederrecht, G. J. (1996). Immunopharmacology of rapamycin. *Annu Rev Immunol, 14*, 483-510.

[99] Hoekstra, M. F. (1997). Responses to DNA damage and regulation of cell cycle checkpoints by the ATM protein kinase family. *Curr Opin Genet Dev, 7*, 170-5.

[100] Wullschleger, S., Loewith, R. & Hall, M. N. (2006). TOR signaling in growth and metabolism. *Cell, 124*, 471-84.

[101] Inoki, K., Ouyang, H., Li, Y. & Guan, K. L. (2005). Signaling by target of rapamycin proteins in cell growth control. *Microbiol Mol Biol Rev, 69*, 79-100.

[102] Peterson, R. T., Beal, P. A., Comb, M. J. & Schreiber, S. L. (2000). FKBP12-rapamycin-associated protein (FRAP) autophosphorylates at serine 2481 under translationally repressive conditions. *J Biol Chem, 275*, 7416-23.

[103] Avruch, J., Belham, C., Weng, Q., Hara, K. & Yonezawa, K. (2001). The p70 S6 kinase integrates nutrient and growth signals to control translational capacity. *Prog Mol Subcell Biol, 26*, 115-54.

[104] Gingras, A. C., Kennedy, S. G., O'Leary, M. A., Sonenberg, N. & Hay, N. (1998). 4E-BP1, a repressor of mRNA translation, is phosphoylated and inactivated by the Akt(PKB) signaling pathway. *Genes Dev, 12*, 502-13.

[105] Holz, M. K., Ballif, B. A., Gygi, S. P. & Blenis, J. (2005). mTOR and S6K1 mediate assembly of the translation preinitiation complex through dynamic protein interchange and ordered phosphorylation events. *Cell, 123*, 569-80.

[106] Jeno, P., Ballou, L. M., Novak-Hofer, I. & Thomas, G. (1988). Identification and characterization of a mitogen-activated S6 kinase. *Proc Natl Acad Sci U S A, 85*, 406-10.

[107] Pause, A., Belsham, G. J., Gingras, A. C., Donze, O., Lin, T. A., Lawrence, J. C., Jr. & Sonenberg, N. (1994). Insulin-dependent stimulation of protein synthesis by phosphorylation of a regulator of 5'-cap function. *Nature, 371*, 762-7.

[108] Gomez, M. R. (1991). Phenotypes of the tuberous sclerosis complex with a revision of diagnostic criteria. *Ann N Y Acad Sci, 615*, 1-7.

[109] van Slegtenhorst, M., de Hoogt, R., Hermans, C., Nellist, M., Janssen, B., Verhoef, S., Lindhout, D., van den Ouweland, A., Halley, D., Young, J., Burley, M., Jeremiah, S., Woodward, K., Nahmias, J., Fox, M., Ekong, R., Osborne, J., Wolfe, J., Povey, S., Snell, R. G., Cheadle, J. P., Jones, A. C., Tachataki, M., Ravine, D., Sampson, J. R., Reeve, M. P., Richardson, P., Wilmer, F., Munro, C., Hawkins, T. L., Sepp, T., Ali, J. B., Ward, S., Green, A. J., Yates, J. R., Kwiatkowska, J., Henske, E. P., Short, M. P., Haines, J. H., Jozwiak, S. & Kwiatkowski, D. J. (1997). Identification of the tuberous sclerosis gene TSC1 on chromosome 9q34. *Science, 277*, 805-8.

[110] (1993). Identification and characterization of the tuberous sclerosis gene on chromosome 16. *Cell, 75*, 1305-15.

[111] van Slegtenhorst, M., Nellist, M., Nagelkerken, B., Cheadle, J., Snell, R., van den Ouweland, A., Reuser, A., Sampson, J., Halley, D. & van der Sluijs, P. (1998). Interaction between hamartin and tuberin, the TSC1 and TSC2 gene products. *Hum Mol Genet, 7*, 1053-7.

[112] Kobayashi, T., Minowa, O., Sugitani, Y., Takai, S., Mitani, H., Kobayashi, E., Noda, T. & Hino, O. (2001). A germ-line Tsc1 mutation causes tumor development and embryonic lethality that are similar, but not identical to, those caused by Tsc2 mutation in mice. *Proc Natl Acad Sci U S A, 98*, 8762-7.

[113] Onda, H., Lueck, A., Marks, P. W., Warren, H. B. & Kwiatkowski, D. J. (1999). Tsc2(+/-) mice develop tumors in multiple sites that express gelsolin and are influenced by genetic background. *J Clin Invest, 104*, 687-95.

[114] Potter, C. J., Huang, H. & Xu, T. (2001). Drosophila Tsc1 functions with Tsc2 to antagonize insulin signaling in regulating cell growth, cell proliferation, and organ size. *Cell, 105*, 357-68.

[115] Goncharova, E. A., Goncharov, D. A., Eszterhas, A., Hunter, D. S., Glassberg, M. K., Yeung, R. S., Walker, C. L., Noonan, D., Kwiatkowski, D. J., Chou, M. M., Panettieri, R. A., Jr. & Krymskaya, V. P. (2002). Tuberin regulates p70 S6 kinase activation and ribosomal protein S6 phosphorylation. A role for the TSC2 tumor suppressor gene in pulmonary lymphangioleiomyomatosis (LAM). *J Biol Chem, 277*, 30958-67.

[116] Inoki, K., Li, Y., Zhu, T., Wu, J. & Guan, K. L. (2002). TSC2 is phosphoylated and inhibited by Akt and suppresses mTOR signalling. *Nat Cell Biol, 4*, 648-57.

[117] Yeh, W. C., Bierer, B. E. & McKnight, S. L. (1995). Rapamycin inhibits clonal expansion and adipogenic differentiation of 3T3-L1 cells. *Proc Natl Acad Sci U S A, 92*, 11086-90.

[118] Polak, P. & Hall, M. N. (2009). mTOR and the control of whole body metabolism. *Curr Opin Cell Biol, 21*, 209-18.

[119] Zhang, H., Stallock, J. P., Ng, J. C., Reinhard, C. & Neufeld, T. P. (2000). Regulation of cellular growth by the Drosophila target of rapamycin dTOR. *Genes Dev, 14*, 2712-24.

[120] Um, S. H., Frigerio, F., Watanabe, M., Picard, F., Joaquin, M., Sticker, M., Fumagalli, S., Allegrini, P. R., Kozma, S. C., Auwerx, J. & Thomas, G. (2004). Absence of S6K1 protects against age- and diet-induced obesity while enhancing insulin sensitivity. *Nature, 431*, 200-5.

[121] Le Bacquer, O., Petroulakis, E., Paglialunga, S., Poulin, F., Richard, D., Cianflone, K. & Sonenberg, N. (2007). Elevated sensitivity to diet-induced obesity and insulin resistance in mice lacking 4E-BP1 and 4E-BP2. *J Clin Invest, 117*, 387-96.

[122] Polak, P., Cybulski, N., Feige, J. N., Auwerx, J., Ruegg, M. A. & Hall, M. N. (2008). Adipose-specific knockout of raptor results in lean mice with enhanced mitochondrial respiration. *Cell Metab, 8*, 399-410.

[123] Fraenkel, M., Ketzinel-Gilad, M., Ariav, Y., Pappo, O., Karaca, M., Castel, J., Berthault, M. F., Magnan, C., Cerasi, E., Kaiser, N. & Leibowitz, G. (2008). mTOR inhibition by rapamycin prevents beta-cell adaptation to hyperglycemia and exacerbates the metabolic state in type 2 diabetes. *Diabetes, 57*, 945-57.

[124] Dann, S. G., Selvaraj, A. & Thomas, G. (2007). mTOR Complex1-S6K1 signaling: at the crossroads of obesity, diabetes and cancer. *Trends Mol Med, 13*, 252-9.

[125] Kimball, S. R. & Jefferson, L. S. (2006). Signaling pathways and molecular mechanisms through which branched-chain amino acids mediate translational control of protein synthesis. *J Nutr, 136*, 227S-31S.

[126] Roos, S., Lagerlof, O., Wennergren, M., Powell, T. & Jansson, T. (2009). Regulation of amino acid transporters by glucose and growth factors in cultured primary human trophoblast cells is mediated by mTOR signaling. *Am J Physiol Cell Physiol,*

[127] Peng, T., Golub, T. R. & Sabatini, D. M. (2002). The immunosuppressant rapamycin mimics a starvation-like signal distinct from amino acid and glucose deprivation. *Mol Cell Biol, 22*, 5575-84.

[128] Dennis, P. B., Jaeschke, A., Saitoh, M., Fowler, B., Kozma, S. C. & Thomas, G. (2001). Mammalian TOR: a homeostatic ATP sensor. *Science, 294*, 1102-5.

[129] Kahn, B. B., Alquier, T., Carling, D. & Hardie, D. G. (2005). AMP-activated protein kinase: ancient energy gauge provides clues to modern understanding of metabolism. *Cell Metab, 1*, 15-25.

[130] Inoki, K., Zhu, T. & Guan, K. L. (2003). TSC2 mediates cellular energy response to control cell growth and survival. *Cell, 115*, 577-90.

[131] Wu, Q., Zhang, Y., Xu, J. & Shen, P. (2005). Regulation of hunger-driven behaviors by neural ribosomal S6 kinase in Drosophila. *Proc Natl Acad Sci U S A, 102*, 13289-94.

[132] Blouet, C., Ono, H. & Schwartz, G. J. (2008). Mediobasal hypothalamic p70 S6 kinase 1 modulates the control of energy homeostasis. *Cell Metab, 8*, 459-67.

[133] Cota, D., Proulx, K., Smith, K. A., Kozma, S. C., Thomas, G., Woods, S. C. & Seeley, R. J. (2006). Hypothalamic mTOR signaling regulates food intake. *Science, 312*, 927-30.

[134] Chang, G. R., Chiu, Y. S., Wu, Y. Y., Chen, W. Y., Liao, J. W., Chao, T. H. & Mao, F. C. (2009). Rapamycin protects against high fat diet-induced obesity in C57BL/6J mice. *J Pharmacol Sci, 109*, 496-503.

[135] Cota, D., Proulx, K. & Seeley, R. J. (2007). The role of CNS fuel sensing in energy and glucose regulation. *Gastroenterology, 132*, 2158-68.

[136] Zhang, W., Zhao, L., Lin, T. R., Chai, B., Fan, Y., Gantz, I. & Mulholland, M. W. (2004). Inhibition of adipogenesis by ghrelin. *Mol Biol Cell, 15*, 2484-91.

[137] Gualillo, O., Lago, F. & Dieguez, C. (2008). Introducing GOAT: a target for obesity and anti-diabetic drugs? *Trends Pharmacol Sci, 29*, 398-401.

[138] Kopelman, P. G. (2000). Obesity as a medical problem. *Nature, 404*, 635-43.

In: Neuroendocrinology Research Developments
Editor: N. S. Penkava and L.R. Haight, pp. 63-78
ISBN: 978-1-60876-983-4
© 2010 Nova Science Publishers, Inc.

Chapter 3

IMPORTANCE OF THE DEVELOPMENTAL-BEHAVIORAL APPROACH TO CLARIFY THE MECHANISM UNDERLYING SOCIALITY IN DOGS

Miho Nagasawa, Kazutaka Mogi *, and Takefumi Kikusui
Scool of Veterinary Medicine, Animal Science and Biotechnology,
Azabu University, Sagamihara 252-5201, Japan
* Corresponding author: E-mail; mogik@azabu-u.ac.jp

1. PRESENT SITUATION OF STUDIES ON SOCIALITY IN DOGS

Dogs (*Canis familiaris*) are believed to be one of the oldest domesticated animals (Serpell, 1995), and undoubtedly, they have naturally adapted to humans and established a niche for themselves in modern human society. Considering the numerous other animals inhabiting the planet, the affinity between humans and dogs can be considered special. Recent comparative cognitive studies, involving the comparison of dogs with wolves (*Canis lupus*) or other species, have suggested that this adaptation of dogs to humans is because of dogs' superior social skills and cognitive ability. For example, when dogs and their owners were subjected to the Strange Situation Test, which was developed to examine the attachment patterns of human infants separated from or reunited with their mothers, dogs behaved differently toward their owners as compared to strangers (Topál, Miklósi, Csányi, & Dóka, 1998). However, the behavior of hand-reared wolves did not differ between their owners and strangers (Topál, Gácsi, Miklósi, Virányi, Kubinyi, & Csányi, 2005). These findings lead us assume that dogs can recognize the difference between their owners and strangers and exhibit specific responses to their owners. In contrast, at least under the conditions of the study, wolves cannot distinguish their owners from strangers or respond differently even if they do recognize their owners. Moreover, dogs can select an object indicated to them with using human signals, such as finger pointing or gazing (Hare, Brown, Williamson, & Tomasello, 2002; Virányi, Gácsi, Kubinyi, Topál, Belényi, Ujfalussy & Miklósi, 2008). Several studies have reported that unlike dogs, wolves cannot respond to human gestures (Hare, Brown,

Williamson, & Tomasello, 2002; Virányi, Gácsi, Kubinyi, Topál, Belényi, Ujfalussy & Miklósi, 2008), although the results of these studies remain controversial (Udell, Dorey & Wynne, 2008). It was also reported that when both dogs and socialized wolves that had been trained to perform a simple manipulation task were presented with an insoluble version of the same task, the dogs gazed at the presenting human, while the socialized wolves did not (Miklósi, Kubinyi, Topál, Gácsi, Virányi, & Csányi, 2003). All these studies indicate that dogs have the ability to acquire a high level of social skills and cognitive ability such as pointing or gazing. Such abilities help dogs engage in nonverbal communicative interactions with humans, and this may be a reason for why dogs but not wolves adapted to human society, although these animals appear similar.

How have dogs acquired this high level of social skills and cognitive ability? The answer to this question has been suggested by an interesting study on the domestication of the fox (*Vulpes vulpes*), a wild canine. This study conducted in Russia succeeded in domesticating foxes by selecting particular characteristics—lack of fear of or aggression toward humans—as the main index. Interestingly, the domesticated foxes could respond to human gestures just as dogs could, whereas non-selected foxes could not (Hare, Plyusnina, Ignacio, Schepina, Stepika, Wrangham, & Trut, 2005). Hare and Tomasello (2005) proposed the hypothesis that specialized social skills and cognitive ability appeared in dogs after the central nervous system of this animal, which mediates fear and aggression, evolved during the process of domestication. The serotonergic neural system, which is related to aggressive behavior or anxiety, was reportedly changed in domesticated foxes compared to non-selected foxes (Popova, Voitenko, Kulikov, & Avgustinovich, 1991). Furthermore, the basal plasma levels of both adrenocorticotrophic hormone and glucocorticoid and the glucocorticoid response to stress were found to be lower in domesticated foxes than non-selected ones; in other words, a decrease in the activity of the hypothalamus-pituitary-adrenal (HPA) axis was also found (Oskina, 1996). Hare and Tomasello (2005) assumed that this attenuation of HPA axis activity might contribute to the inhibition of the fear response or aggressive behavior toward humans. Although the mechanism by which dogs exhibit superior social skills remains largely unknown, the series of experiments on domesticated foxes have provided one possible explanation: the changes of the central nervous system mediating the fear response and aggression or regulating the activity of the HPA axis are involved in the mechanism.

Recently, researchers in the field of neuroscience have developed a keen interest in understanding the neural mechanisms important for social cognition or social behavior, such as affinitive behavior toward others, which have thus far been scientifically vague, since molecules related to social cognition or social behavior are now being identified. From this viewpoint, attempts to explain the special affinity between humans and dogs are also being made. Odendaal & Meintjes (2003) compared the plasma levels of hormones in humans and dogs before and after an interaction between the 2 species, and they found that oxytocin secretion in both was greater after the interaction. Oxytocin was first found as a bioactive nonapeptide that is synthesized in hypothalamic neurons and secreted from the posterior pituitary into the general circulation. Oxytocin contracts the smooth muscles in the uterus or mammary glands during parturition or lactation, respectively. However, recently, another physiological role played by oxytocin -that of a neurotransmitter- has been in focus. In rats (*Rattus norvegicus*), the intracerebroventricular administration of oxytocin enhances grooming behavior, contact with others, and maternal behavior (Pedersen, Caldwell, Drago, Noonan, Peterson, Hood, & Prange, 1988; Witt, Winslow, & Insel, 1992), and it was also reported that the oxytocin concentration in the cerebrospinal fluid is positively correlated with the degree to which social behaviors are manifested (Haller, Makara, Barna, Kovacs, Nagy, & Vecsernyes, 1996). Furthermore, it has been shown that social cognition is impaired in oxytocin gene-knockout mice (*Mus musculus*) (Ferguson, Young, Hearn, Matzuk, Insel, & Winslow, 2000; Winslow & Insel, 2002). Oxytocin and vasopressin, a nonapeptide whose sequence differs from oxytocin by only 2 amino acids, have also been found to be essential for the prairie vole (*Microtus ochrogaster*), a completely monogamous rodent, to maintain the bond of monogamy (Young, Lim, Gingrich, & Insel, 2001; Young & Wang, 2004). In humans, oxytocin level in the plasma of mothers after delivery is positively correlated with maternal behavior toward their infants (Feldman, Weller, Zagoory-Sharon, & Levine, 2007). The plasma levels of oxytocin were decreased in children with autistic disorders (Green, Fein, Modahl, Feinstein, Waterhouse, & Morris, 2001), and a correlation was found between alterations in the oxytocin receptor gene and the susceptibility to autism (Wu, Jia, Ruan, Liu, Guo, Shuang, Gong, Zhang, Yang, & Zhang, 2005). These studies strongly indicate the importance of the oxytocinergic neural system in social behavior and cognition (Donaldson & Young, 2008). Nagasawa, Kikusui, Onaka, & Ohta (2009) focused on the relationship between the level of oxytocin in dog owners and the gazing behavior of the dogs, and they showed that the urinary levels of oxytocin in the dog owners increased after frequent behavioral exchanges initiated by their dog's gaze; this phenomenon was not observed in the case of dogs that initiated behavioral exchanges with their gaze at a low frequency. Moreover, a questionnaire survey, which simultaneously executed to dog owners in the experiment by Nagasawa *et al.* (2009), also showed that former dog owners were more satisfied with their dogs than later dog owners. These results suggested that dogs' gaze not only activated the oxytocinergic neural system in humans but also positively influenced the humans' mental state. Human infants are believed to be able to innately utilize gazing as a social cue (Batki, Baron-Cohen, Wheelwright, Connellan, & Ahluwalia, 2000; Farroni, Csibra, Simion, & Johnson, 2002). The infant's gaze is interpreted by caregivers as a purposeful signal and, as a result of that, caregivers approach infants (Meins, 1997). Similarly, a dog's gaze may function as a social cue. We hypothesize that the specific affinity between human and dogs is synonymous to the mother-infant attachment propounded by Bowlby (1969), that is, as "interspecies attachment" (Nagasawa, Mogi, & Kikusui, 2009). Current studies on comparative cognitive science and neuroscience have strongly indicated that dogs' sociality is characterized by their ability to have the relationship with humans, which may be similar to the association among conspecifics.

2. Importance of Mother-Infant Relationship for Development of Sociality in Dogs

To further understand the sociality of dogs, it is important to blend cognitive science and neuroscience, as in the approach used in the study by Nagasawa et al. (2009). Furthermore, we should not ignore the developmental-behavioral viewpoint, i.e., the influence of the early environment of dogs on their sociality. The importance of this point was first suggested by studies carried out mainly in the 1950s and 1960s by Hebb, and others of the Roscoe B. Jackson Memorial Laboratory (Clarke, Heron, Fetherstonhaugh, Forgays, & Hebb, 1951;

Freedman, King, & Elliot, 1961; Fuller, 1967; Scott & Fuller, 1965; Scott, Stewart, & De Ghett, 1974; Thompson & Heron, 1954). This series of studies mainly proved that contact with human society during development could decrease the fear response of dogs toward humans and improve trainability in adulthood. In the field of veterinary medicine, dogs' antisocial or undesirable behavior toward humans is categorized as dog's 'behavior problems'. Against the background of urbanization and the changed style of dog ownership, these dog behavioral problems have increased and received much attention in recent years. Several investigations conducted in veterinary hospitals to identify the factors affecting the occurrence of these problems have shown the importance of the early developmental environment of dogs. For example, Appleby, Bradshaw, & Casey (2002) researched the relationship between the occurrence rate of behavioral problems in dogs and the period for which as pups, the dogs were in contact with humans. They found that dogs that were not exposed to the human domestic environment until 8 weeks of age were prone to strongly exhibit avoidance behavior toward humans and aggressiveness toward unfamiliar persons during adulthood. These studies strongly suggest that a dog's exposure to human society for the appropriate period is important for the development of the dog's characteristic relationship with humans in adulthood. In this chapter, we propose that to better understand dog's sociality in adulthood, it is also necessary to assess the mother-infant relationship in dogs during the developmental period. Although few studies have been carried out from such a viewpoint, Slabbert & Rasa (1993) found that dogs that had been separated from their mothers and nest sites (but not their littermates) at 6 weeks of age were prone to exhibit loss of appetite and weight and increased distress, mortality, and susceptibility to disease as compared to dogs that had remained at the nest sites with their mothers until 12 weeks of age. Serpell conducted an analysis with an online questionnaire (C-BARQ: Canine Behavioral Assessment and Research Questionnaire) to investigate the association between the age of rehoming with new owners and the temperament in adulthood; this study revealed that dogs that had been separated from their mothers and rehomed before 6 weeks of age were prone to exhibit a hyper stress response and unsocial behavior (personal communication). Overall, it can be inferred that while it is important for dogs to be exposed to human society during the early developmental period for socialization, very early mother-infant separation could cause adverse effects in dogs during adulthood. Recently, studies in rodents have revealed how the relationship between mothers and infants, such as the degree of nursing behavior exhibited by mothers, affects the development of various social behaviors and the oxytocinergic neural system as the basis of social behaviors. However, at present, there are few such studies in dogs. Because the superior social skills and cognitive ability of dogs may be closely related to the fear response, aggressive behavior, and development of the HPA axis, it will be useful for understanding dogs' sociality to identify the developmental period or neural system that is influenced by the relationship between mothers and pups, whereby the characteristic sociality—or the special affinity to humans—can be established in adulthood. In the next section, we will provide a perspective of future developmental-behavioral approaches to clarify the mechanism underlying dogs' sociality, by reviewing the putative theories regarding how the mother-infant relationship affects sociality in adulthood and the neural systems involved.

3. Influence of Conditions in Each Developmental Stage on Sociality

Studies such as those conducted at the Roscoe B. Jackson Memorial Laboratory (Markwell & Thorne, 1987; Scott, Stewart, & De Ghett, 1974) have indicated that the process of development in dogs can generally be divided into 7 stages: the prenatal period; the neonatal period from birth to 2 weeks; the transition period from 2 to 3 weeks; the socialization period from 3 to 12 weeks; the juvenile period, which starts after the socialization period and continues until sexual maturation (6–9 months of age); and the maturation period from sexual maturation until the korontic period, which starts after 7 years of age. In this section, we will review dog development until the juvenile period after weaning, focusing on the relationship between mothers and pups.

3.1. Prenatal Period

Although it is currently unknown whether the fetus is influenced by the physiological state of the mother in dogs, human infants from mothers who had experienced anxiety or stress during pregnancy were reported to have trouble with cognitive ability and emotional expression (Van den Bergh, Mulder, Mennes, & Glover, 2005), and maternal stress during pregnancy was also reported to be associated with a high risk of mental disorders in the offspring, such as schizophrenia (Khashan, Abel, McNamee, Pedersen, Webb, Baker, Kenny, & Mortensen, 2008). In these reports, it could not be denied that these influences to offspring were due to the changes of mother's nursing behavior after delivery, which had affected by anxiety or stressful experiences. However, since cross-fostering pups from prenatally stressed mothers to non-stressed mothers failed to improve the social deficit of the prenatally stressed male offspring in rats, it is very likely that the environment in the prenatal period affects the development of social behaviors in the offspring (Lee, Brady, Shapiro, Dorsa, & Koenig, 2007). In both rodents and humans, prenatal anxiety or stress in mothers caused offspring to exhibit excessive secretion of glucocorticoid from the adrenal cortex on exposure to stress (Gutteling, de Weerth, & Buitelaar, 2005; Koenig, Elmer, Shepard, Lee, Mayo, Joy, Hercher, & Brady, 2005). These findings suggest that the developmental defect in the HPA axis due to the conditions in the prenatal period may be one of the neural mechanisms of impaired sociality in offspring. In rats, hippocampal glucocorticoid receptors have shown to be decreased in offspring whose mothers experienced stress during pregnancy (Barbazanges, Piazza, Le Moal, & Maccari, 1996); therefore, it would appear that the diminished glucocorticoid negative feedback in the hippocampus is associated with the excessive glucocorticoid secretion observed in the offspring. In a cross-fostering study on rats, the offspring from prenatally stressed mothers showed less oxytocin mRNA in the paraventricular nucleus and increased oxytocin receptor binding in the central amygdala (Lee Brady, Shapiro, et al., 2007), which indicates that the development of the oxytocinergic neural system is also impaired by the stress in the prenatal period. With regard to the factors that affect the fetus in mothers exposed anxiety or stress, the "glucocorticoid hypothesis" has proposed, which states that the stress-induced increase in maternal glucocorticoid directly affects the fetus (Barbazanges, Piazza, Le Moal, et al., 1996; Seckl & Meaney, 2004).

However, because 11β-hydroxysteroid dehydrogenase, the enzyme that inactivates glucocorticoid, has been shown to be present in the placenta of many animals including dogs (Sieber-Ruckstuhl, Meli, Boretti, Gonczi, Lutz, & Reusch, 2007), further research will be necessary to identify the prenatal stress-induced factors affecting the fetus.

3.2. Neonatal Period

Neonatal pups mainly approach their mothers by using olfactory information because of the immature state of their visual and auditory systems; at this stage, they cannot urinate or defecate independently. During the neonatal period, pups are completely dependent on their mothers for survival. It has been shown that in rats, animals that have experienced neonatal handling exhibit a lowered response to stress after maturation and can easily adapt to novel environments as compared to those that have not been handled (Levine, 1967). This finding indicates that tactile stimuli to pups are significant for their social development. Meaney and his colleague focused on the maternal behaviors of rats in this period and clarified that offspring nurtured by mothers showing more frequently licking and grooming for the first week postpartum exhibit reduced anxiety and behavioral fearfulness or corticosterone levels in response to stress in adulthood compared to offspring with mothers exhibiting less frequent licking/grooming (Caldji, Tannenbaum, Sharma, Francis, Plotsky, & Meaney, 1998; Liu, Diorio, Tannenbaum, Caldji, Francis, Freedman, Sharma, Pearson, Plotsky, & Meaney, 1997). Moreover, it has been revealed that female pups nurtured by mothers showing high levels of maternal behavior also grew up to be mothers showing frequent grooming (Francis, Diorio, Liu, & Meaney, 1999). The neural mechanism involved in the decreased reactivity to stress in offspring nurtured by good mothers has been suggested to be a result of enhanced glucocorticoid feedback sensitivity, which results from an increase in the hippocampal glucocorticoid receptor (Liu, Diorio, Tannenbaum, et al., 1997). Further, it has also been suggested that the effect of postnatal handling on glucocorticoid receptor expression is mediated by an increase in serotonin activity (Mitchell, Iny, & Meaney, 1990; Smythe, Rowe, & Meaney, 1994). Enhanced maternal behavior is considered to be associated with an increase in oxytocin receptor and estrogen receptor expression in the medial preoptic area; these receptors appear to be important for the manifestation of maternal behavior (Champagne, Weaver, Diorio, Sharma, & Meaney, 2003; Francis, Champagne, & Meaney, 2000). Interestingly, a cross-fostering study showed that the female offsprings' maternal potential was diminished if they were born of a mother showing a high level of maternal behavior but nurtured by a mother showing a low level of maternal behaviors, indicating that the above results were not due to heredity (Francis, Diorio, Liu, et al., 1999). These epigenetic changes could be explained by the following mechanism: the reception of tactile stimuli decreases DNA methylation in the glucocorticoid receptor or estrogen receptor gene in the neonatal period, thereby increasing the expression of these receptors after maturation (Champagne, Weaver, Diorio, Dymov, Szyf, & Meaney, 2006; Weaver, Cervoni, Champagne, D'Alessio, Sharma, Seckl, Dymov, Szyf, & Meaney, 2004). The details of maternal behavior in this period has not been studied yet in dogs, but Fox (1978) reported that pups exposed to various stimuli from birth to 5 weeks of age were found to be more confident, exploratory, and socially dominant than unstimulated controls when tested in novel environments after maturation. It is well estimated that in dogs, maternal behavior in the neonatal period affects the sociality of the offspring in adulthood by altering the development of the HPA axis or oxytocinergic neural system.

Canine neonates begin to suckle just after birth and spend most of their time sleeping or suckling. In this period, because the blood-brain barrier is immature, bioactive peptides transferred from mother's blood to milk, such as oxytocin, can also affect the central nervous system of pups. In rats, sbcutaneous injections of oxytocin to pups on 14 consecutive days after birth were reported to attenuate the glucocorticoid response to stress in adulthood (Sohlstrom, Carlsson, & Uvnas-Moberg, 2000). Carter and her colleague conducted a series of studies in which oxytocin or an oxytocin antagonist was intraperitoneally injected to pups of prairie vole, a biological monogamous, just after birth. These studies showed that manipulation of oxytocin exposure in the neonatal period can influence the onset of partner preference formation or glucocorticoid secretion in response to stress in adulthood (Bales & Carter, 2003; Kramer, Cushing, & Carter, 2003). The results support the hypothesis that oxytocin transferred from the mother via milk has the potential to act on pups' brains and influence the development of the central oxytocin and vasopressin neural systems, both of which may play an important role in the development of sociality (Carter, 2003). In humans, the plasma oxytocin levels in early pregnancy and the postpartum period were positively correlated to a clearly defined set of maternal bonding behaviors (Feldman, Weller, Zagoory-Sharon, et al., 2007). It may be assumed that pups of mothers showing higher levels of maternal behavior could be exposed to oxytocin from the mother via milk, and a similar mechanism may be responsible for the enhanced sociality of offspring nurtured by extremely caring mothers.

3.3. Transition Period

The transition period of about a week is when pups make the transition from complete dependence on their mothers to a somewhat independent state. The period starts with opening of the eyes and the external ear canals, and pups begin reacting to light, moving stimuli, and loud sounds. They exhibit enhanced physical ability and begin to stand and walk, although awkwardly. This period in the case of wild wolf pups corresponds to emergence from the dark den (Frank & Frank, 1982).

3.4. Socialization Period

Many studies conducted in the 1950s–1960s showed that the behavioral responses of adult dogs are influenced by their experiences of social contact with other species, including human, during the socialization period of development. In particular, these studies clarified how dogs' sociality, assessed in terms of their fear response toward humans or trainability, could be influenced by their experiences in this period. As a representative experiment, Freedman et al. (1961) compared different groups of pups who interacted with humans for only a week at 2, 3, 5, 7, and 9 weeks of age with a group isolated from humans until 14 weeks of age (control). At 14 weeks of age, all groups were tested for their responses to a human handler and to being walked on a leash. The pups that had interacted with humans for a week at age 5–9 weeks did not exhibit any fear response to the handler and could easily be trained. On the other hand, the control pups remained fearful and intractable even after many weeks of careful handling and petting. It was also found that non-conspecific encounters do not need to be particularly frequent or protracted for effective socialization. A study showed that pups could be socialized to humans during this period with as little as two 20-minute sessions of exposure per week (Fuller, 1967). Because of these findings, the socialization period was recognized as the limited developmental phase in which pups acquire specific preferences as well as "a critical period"—a concept advocated by Lorenz (1935) that explained the phenomenon of imprinting in birds. At present, this period is treated as the "sensitive period" in which pups find it easier to acquire specific responses and preferences compared to other periods. Scott & Fuller (1965) examined the behavioral responses of pups of different ages to experimenters and found that pups aged between 3 and 5 weeks showed a rapid increase in their tendency to approach and interact socially with even unfamiliar humans. This tendency later decreased gradually, and beyond 12 weeks of age, pups began to show anxiety and the fear response to unknown persons or unfamiliar situations. Therefore, Scott & Fuller concluded that the socialization period was between 3 and 12 weeks of age, and the sensitivity peaked at between 6 and 8 weeks of age. Fox & Stelzner (1966) conducted conditioned aversion experiments in which an electric shock was delivered to pups that interacted with humans at 5, 8, and 12 weeks of age; they observed long-lasting aversive effects only in pups that were given the shock at 8 weeks of age. It was also previously reported that pups tended to have a higher heart rate and exhibit distress vocalization in strange situations between the ages of 6 and 8 weeks (Elliot & Scott, 1961).

It is easy to understand that social contact with humans at 6–8 weeks of age would greatly affect the affinity of dogs to humans in adulthood. Then how do pups of this age acquire a preference or aversion to humans? A clue to the answer to this question may be a phenomenon found in rodent by Moriceau & Sullivan (2006), although the mechanism has not been understood yet in dogs. A series of odor-shock conditionings was conducted with the presentation of peppermint odor to rat pups at 8, 12–15, and 21–23 days after birth. The pups learned odor aversion at 21–23 days of age, and this aversion learning was also observed in adulthood. However, 8-day-old pups adversely learned to prefer the odor paired with the shock. Aversion learning could not be completed in these pups because the HPA axis and amygdala functioned immaturely in them. Since the age of 8 days falls within the stress hyporesponsive period, an electric shock cannot accelerate glucocorticoid secretion, which is necessary for aversion learning in addition to a completely functional amygdala. The detailed mechanism of odor preference as opposed to aversion learning has not been understood yet. However, it was reported that excess noradrenaline is secreted from the locus coeruleus to the olfactory bulb in this period as compared to the period after maturation, and this may responsible for the difference in olfactory function in this period (Moriceau & Sullivan, 2005). The stress hyporesponsive period or olfactory function in this period has not yet been investigated in dogs. However, taking into consideration the findings that (1) canine pups at 3–5 weeks of age tended to approach and contact even unfamiliar persons (Scott and Fuller, 1965) and (2) aversion conditioning was not complete in 5-week-old pups (as determined by an electric shock experiment; Fox & Stelzner, 1966), it could be speculated that the physiological state of dogs at 5 weeks of age might be the same as that of rats at 8 days of age. Furthermore, the most interesting phenomenon was found by Moriceau & Sullivan

(2006) in rats at 12–15 days of age, when breast-feeding has not completely stopped and the pups are just short of being weaned. They found that in this period, aversion learning could be completed to the same extent as that observed at 21–23 days of age since the HPA axis as well as the amygdala is developing, and glucocorticoid secretion has begun in response to electric shock. However, the absence of mothers was required for completion of aversion learning in this period, because the glucocorticoid response to electric shock was inhibited by the presence of the mothers even if they were anesthetized. The phenomenon wherein the response of the HPA axis to stress is diminished by the presence of conspecific animals is known as "social buffering" and is widely recognized in social animals, although the factors or underlying mechanisms involved are not known in detail (Kikusui, Winslow, & Mori, 2006). The age of around 6 to 8 weeks in dogs, considered as the peak of the "sensitive period," corresponds to 12–15 days of age in rats, because these are the respective ages at which breast feeding is reduced but not completely terminated. Therefore, dogs at the peak of the sensitive period may be in a physiological state in which the presence of mothers alters the glucocorticoid response to stimuli and determines the completion of aversion learning against the stimuli. If this hypothesis is true in the case of dogs, it may be useful in simultaneous reciprocal studies: the first study would be a series of experiments on the importance of human contact during the socialization period, and the other would be a study and questionnaire survey showing the impaired sociality of dogs separated from their mothers before 6 weeks of age. As we wait for these future investigations to determine the exact characteristics of the socialization period, this period in dogs may be considered as the period in which pups are not only socialized to humans but also tend to acquire aversion toward humans inversely if they have an unstable relationship with their mother.

Although few studies have experimentally shown that early mother-infant separation during the socialization period affects dogs' sociality in adulthood, many studies on rodent have suggested that social behavior could be affected by early weaning in the late lactation period. For example, in mice weaned at 14 days of age, a week earlier than normal weaning, the response of the HPA axis to stress, anxiety, or aggressiveness is enhanced (Kikusui, Takeuchi, & Mori, 2004; Kikusui, Nakamura, Kakuma, & Mori, 2006; Nakamura, Kikusui, Takeuchi, & Mori, 2008). It has been shown that in these early-weaned mice, glucocorticoid receptor expression in the hippocampus is altered (Kikusui, Nakamura, Kakuma, et al., 2006) ; further, the serotonergic neural system is also impaired, as indicated by the reduced serotonin receptor expression in the hippocampus (Nakamura, Kikusui, Takeuchi, et al., 2008). Although the functional relationship between serotonergic neural system and glucocorticoid receptors in the hippocampus during the late lactation period of mice has not been clarified, serotonin activity may influence glucocorticoid receptor expression in hippocampus in this period, as suggested above with regard to the neonatal period (Mitchell, Iny, & Meaney, 1990; Smythe, Rowe, & Meaney, 1994). In mice, the serotonergic neural system has been shown to start developing from the late lactation period onward, and a period-specific defect in serotonin receptor expression only during the lactation period was found to lead to increased anxiety in adulthood (Gross, Zhuang, Stark, Ramboz, Oosting, Kirby, Santarelli, Beck, & Hen, 2002). These findings have raised the possibility that the degree of development of the serotonergic neural system in the lactation period affects the expression of anxiety in adulthood (Gross & Hen, 2004). In central serotonin or serotonin receptor-deficient mice, the response to aversion stimuli is augmented after aversion learning, and it is difficult to delete fear memories (Dai, Han, Tian, Cao, Xiu, Song, Huang, Xu, Ding,

& Xu, 2008; Klemenhagen, Gordon, David, Hen, & Gross, 2006). In dogs, the process of the development of the serotonergic neural system is unknown; however, many studies have reported that the central serotonergic neural system is abnormal in dogs exhibiting dominant aggressive behavior (Badino, Odore, Osella, Bergamasco, Francone, Girardi, & Re, 2004; Peremans, Audenaert, Coopman, Blanckaert, Jacobs, Otte, Verschooten, van Bree, van Heeringen, Mertens, Slegers, & Dierckx, 2003; Reisner, Mann, Stanley, Huang, & Houpt, 1996). Thus, it is conceivable that the impaired development of the serotonergic neural system may be involved in the poor sociality of early-weaned dogs, as reported by Slabbert & Rasa (1993) and Serpell (personal communication).

3.5. Juvenile Period

In the juvenile period, the physical ability of pups improves dramatically, and sex-specific behavior develops along with the development of gonads. With the initiation of territorial imperative, pups begin to show aggressive behavior such as barking, which can affect the establishment of the special affinity between humans and dogs. Wolf pups start to prowl away from their den at 4–6 months of age (Mech, 1970). Wolves may have a second sensitive period in which they display strong sensitivity to novel or fear-arousing stimuli, because they begin to exhibit explicitly hostile behavior toward unfamiliar intruders in this period (Fentress, 1967; Fox, 1971; Mech, 1970). However, few studies have scientifically assessed whether dogs experience a second sensitive period like wolves.

4. Prospective of the Developmental-Behavioral Approach

With regard to the developmental process in many mammals, it is now strongly established that the early environment represented by the mother-infant relationship, including that in the prenatal period, critically influences the manifestation of sociality of the offspring in adulthood. It has been scientifically demonstrated that the better the mother-infant relationship, the better the sociality of the offspring. In contrast, a poor mother-infant relationship would result in poor sociality of the offspring. However, there are few studies from the viewpoint of the effect of the mother-infant relationship in dogs. It has been recognized that various stimulations during the neonatal period enhance the sociality of dogs in adulthood; therefore, the mechanism in which the mother-infant relationship alters the sociality of offspring is expected to be clarified soon, by analysis of the relationship between affinity/aggression toward humans in adulthood and the quality of maternal behavior such as breastfeeding or grooming during the neonatal period.

Another important issue that remains to be elucidated is the mechanism underlying the special affinity between humans and dogs. It may be necessary to understand how neural changes occur in the socialization period, particularly around 6–8 weeks of age, which is considered as the peak of the sensitive period. It is important to verify whether the phenomenon indicated by Moriceau & Sullivan (2006) in rodents also occurs in dogs. To that end, by analyzing the glucocorticoid response to stress, we should first demonstrate how long the stress hyporesponsive period lasts in the socialization period in dogs and determine whether "social buffering" by the presence of the mother after the stress hyporesponsive period exists in dogs.

It has been suggested that a decrease in the activity of the HPA axis or fear response is involved in the acquisition of superior social skills by dogs. It has been confirmed that in rodents, a good mother-infant relationship in the neonatal period decreases the activity of the HPA axis and the fear response, and in contrast, a poor mother-infant relationship in the socialization period (e.g., early maternal deprivation) enhances the activity of the HPA axis and the fear response. Therefore, determining the relationship between the mother-infant relationship in each developmental period and the social skills after maturation in dogs would be very interesting. Nagasawa, et al. (2009) indicated that dogs could be divided into 2 groups depending on whether they gazed at their owner for long or not. Gaze can be considered to be influenced by the oxytocinergic nerve system, because in humans, nasal administration of oxytocin leads to greater gazing toward the eye region of the face (Guastella, Mitchell, & Dadds, 2008). It has been suggested that in rodents, the development of the oxytocinergic nerve system is altered by the quality of the mother-infant relationship (Francsi et al. 2000, Lee et al. 2007). Taking both these findings into account, it is plausible that the difference in the duration of the dogs' gaze toward humans in Nagasawa, et al. (2009) might be because of a difference in the quality of the mother-infant relationship during the developmental period among dogs. To further clarify dogs' sociality, it is important to blend cognitive science and neuroscience, and conduct an assessment from the viewpoint of the developmental-behavioral approach.

REFERENCES

Appleby, D. L., Bradshaw, J. W. & Casey, R. A. (2002). Relationship between aggressive and avoidance behaviour by dogs and their experience in the first six months of life. *The Veterinary Record*, *150*, 434-438.

Badino, P., Odore, R., Osella, M. C., Bergamasco, L., Francone, P., Girardi, C. & Re, G. (2004). Modifications of serotonergic and adrenergic receptor concentrations in the brain of aggressive canis familiaris. Comparative Biochemistry and Physiology. *Part A, Molecular & Integrative Physiology*, *139*, 343-350.

Bales, K. L., & Carter, C. S. (2003). Developmental exposure to oxytocin facilitates partner preferences in male prairie voles (microtus ochrogaster). *Behavioral Neuroscience*, *117*, 854-859.

Barbazanges, A., Piazza, P. V., Le Moal, M. & Maccari, S. (1996). Maternal glucocorticoid secretion mediates long-term effects of prenatal stress. The Journal of Neuroscience, 16, 3943-3949.

Batki, A., Baron-Cohen, S., Wheelwright, S., Connellan, J., & Ahluwalia, J. (2000). Is there an innate gaze module? evidence from human neonates. Infant Behavior and Development, 23, 223-229.

Bowlby, J. (1969) Attachment and loss: Vol. I. attachment. New York: Basic Books. Caldji, C., Tannenbaum, B., Sharma, S., Francis, D., Plotsky, P. M., & Meaney, M. J. 1998 Maternal care during infancy regulates the development of neural systems mediating the expression of fearfulness in the rat. *Proceedings of the National Academy of Sciences of the United States of America, 95*, 5335-5340.

Carter, C. S. (2003). Developmental consequences of oxytocin. *Physiology & Behavior, 79*, 383-397.

Champagne, F. A., Weaver, I. C., Diorio, J., Dymov, S., Szyf, M. & Meaney, M. J. (2006). Maternal care associated with methylation of the estrogen receptor-alpha1b promoter and estrogen receptor-alpha expression in the medial preoptic area of female offspring. *Endocrinology, 147*, 2909-2915.

Champagne, F. A., Weaver, I. C., Diorio, J., Sharma, S. & Meaney, M. J. (2003). Natural variations in maternal care are associated with estrogen receptor alpha expression and estrogen sensitivity in the medial preoptic area. *Endocrinology, 144*, 4720-4724.

Clarke, R. S., Heron, W., Fetherstonhaugh, M. L., Forgays, D. G. & Hebb, D. O. (1951). Individual differences in dogs: Preliminary report on the effects of early experience. *Canadian Journal of Psychology, 5*, 150-156.

Dai, J. X., Han, H. L., Tian, M., Cao, J., Xiu, J. B., Song, N. N., Huang, Y., Xu, T. L., Ding, Y. Q. & Xu, L. (2008). Enhanced contextual fear memory in central serotonin-deficient mice. *Proceedings of the National Academy of Sciences of the United States of America, 105*, 11981-11986.

Donaldson, Z. R. & Young, L. J. (2008). Oxytocin, vasopressin, and the neurogenetics of sociality. *Science, 322*, 900-904.

Elliot, O. & Scott, J. P. 1961 The development of emotional distress reactions to separation, in puppies. *The Journal of Genetic Psychology, 99*, 3-22.

Farroni, T., Csibra, G., Simion, F. & Johnson, M. H. (2002). Eye contact detection in humans from birth. *Proceedings of the National Academy of Sciences of the United States of America, 99*, 9602-9605.

Feldman, R., Weller, A., Zagoory-Sharon, O. & Levine, A. (2007). Evidence for a neuroendocrinological foundation of human affiliation: Plasma oxytocin levels across pregnancy and the postpartum period predict mother-infant bonding. *Psychological Science, 18*, 965-970.

Fentress, J. C. (1967). Observations on the behavioral development of a hand-reared male timber wolf. *American Zoologist, 7*, 339-351.

Ferguson, J. N., Young, L. J., Hearn, E. F., Matzuk, M. M., Insel, T. R. & Winslow, J. T. (2000). Social amnesia in mice lacking the oxytocin gene. *Nature Genetics, 25*, 284-288.

Fox, M. W. (1971). *Behaviour of wolves, dogs, and related canids*. New York: Harper & Row.

Fox, M. W. (1978). *The dog: Its domestication and behavior*. New York: Garland STPM Press.

Fox, M. W. & Stelzner, D. (1966) Approach/withdrawal variables in the development of social behaviour in the dog. *Animal Behaviour, 14*, 362-366.

Francis, D., Diorio, J., Liu, D. & Meaney, M. J. (1999). Nongenomic transmission across generations of maternal behavior and stress responses in the rat. *Science, 286*, 1155-1158.

Francis, D. D., Champagne, F. C. & Meaney, M. J. (2000). Variations in maternal behaviour are associated with differences in oxytocin receptor levels in the rat. *Journal of Neuroendocrinology, 12*, 1145-1148.

Frank, H. & Frank, M. G. (1982) On the effects of domestication on canine social development and behavior. *Applied Animal Ethology, 8*, 507-525.

Freedman, D. G., King, J. A. & Elliot, O. (1961). Critical period in the social development of dogs. *Science*, *133*, 1016-1017.

Fuller, J. L. (1967). Experiential deprivation and later behavior. *Science*, *158*, 1645-1652.

Green, L., Fein, D., Modahl, C., Feinstein, C., Waterhouse, L. & Morris, M. (2001). Oxytocin and autistic disorder: Alterations in peptide forms. *Biological Psychiatry*, *50*, 609-613.

Gross, C. & Hen, R. (2004). The developmental origins of anxiety. *Nature Reviews Neuroscience*, *5*, 545-552.

Gross, C., Zhuang, X., Stark, K., Ramboz, S., Oosting, R., Kirby, L., Santarelli, L., Beck, S. & Hen, R. (2002). Serotonin1A receptor acts during development to establish normal anxiety-like behaviour in the adult. *Nature*, *416*, 396-400.

Guastella, A. J., Mitchell, P. B. & Dadds, M. R. (2008). Oxytocin increases gaze to the eye region of human faces. *Biological Psychiatry*, *63*, 3-5.

Gutteling, B. M., de Weerth, C. & Buitelaar, J. K. (2005). Prenatal stress and children's cortisol reaction to the first day of school. *Psychoneuroendocrinology*, *30*, 541-549.

Haller, J., Makara, G. B., Barna, I., Kovacs, K., Nagy, J. & Vecsernyes, M. (1996), Compression of the pituitary stalk elicits chronic increases in CSF vasopressin, oxytocin as well as in social investigation and aggressiveness. *Journal of Neuroendocrinology*, *8*, 361-365.

Hare, B., Brown, M., Williamson, C. & Tomasello, M. (2002). The domestication of social cognition in dogs. *Science*, *298*, 1634-1636.

Hare, B., Plyusnina, I., Ignacio, N., Schepina, O., Stepika, A., Wrangham, R. & Trut, L. (2005). Social cognitive evolution in captive foxes is a correlated by-product of experimental domestication. *Current Biology*, *15*, 226-230.

Hare, B. & Tomasello, M. (2005). Human-like social skills in dogs? *Trends in Cognitive Sciences*, *9*, 439-444.

Khashan, A. S., Abel, K. M., McNamee, R., Pedersen, M. G., Webb, R. T., Baker, P. N., Kenny, L. C. & Mortensen, P., B. (2008). Higher risk of offspring schizophrenia following antenatal maternal exposure to severe adverse life events. *Archives of General Psychiatry*, *65*, 146-152.

Kikusui, T., Nakamura, K., Kakuma, Y. & Mori, Y. (2006). Early weaning augments neuroendocrine stress responses in mice. *Behavioural Brain Research*, *175*, 96-103.

Kikusui, T., Takeuchi, Y. & Mori, Y. (2004). Early weaning induces anxiety and aggression in adult mice. *Physiology & Behavior*, *81*, 37-42.

Kikusui, T., Winslow, J. T. & Mori, Y. (2006). Social buffering: Relief from stress and anxiety. Philosophical Transactions of the Royal Society of London. Series B, *Biological Sciences*, *361*, 2215-2228.

Klemenhagen, K. C., Gordon, J. A., David, D. J., Hen, R. & Gross, C. T. (2006). Increased fear response to contextual cues in mice lacking the 5-HT1A receptor. *Neuropsychopharmacology*, *31*, 101-111.

Koenig, J. I., Elmer, G. I., Shepard, P. D., Lee, P. R., Mayo, C., Joy, B., Hercher, E. & Brady, D. L. (2005). Prenatal exposure to a repeated variable stress paradigm elicits behavioral and neuroendocrinological changes in the adult offspring: Potential relevance to schizophrenia. *Behavioural Brain Research*, *156*, 251-261.

Kramer, K. M., Cushing, B. S. & Carter, C. S. (2003). Developmental effects of oxytocin on stress response: Single versus repeated exposure. *Physiology & Behavior*, *79*, 775-782.

Lee, P. R., Brady, D. L., Shapiro, R. A., Dorsa, D. M. & Koenig, J. I. (2007). Prenatal stress generates deficits in rat social behavior: Reversal by oxytocin. *Brain Research*, 1156, 152-167.

Levine, S. (1967). Maternal and environmental influences on the adrenocortical response to stress in weanling rats. *Science*, *156*, 258-260.

Liu, D., Diorio, J., Tannenbaum, B., Caldji, C., Francis, D., Freedman, A., Sharma, S., Pearson, D., Plotsky, P. M. & Meaney, M. J. (1997). Maternal care, hippocampal glucocorticoid receptors, and hypothalamic-pituitary-adrenal responses to stress. *Science*, *277*, 1659-1662.

Markwell, P. & Thorne, C. (1987). Early behavioural development of dogs. *Journal of Small Animal Practice*, *28*, 984-991.

Mech, L. D. (1970). *The wolf: The ecology and behavior of an endangered species*. New York: Natural History Press.

Meins, E. (1997). *Security of attachment and the social development of cognition. essays in developmental psychology*. Philadelphia: Psychology Press.

Miklósi, A., Kubinyi, E., Topál, J., Gácsi, M., Virányi, Z. & Csányi, V. (2003). A simple reason for a big difference: Wolves do not look back at humans, but dogs do. *Current Biology*, *13*, 763-766.

Mitchell, J. B., Iny, L. J. & Meaney, M. J. (1990). The role of serotonin in the development and environmental regulation of type II corticosteroid receptor binding in rat hippocampus. *Developmental Brain Research*, *55*, 231-235.

Moriceau, S. & Sullivan, R. M. (2005). Neurobiology of infant attachment. *Developmental Psychobiology*, *47*, 230-242.

Moriceau, S. & Sullivan, R. M. (2006). Maternal presence serves as a switch between learning fear and attraction in infancy. *Nature Neuroscience*, *9*, 1004-1006.

Nagasawa, M., Kikusui, T., Onaka, T. & Ohta, M. (2009). Dog's gaze at its owner increases owner's urinary oxytocin during social interaction. *Hormones and Behavior*, *55*, 431-441.

Nagasawa, M., Mogi, K. & Kikusui, T. (2009) Attachment between humans and dogs. *Japanease Psychological Research*, *51*, 209-221.

Nakamura, K., Kikusui, T., Takeuchi, Y. & Mori, Y. (2008). Changes in social instigation- and food restriction-induced aggressive behaviors and hippocampal 5HT1B mRNA receptor expression in male mice from early weaning. *Behavioural Brain Research*, *187*, 442-448.

Odendaal, J. S. & Meintjes, R. A. (2003). Neurophysiological correlates of affiliative behaviour between humans and dogs. *Veterinary Journal*, *165*, 296-301.

Oskina, I. N. (1996). Analysis of the functional state of the pituitary-adrenal axis during postnatal development of domesticated silver foxes (vulpes vulpes). *Scientifur*, *20*, 159-167.

Pedersen, C. A., Caldwell, J. D., Drago, F., Noonan, L. R., Peterson, G., Hood, L. E. & Prange, A. J. Jr. (1988). Grooming behavioral effects of oxytocin. pharmacology, ontogeny, and comparisons with other nonapeptides. *Annals of the New York Academy of Sciences*, *525*, 245-256.

Peremans, K., Audenaert, K., Coopman, F., Blanckaert, P., Jacobs, F., Otte, A., Verschooten, F., van Bree, H., van Heeringen, K., Mertens, J., Slegers, G.,& Dierckx, R. (2003). Estimates of regional cerebral blood flow and 5-HT2A receptor density in impulsive, aggressive dogs with 99mTc-ECD and 123I-5-I-R91150. *European Journal of Nuclear Medicine and Molecular Imaging*, *30*, 1538-1546.

Popova, N. K., Voitenko, N. N., Kulikov, A. V. & Avgustinovich, D. F. (1991). Evidence for the involvement of central serotonin in mechanism of domestication of silver foxes. Pharmacology, *Biochemistry, and Behavior*, *40*, 751-756.

Reisner, I. R., Mann, J. J., Stanley, M., Huang, Y. Y. & Houpt, K. A. (1996). Comparison of cerebrospinal fluid monoamine metabolite levels in dominant-aggressive and non-aggressive dogs. *Brain Research*, *714*, 57-64.

Scott, J. P. & Fuller, J. L. (1965). *Genetics and the social behavior of the dog*. Chicago: University of Chicago Press.

Scott, J. P., Stewart, J. M. & De Ghett, V. J. (1974) Critical periods in the organization of systems. *Developmental Psychobiology*, *7*, 489-513.

Seckl, J. R. & Meaney, M. J. (2004). Glucocorticoid programming. *Annals of the New York Academy of Sciences*, *1032*, 63-84.

Serpell, J. (1995). *The domestic dog: Its evolution, behaviour, and interactions with people*. Cambridge: Cambridge University Press.

Sieber-Ruckstuhl, N. S., Meli, M. L., Boretti, F. S., Gonczi, E., Lutz, H. & Reusch, C. E. (2007). Quantitative real-time PCR for the measurement of 11beta-HSD1 and 11beta-HSD2 mRNA levels in tissues of healthy dogs. Hormone and Metabolic Research.Hormon- Und Stoffwechselforschung. *Hormones Et Metabolisme*, *39*, 548-554.

Slabbert, J. M. & Rasa, O. A. (1993). The effect of early separation from the mother on pups in bonding to humans and pup health. *Journal of the South African Veterinary Association*, *64*, 4-8.

Smythe, J. W., Rowe, W., Meaney, M. J. (1994). Neonatal handling alters serotonin turnover and serotonin type 2 receptor density in selected brain regions. *Developmental Brain Research*, *80*, 183-189.

Sohlstrom, A., Carlsson, C. & Uvnas-Moberg, K. (2000). Effects of oxytocin treatment in early life on body weight and corticosterone in adult offspring from ad libitum-fed and food-restricted rats. *Biology of the Neonate*, *78*, 33-40.

Thompson, W. R. & Heron, W. (1954). The effects of restricting early experience on the problem-solving capacity of dogs. *Canadian Journal of Psychology*, *8*, 17-31.

Topál, J., Gácsi, M., Miklósi, Á, Virányi, Z., Kubinyi, E. & Csányi, V. (2005). Attachment to humans: A comparative study on hand-reared wolves and differently socialized dog puppies. *Animal Behaviour*, *70*, 1367-1375.

Topál, J., Miklósi, A., Csányi, V. & Dóka, A. (1998). Attachment behavior in dogs (canis familiaris): A new application of ainsworth's (1969) strange situation test. *Journal of Comparative Psychology*, *112*, 219-229.

Udell, M. A. R., Dorey, N. R. & Wynne, C. D. L. (2008). Wolves outperform dogs in following human social cues. *Animal Behaviour*, *766*, 1767-1773.

Van den Bergh, B. R., Mulder, E. J., Mennes, M. & Glover, V. (2005). Antenatal maternal anxiety and stress and the neurobehavioural development of the fetus and child: Links and possible mechanisms. A review. *Neuroscience and Biobehavioral Reviews*, *29*, 237-258.

Virányi, Z., Gácsi, M., Kubinyi, E., Topál, J., Belényi, B., Ujfalussy, D. & Miklósi, A. (2008). Comprehension of human pointing gestures in young human-reared wolves (canis lupus) and dogs (canis familiaris). *Animal Cognition*, *11*, 373-387.

Weaver, I. C., Cervoni, N., Champagne, F. A., D'Alessio, A. C., Sharma, S., Seckl, J. R., Dymov, S., Szyf, M. & Meaney, M. J. (2004). Epigenetic programming by maternal behavior. *Nature Neuroscience*, *7*, 847-854.

Winslow, J. T. & Insel, T. R. (2002). The social deficits of the oxytocin knockout mouse. *Neuropeptides*, *36*, 221-229.

Witt, D. M., Winslow, J. T. & Insel, T. R. (1992). Enhanced social interactions in rats following chronic, centrally infused oxytocin. *Pharmacology, Biochemistry, and Behavior*, *43*, 855-861.

Wu, S., Jia, M., Ruan, Y., Liu, J., Guo, Y., Shuang, M., Gong, X., Zhang, Y., Yang, X. & Zhang, D. (2005). Positive association of the oxytocin receptor gene (OXTR) with autism in the chinese han population. *Biological Psychiatry*, *58*, 74-77.

Young, L. J., Lim, M. M., Gingrich, B. & Insel, T. R. (2001). Cellular mechanisms of social attachment. *Hormones and Behavior*, *40*, 133-138.

Young, L. J. & Wang, Z. (2004). The neurobiology of pair bonding. *Nature Neuroscience*, *7*, 1048-1054.

In: Neuroendocrinology Research Developments
Editor: N. S. Penkava and L.R. Haight, pp. 79-91
ISBN: 978-1-60876-983-4
© 2010 Nova Science Publishers, Inc.

Chpater 4

K-RAS AND C-MYC MOLECULAR CHANGES FOUND IN PHEOCHROMOCYTOMAS FROM CROATIAN PATIENTS

Nives Pećina-Šlaus[1,2*], Reno Hrašćan[3], Tamara Nikuševa-Martić[1,2] and Božo Krušlin[4]

[1]Laboratory of Neurooncology, Croatian Institute for Brain Research, School of Medicine University of Zagreb, Šalata 12, HR-10000 Zagreb;
[2] Department of Biology, School of Medicine, University of Zagreb, Zagreb, Croatia;
[3]Department of Biochemical Engineering, Faculty of Food Technology and Biotechnology, University of Zagreb, Pierottijeva 6, HR-10000 Zagreb
[4]Ljudevit Jurak Department of Pathology, University Hospital "Sisters of Charity", Vinogradska 29, HR-10000 Zagreb, Croatia.

ABSTRACT

Pheochromocytomas are neuroendocrine tumors that may be either sporadic or manifestation of a familial cancer syndromes and are derived from neural-crest. In the present study oncogenes — *k-ras* and *c-myc* were investigated in sporadic human pheochromocytomas in order to identify their involvement. The aim of their investigation was to identify new molecular targets of neuroendocrine carcinogenesis.

Pheochromocytoma samples were tested for activating point mutations of *k-ras* and to the levels of k-Ras and c-Myc protein expression by immunohistochemistry.

The results of their analysis showed that point mutations of *k-ras* were frequent changes, namely 88.9% of pheochromocytomas harbored activating *k-ras* mutations in codon 12. The k-Ras and c-Myc proteins were up regulated in the pheochromocytomas we investigated. Sixty-one point five percent of samples had moderate upregulation of k-Ras, while strong expression of k-Ras proteins was not observed in any of their pheochromocytoma case. Increased levels of Myc protein were detected in 92.3% of

* Correspondence to: E-mail: nina@mef.hr, tel. +385 1 46 21 140, fax:+385 1 45 90199; +385 1 49 20 050; +385 1 45 96 942

cases. Strong upregulation was observed in 6 pheochromocytoma samples and also in the investigated lymph node metastasis (53.8%). Five out of 10 samples with activating *k-ras* mutation had upregulated levels of both k-Ras and c-Myc.

Their findings on upregulation of *k-ras* and *c-myc* oncogenes expression in pheochromocytoma samples may indicate their collaborative involvement in tumorigenesis and may contribute to better understanding of pheochromocytoma molecular profile.

Keywords: pheochromocytoma, oncogenes, k-ras, c-myc, signal transduction pathways

INTRODUCTION

As with other tumors, the formation of pheochromocytoma is the result of multiple consecutive genetic changes that represent a critical factor in tumor formation and later on progression. In recent years new data have been obtained on the genetics of neural crest derived tumors such as pheochromocytoma [1-7], and many genes have been implicated in genesis of pheochromocytomas.

The genome of tumor cells is affected by two crucial types of changes: the accumulation of somatic mutations and the acquisition of genomic instability. The usual incidence rate of spontaneous somatic mutations is much lower to the rates of genetic changes observed in tumor cells and this increased frequency is the result of genomic instability that characterizes such cells. Their knowledge of the etiology and pathogenesis of pheochromocytoma still needs to be elucidated although great progress has been achieved along with the increasing discoveries in molecular biology and molecular medicine.

Novel findings indicate that besides different protooncogenes and tumor suppressor genes, mitochondrial complex II genes are also involved. Succinate dehydrogenase (SDH) is a complex II in the mitochondrial respiratory chain and consists of four subunits. Two subunits are especially interesting for genetics of neural crest derived tumors, the one encoded with *SDHB*, and the one encoded with *SDHD* gene. Germline mutations in *SDHB* and *SDHD* genes have been found to be responsible for susceptibility to head and neck paraganglioma and pheochromocytoma [8, 9] Hereditary pheochromocytomas more often demonstrate *SDHB* mutations, while carriers with *SDHD* mutations more often have hereditary head and neck paragangliomas [10,11]. Nevertheless, the final list of genes involved in pheochromocytoma is still incomplete.

From the clinical view pheochromocytomas are neural-crest derived neuroendocrine tumors that produce catecholamines and originate from chromaffin cells of adrenal medulla or extra-adrenal paraganglia. They can cause endocrine hypertension by oversecretion of catecholamines. Pheochromocytomas are mostly located in the adrenal medulla, but also in the ganglia of the sympathetic nervous system. These extra-adrenal pheochromocytomas occur in 15% of cases [2]. Although, they typically follow a benign course, about 10% of the pheochromocytoma cases are malignant [3]. Forty percent of cases of the malignant tumor localize in the extra-adrenal tissues [1, 2]. Pheochromocytomas may be either sporadic or a manifestation of a familial cancer syndrome. For instance, Multiple Endocrine Neoplasia type 2 (MEN 2), von Hippel-Lindau (VHL) disease, or neurofibromatosis type 1 (NF 1) all include pheochromocytomas in their clinical picture.

Specific genetic alterations have been found to be associated with hereditary-predisposition [4, 5, 12]. Ninety-five percent of investigated patients with MEN 2 have germline mutations in the *ret* protooncogene [3, 13]. Expression of *ret,* a receptor tyrosine kinase protein, is fundamental for appropriate migration, development, and differentiation of neuroendocrine cells originating from neural crest. Von Hippel-Lindau-associated pheochromocytomas exhibit mutations in the *VHL* tumor suppressor gene [14, 15] and patients with NF-associated pheochromocytoma show loss of the wild-type allele of the *NF1* tumor suppressor gene [3, 16-18].

On the other hand, the genetic basis of sporadic pheochromocytoma is unclear, and much work is still required to determine the final list of genes involved, as well as the point in time of their activation/inactivation. Although it was suspected that the *ret* protooncogene may also be involved in the pathophysiology of sporadic pheochromocytoma [19], only about 8% of cases show *ret* protooncogene mutation. The mutations of the *VHL* and *NF1* genes are also uncommon [11, 20].

There are indications that multiple signaling pathways and diverse genetic components might be involved in the molecular mechanisms that lead to the development of sporadic pheochromocytoma [21]. The involvement of two classical proto-oncogenes, such as *k-ras* and *c-myc*, in sporadic pheochromocytoma initiation and development have not been enough investigated.

K-ras is a well known oncogene whose mutations occur frequently in cancer. The first experiments on mouse NIH 3T3 fibroblasts revealed the ras family members as the transforming genes and identified their human homologs [22]. The human ras family numbers three proto-oncogenes, *cH-ras, cK-ras* and *N-ras* and they share a great sequence similarity. Ras proteins are localized in the inner cytoplasmic membrane and have function in binding GDP and GTP showing GTPase activity [23]. Ras proteins are activated by signals originated in surface receptors, sending the signals downstream through diverse routes and pathways.

New research indicates that genes of the *ras* family which encode guanine nucleotide-binding proteins, have potential involvement in neuroendocrine tumors [24, 25]. Activated Ras stimulates serin/threonine kinase cascade, including molecules Raf1, Mek, and Erk. Ras proteins regulate cellular proliferation and differentiation, and activating mutations of *ras* are commonly associated with human tumors. Interaction of Ras protein with neurofibromin, product of NF1 gene, stimulates intrinsic GTPase activity of Ras, suggesting that NF1 protein may function as a negative regulator of Ras protein [26].

c-myc is a prototype oncogene, one of the most famous one and the one that activates a wide variety of target genes. A significant number of Myc-induced genes encode positive regulators of the cell cycle (for example CDK4, Cyclin E1 and Cyclin D2). c-Myc is a famous transcription factor consisting of helix-loop-helix motive that binds directly to DNA. c-Myc activities on its molecular targets are biologically very diverse. Myc activity derives cells into proliferation, and this involvement has been proposed after studying its expression following growth stimulation of tumor with different growth factors [27, 28]. Myc can also block differentiation in a number of model systems. Myc mutations are associated with a variety of human tumors, moreover amplification, and chromosomal translocations of *c-myc* that usually result in constitutive expression of its protein are also common in tumors [29].

The association of *k-ras* and *c-myc* was established long time ago [30, 31]. The interesting cooperation of those oncogenes was first described in the transformation of rodent primary fibroblasts. The result of Myc-Ras cooperation is the cellular transformation and oncogenesis. It has been [31, 32] that Ras enhanced the accumulation of Myc and enhances its activity in a way that it stabilizes its protein product. Half-life of c-Myc protein is much longer due to its stabilization by k-Ras. In normal circumstances, or at least when produced without mitogenic signals, Myc has a very short life in the cell. It has been suggested that Ras inhibits the proteasome degradation of Myc and that is how it stabilizes the transcriptionally active Myc protein.

The aim of their investigation was to identify new molecular targets of neuroendocrine carcinogenesis. We analyzed changes in sporadic pheochromocytoma with regards to the roles of two oncogenes — *k-ras* and *c-myc*. Pheochromocytoma samples were tested for activating point mutations of *k-ras* and to the level of k-Ras and c-Myc protein expression.

MATERIALS AND METHODS

Patients and Tumor Material. Twelve sporadic pheochromocytomas, together with 12 autologous normal adrenal tissues and one lymph node metstasis, were collected from The Department of Pathology, Sisters of Charity University Hospital, Zagreb, Croatia. The diagnosis of pheochromocytoma was suspected based on the clinical phenotype of paroxysmal tachycardia and uncontrolled hypertension associated with bouts of sweating. It was confirmed by measuring the 24 hours urinary metanephrines, which were more that 100-fold the normal values. A highly vascularized adrenal mass was detected by ultrasonography, computed tomography, selective arteriography (renal and suprarenal blood vessels) and octreotide scan. Pheochromocytomas with a diameter higher than 10 cm and suspected to malignancy were removed using conventional laparotomy. For tumors smaller than 5 cm laparoscopic adrenalectomy was done. The key parameter of malignancy was the presence of metastases in local lymph nodes and liver, local invasion of surrounding soft tissue, as well as lesions with a diameter higher than 2 cm. Other parameters included angioinvasion and proliferation index (>2%). The cases we studied were consecutive and not specifically selected. They were analyzed as they appeared in the clinical practice during the last 10 years. Tumor tissue was in all cases from the primary except one from a metastatic site.

The samples were formalin-fixed and paraffin-embedded. Among those 12 cases, 10 were benign and 2 malignant. All samples were located in the adrenal medulla and were unilateral. The age of patients varied from 28 to 66 years (mean age = 44.7), and there were 9 females and 3 males. The histopathological classification was pheochromocytoma.

The local Ethical Committee approved their study and all the patients gave their informed consent.

DNA extraction. For each specimen, 20 μm paraffin section was prepared for DNA extraction. In addition, 4 μm section was stained with hemalaun-eosin to identify the tumor and normal tissue areas.

Tumor samples used for DNA isolation were parts of the obvious tumor mass. Prior to DNA extraction, the pheochromocytoma samples were microdissected, so that the DNA extraction could be performed exclusively on tumor cells.

Twenty-micrometer paraffin sections were separated from the slide, transferred to a microtube and repeatedly extracted with xylene for a couple of hours. The tissue was then rinsed with absolute ethanol and incubated for two days at 37°C in digestion buffer (50 mM Tris-HCl, 1 mM EDTA, 0.5% Tween 20, pH 8.5) together with proteinase K. The digestion was stopped by heating the mixture for 10 min at 95°C [33].

One sample investigated was immediately frozen in liquid nitrogen and transported to the laboratory, together with 5 ml of corresponding blood sample in order to compare the amounts of DNA extracted from fresh tissue to the DNA from paraffin blocks and to optimize PCR reactions. Approximately 0.5 g of this tumor tissue was homogenized with 1 ml extraction buffer (10 mM Tris-HCl, pH 8.0; 0.1 M EDTA, pH 8.0; 0.5% sodium dodecyl sulfate) and incubated with proteinase K (final concentration 100 μg/ml; Sigma, USA) overnight at 37°C. Phenol chloroform extraction and ethanol precipitation followed. The corresponding blood sample was lysed with 7 ml distilled water and centrifuged (15 min/5000 g). The pellet was then processed as for DNA extraction from the tissue sample.

Detection of mutations in k-ras gene. Mutation in *k-ras* at codon 12 was detected by the primer-mediated, mutant-enriched PCR-RFLP method described by Levi *et al.* [34]. This technique employs two PCR amplification stages. First, the *k-ras* exon 1 was amplified using a mismatched (+) primer 5'-ACTGAATATAAACTTGTGGTAGTTGGACCT-3' which generated a BstNI restriction site in combination with the wild type allele of *k-ras* codon 12. Primer 5'-TCAAAGAATGGTCCTGGACC-3' served as a (-) primer in this first PCR. Incubation of a 157-bp product of the first PCR with the restriction enzyme BstNI cleaves amplified wild type alleles to 14-, 29-, and 114-bp fragments, and leaves the amplified alleles with mutation in codon 12 of *k-ras* intact (14- and 143-bp fragments). The product of the first PCR contains two BstNI restriction sites if codon 12 is normal and only one if codon 12 is mutated. In the second PCR, the noncleaved fragments are then reamplified to enhance specificity. In this second PCR, the same (+) primer is used, and a different (-) primer 5'-TAATATGTCGACTAAAACAAGATTTACCTC-3'. Incubation of a 135-bp product of the second PCR with BstNI cleaves the wild type alleles into two fragments (29- and 106-bp). Mutation in *k-ras* codon 12 results in 135-bp fragments that do not have BstNI restriction site. The reaction mixture for *k-ras* exon 1 amplification was: 5 pmol of each primer, 2.5 mM of each dNTP, 100 ng DNA (1 μl of the BstNI incubation mix for the second PCR), 0.25 U Taq polymerase, 1.5 mM $MgCl_2$, 10x reaction buffer. PCR conditions were: 3 min/96°C, 30 sec/96°C, 30 sec/56°C, 30+1 sec/72°C, 10 min/72°C, 35 cycles. PCR aliquots (10-20 μl) were digested with 4 U BstNI (NewEngland BioLabs) at 60°C for 12 hours. Fragments were analyzed on 3% NuSieve agarose gels containing ethidium-bromide.

Immunohistochemistry. Immunohistochemistry (IHC) was performed in order to establish the level of c-Myc and k-Ras protein expression. The samples were formalin-fixed, paraffin-embedded, and 4-μm thick sections were placed on Capillary gap microscope slides (DakoCytomation, Denmark). The sections were immunostained using the biotin–avidin–horseradish peroxidase method. Deparaffinized and rehydrated sections were microwaved in Dako Target Retrieval Solution (Dako Corporation, USA) three times for 5 min at 800 W to unmask epitopes. To block endogenous peroxidase activity, we fixed the cells in methanol containing 3% H_2O_2. Non-specific binding was blocked by the application of normal mouse serum for 30 min in a humid chamber. Slides were blotted and the primary antibody at optimized dilution of 1:100 was applied for 30 min at room temperature. The antibodies used were mouse monoclonal antibodies raised to human c-Myc protein (diluted 1 : 100 in PBS/0.1% BSA) (Oncogene Science) and mouse monoclonal antibodies raised to human k-Ras (Oncogene Science). After incubation, the slides were washed three times in phosphate-buffered saline/goat serum. Secondary LINK antibody was applied for 25 min. The washing was repeated, and the slides were incubated with streptavidin horseradish peroxidase for another 25 min. Secondary antibodies were rabbit to mouse immunoglobulins (Dako) and the chromogen was DAB. All chemicals were from DakoCytomation.

The positive control for the IHC assay was normal adrenal gland medulla. Negative controls were samples that underwent same staining procedure with the exclusion of the primary antibodies. The analysis of the labeling was performed by two independent observers, i.e. blinded pathologists, experts in the field on an Olympus BH-2 microscope.

For each tumor the c-Myc and k-Ras positive cells were evaluated in at least four randomly selected areas. Each section was assessed independently by two observers, i.e. blinded pathologists, experts in the field. Weak expression was labeled as +, moderate expression as ++, and strong expression as +++. There was 95% initial agreement between the observers.

RESULTS

Genetic studies were performed for the presence of activating point mutations of *k-ras* oncogene. Mutations in *k-ras* at codon 12 were detected by two PCR amplification stages. The product of the first PCR contained two BstNI restriction sites if codon 12 is normal and only one if codon 12 is mutated. Incubation of the first PCR product with the BstNI cleaved wild type alleles to 14-, 29-, and 114-bp fragments, but left the alleles with mutation in codon 12 of *k-ras* intact (14- and 143-bp fragments). In the second PCR, the non-cleaved fragments were then reamplified to enhance specificity. Incubation of the second PCR product with BstNI cleaved the wild type alleles into two fragments (29- and 106-bp), while alleles with mutation in *k-ras* codon 12 did not have the BstNI restriction site and 135-bp fragments was visible on the gel.

The results of their analysis showed that point mutations of *k-ras* were frequent changes. Eight out of nine pheochromocytomas available for the genetic analysis harbored *k-ras* mutation in codon 12 (88.9%). Six benign pheochromocytomas and 2 malignant pheochtomocytoma had *k-ras* mutations (Table 1). The related lymph node metastasis also harbored activating point mutation of *k-ras* oncogene. Analysis showed that, in some tumor samples, the mutation involved only one *k-ras* allele since besides 135-bp band additional as 106-bp band appeared on 3% NuSieve agarose gel after the second amplification and restriction stage (Figure 1).

In order to determine whether *k-ras* changes at the genetic level have consequences at the protein level in their sporadic pheochromocytoma samples, the expression of k-Ras proteins was investigated by IHC. Normal levels of k-Ras staining in adrenal tissue were scored as +, and the protein was located in the inner cytoplasmic membrane or inside the cytoplasm. Immunostaining showed that 8 (metastasis included) out of 13 samples (61.5%) had moderate upregulation of k-Ras expression. Five out of 9 samples (55.6%) with activating *k-ras* mutations were accompanied with the moderate upregulation of k-Ras protein expression as shown in Table 1. Strong expression (+++) of k-Ras proteins was not observed in any of their pheochromocytoma cases.

Since the Myc-Ras cooperation is a well known phenomenon on cellular transformation and oncogenesis their samples were also tested to the levels of expression of the c-Myc protein by IHC. Normal levels of c-Myc staining in normal adrenal gland tissue were scored as +, and the protein was located in the nucleus or inside the cytoplasm. Altogether (metastasis included), 12 samples out of 13 (92.3%) showed increased levels of Myc protein in comparison to normal adrenal tissue, as shown in Figure 3. Strong upregulation was observed in 6 pheochromocytoma samples and also in the investigated lymph node metastasis (53.8%). Five out of 10 samples with activating *k-ras* mutation had upregulated levels of both k-Ras and c-Myc expression.

Due to the small number of cases we were not able to establish statistically relevant association between increased expressions of k-Ras and c-Myc, but nevertheless noticed that 61.5% of samples with upregulated k-Ras also showed upregulated levels of c-Myc.

The findings on the mutations and protein levels are shown in Table 1. Immunostaining of k-Ras proteins is demonstrated in Figure 2 and c-Myc proteins in Figure 3.

Their results on upregulation of both *k-ras* and *c-myc* oncogenes expression in pheochromocytoma samples may indicate their collaborative involvement in tumorigenesis.

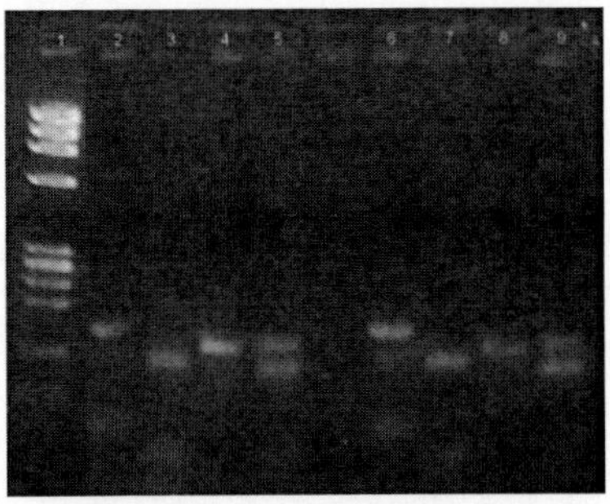

Figure 1. Point mutation in the *k-ras* gene at codon 12. 3% NuSieve agarose gel containing ethidium-bromide. Lane 1: DNA marker ΦX174/Hae III; lanes 2-5: malignant pheochromocytoma (patient no. 9); lanes 6-9: lymph node metastasis (patient no. 9). Lanes 2 and 6: first PCR amplification stages (157-bp fragment); lanes 3 and 7: incubation of the first PCR products with BstNI (114-bp fragments are visible); lanes 4 and 8: second PCR amplification stages (135-bp fragment); lane 5: incubation of the second PCR product with BstNI (106-bp fragment, wild type allele; and 135-bp fragment, allele with mutation in codon 12); lane 9: incubation of the second PCR product with BstNI (106-bp fragment, wild type allele; and 135-bp fragment, allele with mutation in codon 12).

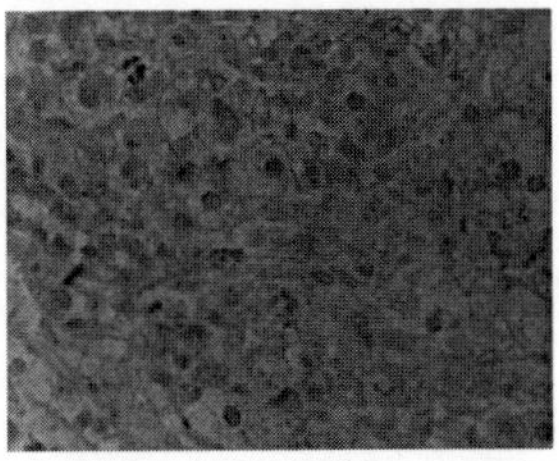

Figure 2. Immunohistochemistry showing moderate expression of k-Ras protein in a malignant pheochromocytoma (patient no. 5). The protein is localized in inner cytoplasmic membranes or inside cytoplasms of cells (400X).

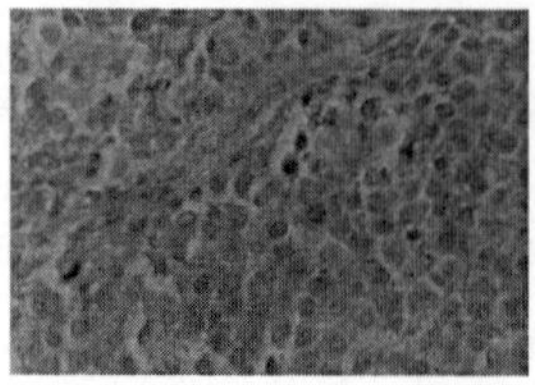

Figure 3. Immunohistochemistry showing moderate expression of c-Myc protein in a malignant pheochromocytoma (patient no. 5). The protein is localized in nuclei or inside cytoplasms of cells (400X).

Table 1. *k-ras* and *c-myc* in phaeochromocytomas. Activating mutations of *k-ras* gene and immunohistochemistry analysis (IHC) of c-Myc and k-Ras products in pheochromocytomas

Patient No.	Tumour	k-ras mutation	k- ras ekspression	c-myc expression
1	Benign pheochromocytoma	+	++	++
2	Benign pheochromocytoma	+	+	+
3	Benign pheochromocytoma	-	++	+++
4	Benign pheochromocytoma	+	+	+++
5*	Malignant pheochromocytoma	+	++	++
6	Benign pheochromocytoma	+	+	+++
7	Benign pheochromocytoma	+	+	++
8	Benign pheochromocytoma	+	++	+++
9*	Malignant pheochromocytoma	+	++	+++
9**	Lymph node metastasis	+	++	+++
10	Benign pheochromocytoma	ND	++	++
11	Benign pheochromocytoma	ND	++	++
12	Benign pheochromocytoma	ND	+	+++

adrenal gland IHC for both proteins = +

+ = normal expression, ++ = moderate expression, +++ = strong expression; *malignant; **metastasis from malignant case; ND = not determined.

Discussion

Many human tumors express high levels of Myc protein. This nuclear protein modulates the expression of many target genes. Although it has been shown that oncogenic activation of *c-myc* alone has the consequence of uncontrolled proliferation, it seems that for full cellular transformation *c-myc* requires additional oncogenic partners. Myc protein acts as transcription factor when coupled with protein Max. Max has a constant cellular expression. It can couple with Myc and promote transcription of specific target genes, but can also couple with protein Mad, and than those coupled molecules will form a transcription repressor [31]. In short - controlling the levels of Myc is very important for proper cellular function.

Genetic alterations underlying tumorigenesis have been described so far for only a limited number of neuroendocrine tumors. Moreover, it seems that sporadic tumors and those syndrome-associated are governed by different genetic events. Further susceptibility genes remain to be identified. Structural changes in *k-ras* gene found in their investigated pheochromocytoma sample indicate that Ras-Raf-Mek-Erk pathway may have a role in pheochromocytoma development.

The data presented in this study demonstrate that high percent of pheochromocytomas contained an activating point mutation in codon 12 of the *k-ras* gene. In their previous work mutations in *k-ras* were also identified in malignant and benign insulinomas [35, 36]. The number of neuroendocrine tumor cases investigated in these papers is rather small and even in the light of new results on pheochromocytoma does not permit to conclude whether the mutations are directed to benign or malignant cases.

Reports in the literature on *ras* involvement in pheochromocytomsa are contradictory. There are data published by several authors [37, 38] who found no evidence for *ras* mutations in primary human pheochromocytomas. On the other hand, novel reports [25, 39] indicate that activation of Ras favors pheochromocytoma formation.

Next, we demonstrated that *k-ras* changes at the genetic level have consequences at the protein level in their sporadic pheochromocytoma samples. k-Ras protein expression was moderately upregulated in 61.5% of cases of which 55.6% of samples harbored activating *k-ras* mutation. Strong expression of k-Ras proteins was not observed. This was not the case with the expression of c-Myc where strong upregulation was observed in 53.8% of cases. It seemed that activating mutations of *k-ras* have stronger impact on protein levels of c-Myc than on the expression of k-Ras. Increased levels of Myc protein were shown in 92.3% of their total sample investigated.

The increased levels of Myc protein expression in pheochromocytoma as compared to normal adrenal tissue was an interesting finding, and consistent with the results of other authors. Goto *et al.* [40] found the expression of *c-fos* and *c-myc* transcripts in pheochromocytoma to be constitutive. Since benign pheochromocytomas are characterized by cells with near absence of mitoses, their results on high Myc levels might indicate the appearance of proliferative signals that precede malignant phenotype. The only sample that did not show increased c-Myc expression in comparison to normal adrenal tissue (patient no. 2) harbored a point mutation in the *ret* oncogene [36]. This suggests that another carcinogenic pathway might be targeted in this sample.

We have to consider the possibility of Myc-Ras cross-talk in their pheochromocytoma samples and reflect on the impact their results could have on differentiation in pheochromocytoma cells. It has been shown that Ras enhances the accumulation of Myc activity by stabilizing the Myc protein. Sears et al, 1999 [31] proposed that the collaboration of Myc-Ras results in ability of Ras to enhance the accumulation of transcriptionally active Myc protein. Although when acting alone both Myc and Ras are insufficient for cellular transformation, their co-expression initiates multiple cell stimulatory activities, induces S phase and gains ability to transform cells. Constitutive overexpression of Myc proteins in cultured cells and in transgenic animals has been shown to block differentiation and induces neoplastic transformation [41, 42]. The mechanisms through which Myc inhibits differentiation are unclear. Nevertheless, it has been suggested that it is done by stimulating cell cycle progression based on the fact that terminal differentiation is often accompanied with cell cycle arrest.

Several reports [43-45] indicate that Ras can induce differentiation of pheochromocytoma cells. It has also been shown in other reports that the most common response to Ras ectopic expression in cell lines is their differentiation. Although there are numerous studies on *myc - ras* oncogene cooperation in cellular transformation [31, 46], their cooperative role in differentiation mechanisms are rarely studied. One of the papers that corrected this injustice is a very interesting paper by Vaqué et al, 2008 [32]. The authors demonstrated that the expression of c-Myc inhibits Ras mediated differentiation in PC 12 pheochromocytoma derived cells. In response to nerve growth factor, PC 12 cells differentiate into a sympathetic neuron-like phenotype. Nerve growth factor activates Ras and the consecutive differentiation is dependent on the activation of Ras-Erk pathway. Myc, on the other hand, impaired the neuronal-like differentiation induced by Ras through mechanism involving the repression of c-Jun. The authors showed that Myc can inhibit he activation of the differentiation program that is activated by Ras in these cells.

Since the majority of the pheochromocytoma samples investigated in their study were benign and well-differentiated, as is typical with this tumor type, it is possible that their findings on high levels of Myc expression suggest that Myc antagonizes Ras –mediated differentiation. Maintaining high levels of Myc protein may be a prerequisite for block of differentiation and consequent pheochromocytoma progression.

Finally, one must not rule out the additional genetic and epigenetic events that might have happened in their samples. Their previous work detected microsatellite genetic instabilities in pheochromocytoma indicating that mismatch repair may be targeted in pheochromocytoma [47, 48].

Evidence of involvement of different signaling pathways that have the same physiological consequences are very important for understanding the development of pheochromocytoma.

Future Perspectives

It is obvious that *myc* and *ras* are relevant targets for studying molecular changes in pheochromocytoma. The question weather Myc-Ras cross-talk in their pheochromocytoma samples reflect on the differentiation in pheochromocytoma cells and have a role in pheochromocytoma development and progression is also very tempting and should be considered for future work.

It would be interesting to explain molecular mechanisms responsible for collaborative effects of Myc-Ras in pheochromocytoma that are still very much unknown. Future studies need to confirm the functional changes of Myc-Ras molecular interplay by analyzing their mRNA levels.

Further investigation regarding those molecules on a bigger sample should also be performed in order to confirm their suggestions. In future studies it would also be relevant to obtain data on the expression of other Ras-Raf-Mek-Erk pathway components and the role they may have in pheochromocytoma development.

ACKNOWLEDGMENTS

This work was supported by grants 108-1081870-1905 and 058-0582261-2246 from Ministry of Science Sports and Education, Republic of Croatia.

REFERENCES

[1] Koch, CA; Vortmeyer, AO; Huang, SC; Alesci, S; Zhuang, Z; Pacak, K. Genetic aspects of pheochromocytoma. *Endocr Regul*, 2001, 35, 43-45.

[2] Nakao, K; Itoh, H; Takaya, K. Current topics in pheochromocytoma. *Biomed Pharmacother*, 2000, 54, 124-128.

[3] Maher, ER; Eng, C. The pressure rises: update on the genetics of pheochromocytoma. *Hum Mol Genet*, 2002, 11, 2347-2354.

[4] Dannenberg, H; Komminoth, P; Dinjens, WN; Speel, EJ; de Krijger, RR. Molecular genetic alterations in adrenal and extra-adrenal pheochromocytomas and paragangliomas. *Endocr Pathol*, 2003, 14, 329-350.

[5] Gimm, O; Koch, CA; Januszewicz, A; Opocher, G; Neumann, HP. The genetic basis of pheochromocytoma. *Front Horm Res*, 2004, 31, 45-60.

[6] Ohta, S; Lai, EW; Pang, ALY; Brouwers, FM; Chan, WY; Eisenhofer, G; *et al.* Downregulation of metastasis suppressor genes in malignant pheochromocytoma. *Int J Cancer* 2005, 114, 139-143.

[7] Karagiannis, A; Mikhailidis, DP; Athyros, VG; Harsoulis, F. Pheochromocytoma: an update on genetics and management. *Endocr Relat Cancer*, 2007, 14, 935-956.

[8] Aguiar, RCT; Cox, G; Pomeroy, SL; Dahia, PLM. Analysis of the SDHD gene, the susceptibility gene for familial paraganglioma syndrome (PGL1), in pheochromocytomas. *J Clin Endocrinol Metab*, 2001, 86, 2890-2894.

[9] Astuti, D; Morris, M; Krona, C; Abel, F; Gentle, D; Martinsson, T; *et al.* Investigation of the role of SDHB inactivation in sporadic pheochromocytoma and neuroblastoma. *Br J Cancer*, 2004, 91, 1835-1841.

[10] Pawlu, C; Bausch, B; Neumann, HP. Mutations of the SDHB and SDHD genes. *Fam Cancer*, 2005, 4, 49-54.

[11] Dahia, PL. Evolving concepts in pheochromocytoma and paraganglioma. *Curr Opin Oncol*, 2006, 18, 1-8.

[12] Tischler, AS. Molecular and cellular biology of pheochromocytomas and extra-adrenal paragangliomas. *Endocr Patho*, 2006, 17 321-328.

[13] Eng, C; Crossey, PA; Mulligan, LM; Healey, CS; Houghton, C; Prowse, A; *et al.* Mutations in the RET proto-oncogene and the von Hippel-Lindau disease tumor suppressor gene in sporadic and syndromic pheochromocytomas. *J Med Genet*, 1995, 32, 934-937.

[14] Friedrich, CA. Genotype-phenotype correlation in von Hippel-Lindau syndrome. *Hum Mol Genet*, 2001, 10, 763-767.

[15] Neumann, HP; Hoegerle, S; Manz, T; Brenner, K; Iliopoulos, O. How many pathways to pheochromocytoma. *Semin Nephrol*, 2002, 22, 89-99.

[16] Xu, W; Mulligan, LM; Ponder, MA; Liu, L; Smith, BA; Mathew, CG; *et al.* Loss of NF1 alleles in pheochromocytomas from patients with type I neurofibromatosis. *Genes Chromosomes Cancer*, 1992, 4, 337-342.

[17] Gutmann, DH; Geist, RT; Rose, K; Wallin, G; Moley, JF. Loss of neurofibromatosis type 1 (NF1) gene expression in pheochromocytomas from patients without NF1. *Genes Chromosomes Cancer*, 1995, 13, 104-109.

[18] Bausch, B; Borozdin, W; Mautner, VF; Hoffmann, MM; Boehm, D; Robledo, M; *et al.* Germline *NF1* mutational spectra and loss of heterozygosity analyses in patients with pheochromocytoma and neurofibromatosis type 1. *J Clin Endocrinol Metab*, 2007, 92, 2784-2792.

[19] Le Hir, H; Colucci-D'Amato, LG; Charlet-Berguerand, N; Plouin, PF; Bertagna, X; de Franciscis, V; *et al.* High levels of tyrosine phosphorylated proto-Ret in sporadic pheochromocytomas. *Cancer Res*, 2000, 60, 1365-1370.

[20] Brauch, H; Hoeppner, W; Jähnig, H; Wöhl, T; Engelhardt, D; Spelsberg, F; *et al.* Sporadic pheochromocytomas are rarely associated with germline mutations in the vhl tumor suppressor gene or the ret protooncogene. *J Clin Endocrinol Metab*, 1997, 82, 4101-4104.

[21] Bender, BU; Gutsche, M; Gläsker, S; Müller, B; Kirste, G; Eng, C; *et al.* Differential genetic alterations in von Hippel-Lindau syndrome-associated and sporadic pheochromocytomas. *J Clin Endocrinol Metab*, 2000, 85, 4568-4574.

[22] Bos, JL. Ras oncogenes in human cancer: a review, *Cancer Res* 1989, 49, 4682-4689.

[23] Denayer, E; de Ravel, Th; Legius, E. Clinical and molecular aspects of RAS related disorders. *J Med Genet*, 2008, 45, 695-703.

[24] Ghaneh, P; Costello, E; Neoptolemos, JP. Biology and management of pancreatic cancer. *Gut*, 2007, 56, 1134-1152.

[25] Geli, J; Kiss, N; Lanner, F; Foukakis, T; Natalishvili, N; Larsson, O; *et al.* The Ras effectors NORE1A and RASSF1A are frequently inactivated in pheochromocytoma and abdominal paraganglioma. *Endocr Relat Cancer*, 2007, 14, 125-134.

[26] Martin, GA; Viskochil, D; Bollag, G; McCabe, PC; Crosier, WJ; Haubruck, M; *et al.* The GAP-related domain of the neurofibromatosis type 1 gene product interacts with Ras p21. *Cell,* 1990, 63, 843-849.

[27] Pelengaris, S; Khan, M. The many faces of c-MYC. *Arch Biochem Biophys*, 2003, 416, 129-136.

[28] Herold, S; Herkert, B; Eilers, M. Facilitating replication under stress: an oncogenic function of MYC? *Nat Rev Cancer*, 2009, 9, 441-444.

[29] Poljak, LJ; Pećina, N; DŽubur, A; Užarević, B; Vitale, B; Pavelić, K. Modulation of p62 *c-myc* expression in a single case of non-T acute lymphoblastic leukemia (ALL) assessed by image analyser. *Tumordiagn. u. Ther*, 1993, 14, 158-162.

[30] Land, H; Parada, LF; Weinberg, RA. Tumorigenic conversion of primary embryo fibroblasts requires at least two cooperating oncogenes. *Nature*, 1983, 304, 596-602.

[31] Sears, R; Leone, G; DeGregori, J; Nevins, JR. Ras enhances Myc protein stability. *Mol Cell*, 1999, 3, 169-179.

[32] Vaqué, JP; Fernández-García, B; García-Sanz, P; Ferrandiz, N; Bretones, G; Calvo, F; *et al.* c-Myc inhibits Ras-mediated differentiation of pheochromocytoma cells by blocking c-Jun up-regulation. *J Mol Cancer Res*, 2008, 6, 325-339.

[33] Cawkwell, L; Quirke, P. Direct multiplex amplification of DNA from a formalin fixed, paraffin wax embedded tissue section. *Mol Pathol*, 2000, 53, 51-52.

[34] Levi, S; Urbano-Ispizua, A; Gill, R; Thomas, DM; Gilbertson, J; Foster, C; *et al.* Multiple *K-ras* codon 12 mutations in cholangiocarcinomas demonstrated with a sensitive polymerase chain reaction technique. *Cancer Res*, 1991, 51, 497-3502.

[35] Pavelić, K; Hrašćan, R; Kapitanović, S; Karapandža, N; Vraneš, Z; Belicza, M; *et al.* Multiple genetic alterations in malignant metastatic insulinomas. *J Pathol*, 1995, 177, 395-400.

[36] Hrašćan, R; Pećina-Šlaus, N; Nikuševa Martić, T; Franekić Čolić, J; Gall-Trošelj, K; Pavelić, K; *et al.* Analysis of selected genes in neuroendocrine tumours: insulinomas and pheochromocytomas. *J Neuroendocrinol*, 2008, 20, 1015-1022.

[37] Moley, JF; Brother, MB; Wells, SA; Spengler, BA; Biedler, JL; Brodeur, GM. Low frequency of *ras* gene mutations in neuroblastomas, pheochromocytomas, and medullary thyroid cancers. *Cancer Res*, 1991, 51, 1596-1599.

[38] Moul, JW; Bishoff, JT; Theune, SM; Chang, EH. Absent *ras* gene mutations in human adrenal cortical neoplasms and pheochromocytomas. *J Urol*, 1993, 149, 1389-1394.

[39] Mannelli, M; Simi, L; Gaglianò, MS; Opocher, G; Ercolino, T; Becherini, L; *et al.* Genetics and biology of pheochromocytoma. *Exp Clin Endocrinol Diabetes*, 2007, 115, 160-165.

[40] Goto, K; Ogo, A; Yanase, T; Haji, M; Ohashi M; Nawata, H. Expression of c-fos and c-myc proto-oncogenes in human adrenal pheochromocytomas. *J Clin Endocrinol Metab*, 1990, 70, 353-357.

[41] Compere, SJ; Baldacci, P; Sharpe, AH; Thompson, T; Land, H; Jaenisch, R. The ras and myc oncogenes cooperate in tumor induction in many tissues when introduced into midgestation mouse embryos by retroviral vectors. *Proc Natl Acad Sci U S A*, 1989, 86, 2224-2228.

[42] Sinn, E; Muller, W; Pattengale, P; Tepler, I; Wallace, R; Leder, P. Coexpression of MMTV/v-Ha-ras and MMTV/c-myc genes in transgenic mice: synergistic action of oncogenes in vivo. *Cell*, 1987, 49, 465-475.

[43] Bar-Sagi, D; Feramisco, JR. Microinjection of the ras oncogene protein into PC12 cells induces morphological differentiation. *Cell*, 1985, 42, 841-848.

[44] Noda, M; Ko, M; Ogura, A; Liu, DG; Amano, T; Takano, T, *et al.* Sarcoma viruses carrying ras oncogenes induce differentiation-associated properties in a neuronal cell line. *Nature,* 1985, 318, 73-75.

[45] Guerrero, I; Wong, H; Pellicer, A; Burstein, DE. Activated N-ras gene induces neuronal differentiation of PC12 rat pheochromocytoma cells. *J Cell Physiol*, 1986, 129, 71-76.

[46] Leone, G; DeGregori, J; Sears, R; Jakoi, L; Nevins, JR. Myc and Ras collaborate in inducing accumulation of active cyclin E/Cdk2 and E2F. *Nature*, 1997 , 387, 422-426.

[47] Pećina-Šlaus, N; Nikuševa-Martić, T; Gall-Trošelj, K; Radić, K; Hrašćan, R. Replication error-positive samples found in pheochromocytomas. *In Vivo*, 2005, 19, 359-365.

[48] Blanes, A; Sanchez-Carrillo, JJ; Diaz-Cano, SJ. Topographic molecular profile of pheochromocytomas: role of somatic down-regulation of mismatch repair. *J Clin Endocrinol Metab*, 2006, 91, 1150-1158.

In: Neuroendocrinology Research Developments
Editor: N. S. Penkava and L.R. Haight, pp. 93-104
ISBN: 978-1-60876-983-4
© 2010 Nova Science Publishers, Inc.

Chapter 5

Brain Sex Differentiation – Are Sex Hormones the Only Answer?

Gregor Majdic[*]
Center for Animal Genomics, Veterinary Faculty, University of Ljubljana,
Gerbiceva 60, 1000 Ljubljana, Slovenia

Abstract

Mammalian sex determination is dependent on a proper function of small gene on the smallest chromosome – Sry. Sry triggers the development of tesis in the male, and subsequently, hormonal secretions by the fetal testis are responsible for the proper development of male sexual organs, while in female, sexual development takes place in the absence of any hormonal exposure. Similar mechanisms of hormonal sex differentiation have been proposed for the development of sex differences in the mammalian brain with one important difference. While testosterone (and its derivative dihydrotestosterone) is the main steroid hormone responsible for the proper development of secondary sexual organs, brain sexual differentiation (at least in rodents) towards male depends on the conversion of testosterone to estradiol by cytochrome P450 aromatase, expressed locally in the brain. However, several studies in recent years have suggested that not all sex differences in the brain are dependent on the exposure to sex steroid hormones. Probably still the most compelling evidence came from birds, more specifically from gynandromorphic zebra finch, described by Arnold and co-workers in 2003. This bird, half male, half female, is showing characteristics of one sex on one side of the body and characteristics of the other sex on the other side of the body. And this does not go only for a plumage, but also for the expression of genes in the brain, where expression of female specific transcripts was detected only in the female half of the brain and expression of male specific transcripts in the male part of the brain. In this case, such differences in gene expression certainly cannot be explained by the action of hormones, as hormones are transported by blood and cannot reach only half of the brain. Therefore, there must be other causes for brain sexual differentiation (and perhaps other organ systems) beside sex steroid hormones. To study hormone independent sex differences in

[*] Corresponding author: Email: gregor.majdic @vf.uni-lj.si

mammals, two mice models have been recently developed. Four core genotype (FCG) mice are mice with manipulated Sry gene where genetic sex is not the same as gonadal sex (XY females, XX males). Another valuable model is SF-1 knockout mice, in which gonads regress very early during development, before gonads start to secrete steroid hormones. These mice are therefore never exposed to any endogenous sex steroids and therefore represent a unique model to study sex differences that must develop due to differences in sex chromosome complements.

In the present review, recent results obtained by studies using mostly these two mice models, will be described along with other evidence for sex differences in the brain that develop in the absence of hormone exposure.

INTRODUCTION

Men and women differ. We all know that. Just by looking at the crowd of humans we can spot obvious differences between males and females. Males are usually larger, have hoarser voice, facial hair and more muscular body while females have breasts, lack facial hair and have usually so called feminine body with narrow waist and broader hips and chest. Of course, males and females also differ in appearance of their external and internal sexual organs. But do the differences end here? According to many studies we can now confidently say no. There are many other differences beside differences connected with sexual reproduction. Studies in recent years and decades have demonstrated differences in such diverse biological phenomena as wound healing (Gilliver, S. C. et al. 2008), drug detoxication in liver (Clodfelter, K. H. et al. 2006), and perhaps most importantly, differences in the brain, which are no longer considered to be a myth but are believed to be present, are important for explaining many physiological and patophysiological processes occurring in their bodies .(Diamond, M. 2009) From clinical point of view it is very important to bear in mind that many different diseases show different prevalence between sexes, and these disparities could not be explained only by differences in lifestyle (idea that has been supported by some in the case of lung cancer). Many psychiatric disorders also show sex bias. For example, major depressive disorder, anxiety and eating disorders are much more prevalent in women, while schizophrenia, autism and attention deficit disorder are diagnosed more often in men (Davies, W. and Wilkinson, L. S. 2006). Because of these clinical implications, studies of sex differences are not only of academic interest, but have important implications for clinical practice, which will, undoubtedly, became even more important in future years with the development of pharmacogenomics.

MAMMALIAN SEXUAL DIFFERENTIATION

In most animals (and even plants) two sexes exist. Nobody has yet come with conclusive answer why sexual reproduction, although it is mostly believed and accepted that sexual reproduction offers an easy way to gene variation, which consequently helps surviving species in hostile environment by easier adaptation to environmental challenges. Somewhat surprisingly, different groups of animals developed very different strategies for sexual differentiation. Most insects determine sex by the number of sex chromosomes, reptiles by the environmental temperature during embryonic development while birds and mammals posses two sex chromosomes that determine development of male or female sex (Manolakou, P. et al. 2006). However, there is an important difference as in birds, males are homozygous for sex chromosomes (ZZ) and females are heterozygouts (ZW) (Smith, C. A. 2007) while in mammals, females are homozygous with two X chromosomes and males heterozygous with XY chromosomes. In mammals, Y chromosome is by far the smallest of all chromosomes. It poses an SRY gene, which is both sufficient and necessary for development of male phenotype. SRY gene, first cloned in 1991 is small gene belonging to the group of high mobility group of proteins. Different studies have demonstrated that SRY alone is sufficient to trigger testis development (Berta, P. et al. 1990; Koopman, P. et al. 1991). Once testis is formed, hormones secreted from the testis govern subsequent development of male phenotype with antimullerian hormone (AMH/ MIS) being responsible for regression of female reproductive organs and steroid hormone testosterone being responsible for development of male secondary sexual organs. In females, ovaries remain relatively inactive until after birth and female secondary sexual organs develop in the absence of any hormonal exposure, what was clearly demonstrated by different clinical cases as well as in animal studies where even in complete absence of gonads (either ovary or testis) female secondary reproductive organs develop (Gilbert, S. F. 1994).

Reproductive development could be divided into two phases. Initial phase occurs during development in utero and comprises of gonadal differentiation and development of secondary sexual organs (penis, scrotum, accessory glands in males and clitoris, vagina, uterus and oviduct in females). This phase is followed by quiescent period during childhood. During puberty, second phase of sexual development occurs with hormones secreted from gonads (this time both from ovaries and testes) triggering sexual maturation and appearance of secondary sexual characteristics such as breasts and wide hips in females, facial hair, muscular body and hoarse voice in males. In addition, several recent studies have also shown that sexual hormones also influence brain development and that several changes occur in the brain during puberty due to exposure to large amount of sex steroid hormones (Schulz, K. M. et al. 2009).

SEXUAL DIFFERENTIATION OF THE BRAIN

Brain is central processing unit of their organism. Brain thus control and govern all processes in the living organism including reproduction. Therefore, it is not surprisingly or unexpectedly to know that sex differences exist also in the mammalian brain. This has been known for many decades with most differences being described in parts of limbic system, mostly in the hypothalamus and preoptic area, two areas closely connected with the function of the reproductive system (Becker, J. B. et al. 2007). The classical view of brain sexual differentiation is built around the dogma that hormones secreted by gonads are solely responsible for differences in the brain between sexes. This hypothesis originated in 1959 when Phoenix, Goy, Gerall and Young published now classical study showing that prenatal administration of testosterone to female guinea pigs induced masculinized behavior in adult female guinea pigs (Phoenix, C. H. et al. 1959). The importance of sex steroid hormones for differences in sexual behavior was acknowledged prior to this publication, although before

1959 it was believed that all actions of sex steroids are activational effects and not organizational. Study by Phoenix et al. (Phoenix, C. H. et al. 1959) therefore for the first time showed that prenatal exposure to sex steroid testosterone could permanently alter brain function. Female guinea pigs that were given testosterone prenataly displayed masculinized behavior as adults, long after testosterone treatment, what could only resulted from permanent effect of testosterone on developing brain. Study by Phoenix et al. of course did not provide all important answers such as which hormone at what time and in what part of the brain is responsible for the sexual differentiation of the brain. Nevertheless, this study was of outmost importance as the first study showing that hormones could permanently alter brain structure and function. In the fifty years after this discovery, many questions about organizational effects of sex steroid hormones have been answered. We now know that at least in rodent brains, estradiol and not testosterone is responsible for the masculinization of the brain. Testosterone, secreted from the testes in male fetuses is transported into the brain, where it is converted into estradiol by cytochrome P450 aromatase, locally expressed in different parts of the brain (Harada, N. 1993; Lephart, E. D. 1996). While female fetuses are not exposed to testosterone from their gonads, they are still exposed to estradiol from their mothers. To prevent masculinization of the female brain, large amounts of alpha-fetoprotein are present in the blood of female fetuses, which could bind estradiol and thus preventing it from entering into the brain (Bakker, J. et al. 2006). Studies in last decades have also indentified many areas of the brain that are altered during development due to exposure to sex steroids, not only areas closely connected with reproduction, but also in the areas important for emotional responses such as amygdala and even other areas such as hippocampus and cerebellum (McCarthy, M. M. and Konkle, A. T. 2005; Galea, L. A. et al. 2006; Cooke, B. M. et al. 2007; Dean, S. L. and McCarthy, M. M. 2008). One of the best known and studied examples is sexually dimorphic nucleus in the preoptic area (SDN), first identified by Gorski et colleagues in the late 70-ties (Gorski, R. A. et al. 1980). This nucleus is larger in males than in females and is believed to be important for male sexual behavior although its precise role is not yet known. SDN has been identified in different species such as sheep (Roselli, C. E. et al. 2004), macaque (Vasey, P. L. and Pfaus, J. G. 2005) and even humans (Swaab, D. F. et al. 1992; Swaab, D. F. et al. 1995). Formation of SDN is dependent on the neonatal exposure to sex steroids as shown by many different studies (Jacobson, C. D. et al. 1981; Dohler, K. D. et al. 1984; Roselli, C. E. et al. 2007) including their own recent study in SF-1 knockout mice (Budefeld, T. et al. 2008). Two other areas in the mammalian brain that are sexually dimorphic are ventromedial hypothalamic nucleus and bed nucleus of stria terminals (Matsumoto, A. and Arai, Y. 1983; al-Shamma, H. A. and De Vries, G. J. 1996; Dugger, B. N. et al. 2007). Both areas are involved in the regulation of sexual behavior and it is thus not surprisingly that these two areas are different in males and females. Perhaps more interesting are reports about sex differences in cerebellum and hippocampus (McCarthy, M. M. and Konkle, A. T. 2005; Galea, L. A. et al. 2006; Dean, S. L. and McCarthy, M. M. 2008). These two areas are not involved in the regulation of reproductive behavior, nevertheless, several studies have shown that sexual dimorphism exist also in hippocampus and cerebellum. Considering the function of these two areas, it is less surprisingly to find sex differences in morphology and gene expression. Hippocampus is considered to be involved in memory and spatial orientation, and spatial orientation in humans is now considered to be one of the important sexually dimorphic traits (Manson, J. E. 2008). As for cerebellum, several different human diseases such as autism and attention deficit disorder that show strong sexual dimorphism are thought to originate from the dysfunction of cerebellum (Dean, S. L. and McCarthy, M. M. 2008). Therefore, it is not surprisingly to find sex differences also in these two areas.

Do Sex Chromosomes Affect Sexual Differentiation of the Brain?

Many studies in the last 50 years since the publication of the paper by Phoenix et al. (Phoenix, C. H. et al. 1959) have shown the importance of sex steroid hormones for brain sexual differentiation. It is now clearly established that sex steroids have important role in brain development in different periods, not only prenataly but also postnatally, during puberty and even in adult life in both animals and humans. However, there was always a question lurking in the dark whether all sex differences in the brain could be explained by one unifying theory about organizational effects of sex steroids. The idea that sex chromosomes could also play a role in brain sexual differentiation was for sometime sidelined because some studies have shown that normal XX females could be completely masculinized (for some phenotypes) if treated with testosterone at appropriate time periods, and likewise, normal XY males could be completely feminized for some phenotypes if fetal testosterone production or action is blocked (Dohler, K. D. et al. 1984; Nordeen, E. J. et al. 1985). However, in the early nineties, several studies suggested that sex steroid hormones might not be the whole answer to sexual differentiation (Reisert, I. et al. 1989; Kolbinger, W. et al. 1991; Reisert, I. and Pilgrim, C. 1991; Beyer, C. et al. 1992). In the last decade, several studies indeed provided evidence for hormone independent brain sexual differentiation. One of the most compelling pieces of evidence came from the laboratory of Art Arnold where they discovered so called gynandomorphic zebrafinch, a bird that is half male and half female, precisely divided through the midline of the body (Agate, R. J. et al. 2003). Not only was plumage of this bird on one side showing male pattern and on the other female pattern, but brain gene expression showed peculiar pattern with female specific genes being expressed only in one side of the brain and male specific genes on the other side. This clearly could not have been the consequence of hormone action as hormones, transported by blood, could not reach only one half of the body.

Mammalian Models for Studying Hormone Independent Brain Sexual Differentiation

Several approaches have been used to study sex differences in the brain that develop in the absence of hormone exposure. One approach is to study fetal brain development early during development, before gonads develop and start to produce sex steroid hormones. This approach was used in several studies and has provided evidence that some sex differences do occur very early during development, before fetuses are exposed to endogenous sex steroid hormones. Study by Kolbinger et al. (Kolbinger, W. et al. 1991) demonstrated sex differences in dopaminergic neurons in rat fetuses already on day 14.5 p.c. while genomic study by

Dewing et al. (Dewing, P. et al. 2003) identified over 50 genes whose expression differed between male and female mouse brain on day 10.5 p.c., well before gonads start to produce sex steroids. However, of real importance would be studies that would demonstrate hormone independent sex differences in adult animals, either in brain morphology or behavior. To achieve this goal, two different models, each with advantages and disadvantages, have been developed.

Four Core Genotype Mice

A very useful model for studying genetic differences between sexes is so called four core genotype (FCG) mice model. In these mice, *sry* gene has been manipulated (translocated or mutated) to produce normal XY males, normal XX females, XX males (*sry* gene translocated to autosome) and XY females (*sry* gene mutated) (De Vries, G. J. et al. 2002). In the XY females and XX males genetic sex does not correspond with phenotypic sex and therefore, relative contribution of sex chromosomes and sex hormones could be studied. This is the most studied model for hormone independent brain sexual differentiation so far, and several studies have shown some differences that could not be attributed to sex hormones but must arise due to differences in sex chromosomes. Initial studies with FCG mice did not reveal any differences that could be attributed to the effect of sex chromosomes for different parameters such as male sexual behavior, cell numbers in hypothalamic anteroventral periventricular nucleus (AVPV), the size of the spinal nucleus of the bulbocavernosus (SNB), cortical thickness and progesterone receptor expression in the preoptic area (POA) (Markham, J. A. et al. 2003; Wagner, C. K. et al. 2004). These studies therefore confirmed classical organizational-activational-hypothesis of brain sexual differentiation. However, arginin vasopressin (AVP) immunoexpression in the lateral septum (LS), which is also known to be sexually dimorphic, differed between XY and XX mice of same phenotypic sex suggesting that this difference is partially dependent on sex chromosomes (De Vries, G. J. et al. 2002; Gatewood, J. D. et al. 2006). Further studies revealed even stronger evidence that sex chromosomes do account for some sex differences between male and female mice. When mesencephalic cells were dissociated from 14.5 days old mouse embryos and cultured, more dopamine producing cells (I.E. tyrosin hydroxlase expressing cells) developed in cultures from XY embryos than in those from XX embryos (Carruth, L. L. et al. 2002), what confirmed the results from previous studies (Reisert, I. et al. 1989; Kolbinger, W. et al. 1991). Adult FCG mice were also tested for male to male aggressive behavior (after testosterone treatment of adult gonadectomized mice) and XY females were more aggressive than XX females while there was no difference between XY and XX males (Gatewood, J. D. et al. 2006). Furthermore, there were differences in nociception, parental behavior and habit formation that could not be attributed to sex hormones but have to be consequences of sex chromosomes (Quinn, J. J. et al. 2007; Gioiosa, L. et al. 2008; Gioiosa, L. et al. 2008; McPhie-Lalmansingh, A. A. et al. 2008). Perhaps most interestingly, FCG mouse model was also applied to studies of incidence and progression of autoimmune diseases, a very important issue as most autoimmune diseases in humans including multiple sclerosis and systemic lupus erhytematosus have a strong sex difference in prevalence. XX mice showed much stronger autoimmune responses than XY mice and although organizational/activational effect of sex steroid hormones do account to some extent for observed sex differences, a study by Smith-Bouvier et al. (Smith-Bouvier, D. L. et al. 2008) strongly suggest that sex chromosomes also play an important role in development of the differences between sexes in incidence and progression of autoimmune diseases.

Steroidogenic Factor 1 Knockout Mice

Steroidogenic factor 1 (SF-1) was initially discovered as a transcription factor regulating expression of different steroidogenic enzymes (Parker, K. L. and Schimmer, B. P. 1997). Further studies, however, revealed it's much wider role in the development and function of endocrine system as SF-1 knockout mice are born without gonads and adrenal glands, have disorganized ventromedial hypothalamic nucleus and unfunctional gonadotrope cells in the pituitary (Luo, X. et al. 1994; Ikeda, Y. et al. 1995). In SF-1 knockout mouse embryos, genital ridges form normally on day 10.5 p.c. (Luo, X. et al. 1994). However, almost immediately after formation of genital ridges, cells became apoptotic and by day 12.5 p.c., genital ridges completely disappear. As steroidogenesis in the fetal mouse testis starts only after day 12.5 p.c., these mice are never exposed to any endogenous sex steroid hormones. SF-1 knockout mice are born completely sex reversed; both XX and XY pups show female phenotype. Since SF-1 knockout mice are never exposed to any sex steroid hormones, they are another very useful model to study hormone independent development of sex differences in the brain. SF-1 knockout model differ from FCG model in one very important way: FCG mice develop gonads independently from chromosomal sex and are thus still exposed to sex steroid hormones during neonatal and pubertal development, even though secreted hormones do not correspond to their chromosomal sex. Sex steroid hormones could therefore still influence brain development and could perhaps even mask or overcome some sex differences that would develop in complete absence of hormones. SF-1 knockout mice are, in contrast to FCG mice, never exposed to any endogenous sex steroid hormones and thus provide a unique model allowing searching for sex differences that develop in true hormoneless environment. Initial studies with SF-1 knockout mice, like studies with FCG mice, did not reveal any major differences between sexes. As expected, sexually dimorphic nucleus was not present in either XX or XY SF-1 knockout mice, confirming that prenatal exposure to testosterone is necessary for the development of this nucleus. Immunocytochemical studies did reveal some sex differences present in both WT and SF-1 knockout mice such as number of calbindin immunopositive cells in the ventromedial hypothalamus and neural nitric oxide synthase in the AVPV (Budefeld, T. et al. 2008). However,sex difference in AVP expression in LS was not confirmed, suggesting that other factors and not just sex chromosomes influence expression of AVP in LS. Recent studies with SF-1 knockout mice revealed very interesting observation in female sex behavior. Unlike in rats, WT mice of both sexes are capable of showing female sexual behavior (lordosis) when treated with estradiol and progesterone. In their studies we found that although mice from all four (WT male, WT female, SF-1 knockout male, SF-1 knockout female) groups did show lordosis, there was a large difference in lordosis quotient between WT male and female mice, with, as expected, WT female mice showing much stronger lordotic response when stimulated by a WT stud male. SF-1 knockout mice of both sexes also showed lordosis, although it was not as strong as in WT females, suggesting that developmental exposure to sex steroids is important also for proper development of lordotic behavior in adult mice. However, most interestingly, there was a significant sex difference in lordosis quotient between XX and XY SF-1 knockout mice suggesting that this behavioral trait is at least partially influenced by sex chromosomes. Similarly to FCG mice, small sex differences were also found in parental and some social behaviors between XX and XY SF-1 knockout mice, suggesting the effect of sex chromosomes.

CONCLUSIONS

Differences in the brain between human males and females have always been a controversial issue. From early (unfounded) suggestions that male brains are bigger than female's, the science of brain sexual differentiation has progressed majorly. Many studies in different animal models during the last 50 years have convincingly shown that brains do differ between sexes, and not only in regions connected with the regulation of reproductive physiology and behavior, but also in other areas such as amygdala, hippocampus and cerebellum. Nevertheless, many clinicians have opposed the idea of prenatal sexual development in humans and have strongly supported the view that human babies are born neurologically neutral (Diamond, M. 2009) and that only nurture during infancy is responsible for development of typical male or female behavioral traits. However, during the last decades, accumulating evidence coming also from different human patients have convinced most, if not all, that differences in the human brain do exist, and these differences most likely account for differences in the behavior between men and women. While it is universally accepted that sex steroids during prenatal, postnatal, pubertal development and perhaps even adult life have a major role in the development of sex differences, one important question still remains largely unanswered. Are the sex steroid hormones the only answer to brain sexual differentiation or perhaps, there is also a role for sex chromosomes? Accumulating evidence from expression of testis determining Y chromosome specific gene SRY/Sry in the brain to the results of recent studies by FCG and SF-1 knockout mice is providing more and more convincing answers that sex chromosomes do contribute to the development of sex differences in the brain and behavior. In the years ahead, their knowledge of brain sexual differentiation will grow and undoubtedly, at some point, we will understand how sex hormones and sex chromosomes interplay to cause differences in brain and behavior. Perhaps even more importantly, with new techniques such as functional MRI and PET we are gaining tools to get better insights also into the human brain. We can therefore expect also a major progress in understanding development of sex differences in human brain, to find out whether they follow the same pattern as in animal models (what to some extent undoubtedly do) or what are the specifics of brain sexual differentiation of their own species.

Acknowledgment

Gregor Majdic is supported by grants from NIH TW005922, ARRS (Slovenian research agency) P4-0053 and ICGEB (GM).

REFERENCES

Agate, R. J., Grisham, W., Wade, J., Mann, S., Wingfield, J., Schanen, C., Palotie A. & Arnold, A. P. (2003). "Neural, not gonadal, origin of brain sex differences in a gynandromorphic finch." *Proc Natl Acad Sci U S A, 100(8)*, 4873-8.

al-Shamma, H. A., & De Vries, G. J. (1996). "Neurogenesis of the sexually dimorphic vasopressin cells of the bed nucleus of the stria terminalis and amygdala of rats." *J Neurobiol, 29(1)*, 91-8.

Bakker, J., De Mees, C., Douhard, Q., Balthazart, J., Gabant, P., Szpirer J. & Szpirer, C. (2006). "Alpha-fetoprotein protects the developing female mouse brain from masculinization and defeminization by estrogens." *Nat Neurosci, 9(2)*, 220-6.

Becker, J. B., Berkley, K. J., Geary, N., Hampson, E., Herman, J. P. & Young, E. (2007). *Sex differences in the brain: From Genes to Behavior.* Oxford New York, Oxford university press.

Berta, P., Hawkins, J. R., Sinclair, A. H., Taylor, A., Griffiths, B. L., Goodfellow, P. N. & Fellous, M. (1990). "Genetic evidence equating SRY and the testis-determining factor." *Nature, 348*, 448-450.

Beyer, C., Eusterschulte, B., Pilgrim C. & Reisert, I. (1992). "Sex steroids do not alter sex differences in tyrosine hydroxylase activity of dopaminergic neurons in vitro." *Cell Tissue Res, 270(3)*, 547-52.

Budefeld, T., Grgurevic, N., Tobet, S. A. & Majdic, G. (2008). "Sex differences in brain developing in the presence or absence of gonads." *Dev Neurobiol, 68(7)*, 981-95.

Carruth, L. L., Reisert, I. & Arnold, A. P. (2002). "Sex chromosome genes directly affect brain sexual differentiation." *Nat Neurosci*, 5(10), 933-4.

Clodfelter, K. H., Holloway, M. G., Hodor, P., Park, S. H., Ray, W. J. & Waxman, D. J. (2006). "Sex-dependent liver gene expression is extensive and largely dependent upon signal transducer and activator of transcription 5b (STAT5b): STAT5b-dependent activation of male genes and repression of female genes revealed by microarray analysis." *Mol Endocrinol, 20(6)*, 1333-51.

Cooke, B. M., Stokas, M. R. & Woolley, C. S. (2007). "Morphological sex differences and laterality in the prepubertal medial amygdala." *J Comp Neurol, 501(6)*, 904-15.

Davies, W. & Wilkinson, L. S. (2006). "It is not all hormones: alternative explanations for sexual differentiation of the brain." *Brain Res, 1126(1)*, 36-45.

De Vries, G. J., Rissman, E. F., Simerly, R. B., Yang, L. Y., Scordalakes, E. M., Auger, C. J., Swain, A., Lovell-Badge, R., Burgoyne, P. S., Arnold, A. P. (2002). "A model system for study of sex chromosome effects on sexually dimorphic neural and behavioral traits." *J Neurosci, 22(20)*, 9005-14.

Dean, S. L. & McCarthy, M. M. (2008). "Steroids, sex and the cerebellar cortex: implications for human disease." *Cerebellum, 7(1)*, 38-47.

Dewing, P., Shi, T., Horvath, S. & Vilain, E. (2003). "Sexually dimorphic gene expression in mouse brain precedes gonadal differentiation." *Brain Res Mol Brain Res, 118(1-2)*, 82-90.

Diamond, M. (2009). "Clinical implications of the organizational and activational effects of hormones." *Horm Behav, 55(5)*, 621-32.

Dohler, K. D., Coquelin, A., Davis, F., Hines, M., Shryne, J. E. & Gorski, R. A. (1984). "Pre- and postnatal influence of testosterone propionate and diethylstilbestrol on differentiation of the sexually dimorphic nucleus of the preoptic area in male and female rats." *Brain Res, 302(2),* 291-5.

Dugger, B. N., Morris, J. A., Jordan, C. L. & Breedlove, S. M. (2007). "Androgen receptors are required for full masculinization of the ventromedial hypothalamus (VMH) in rats." *Horm Behav, 51(2)*, 195-201.

Galea, L. A., Spritzer, M. D., Barker, J. M. & Pawluski, J. L. (2006). "Gonadal hormone modulation of hippocampal neurogenesis in the adult." *Hippocampus, 16(3)*, 225-32.

Gatewood, J. D., Wills, A., Shetty, S., Xu, J., Arnold, A. P., Burgoyne P. S. & Rissman, E. F. (2006). "Sex chromosome complement and gonadal sex influence aggressive and parental behaviors in mice." *J Neurosci, 26(8)*, 2335-42.

Gilbert, S. F. (1994). *Developmental Biology.* Subderland, Massachusetts, Sinauer Associates, Inc.

Gilliver, S. C., Ruckshanthi, J. P., Hardman, M. J., Nakayama T. & Ashcroft, G. S. (2008). "Sex dimorphism in wound healing: the roles of sex steroids and macrophage migration inhibitory factor." *Endocrinology, 149(11)*, 5747-57.

Gioiosa, L., Chen, X., Watkins, R., Klanfer, N., Bryant, C. D., Evans, C. J. & Arnold, A. P. (2008). "Sex chromosome complement affects nociception in tests of acute and chronic exposure to morphine in mice." *Horm Behav, 53*(1), 124-30.

Gioiosa, L., Chen, X., Watkins, R., Umeda, E. A. & Arnold, A. P. (2008). "Sex chromosome complement affects nociception and analgesia in newborn mice." *J Pain, 9(10)*, 962-9.

Gorski, R. A., Harlan, R. E., Jacobson, C. D., Shryne, J. E. & Southam, A. M. (1980). "Evidence for the existence of a sexually dimorphic nucleus in the preoptic area of the rat." *J Comp Neurol, 193(2)*, 529-39.

Harada, N. (1993). "[Estrogen synthetase (P-450. aromatase) as a regulatory factor concerning sexual differentiation of brain and sexual behavior--physiological functions and regulation of gene expression of aromatase]." *Seikagaku, 65(2)*, 67-85.

Ikeda, Y., Luo, X., Abbud, R., Nilson, J. H. & Parker, K. L. (1995). "The nuclear receptor steroidogenic factor 1 is essential for the formation of the ventromedial hypothalamic nucleus." *Mol Endocrinol, 9(4)*, 478-86.

Jacobson, C. D., Csernus, V. J., Shryne, J. E. & Gorski, R. A. (1981). "The influence of gonadectomy, androgen exposure, or a gonadal graft in the neonatal rat on the volume of the sexually dimorphic nucleus of the preoptic area." *J Neurosci, 1(10)*, 1142-7.

Kolbinger, W., Trepel, M., Beyer, C., Pilgrim, C. & Reisert, I. (1991). "The influence of genetic sex on sexual differentiation of diencephalic dopaminergic neurons in vitro and in vivo." *Brain Res, 544(2)*, 349-52.

Koopman, P., Gubbay, J., Vivian, N., Goodfellow, P. N. & Lovell-Badge, R. (1991). "Male development of chromosomally female mice transgenic for Sry." *Nature, 351*, 117-121.

Lephart, E. D. (1996). "A review of brain aromatase cytochrome P450." *Brain Res Brain Res Rev, 22(1)*, 1-26.

Luo, X., Ikeda Y. & Parker, K. L. (1994). "A cell-specific nuclear receptor is essential for adrenal and gonadal development and sexual differentiation." *Cell, 77*, 481-490.

Manolakou, P., Lavranos G. & Angelopoulou, R. (2006). "Molecular patterns of sex determination in the animal kingdom: a comparative study of the biology of reproduction." *Reprod Biol Endocrinol, 4*, 59.

Manson, J. E. (2008). "Prenatal exposure to sex steroid hormones and behavioral/cognitive outcomes." *Metabolism, 57* Suppl 2: S16-21.

Markham, J. A., Jurgens, H. A., Auger, C. J., De Vries, G. J., Arnold, A. P. & Juraska, J. M. (2003). "Sex differences in mouse cortical thickness are independent of the complement of sex chromosomes." *Neuroscience, 116(1)*, 71-5.

Matsumoto, A. & Arai, Y. (1983). "Sex difference in volume of the ventromedial nucleus of the hypothalamus in the rat." *Endocrinol Jpn, 30(3)*, 277-80.

McCarthy, M. M. & Konkle, A. T. (2005). "When is a sex difference not a sex difference?" *Front Neuroendocrinol, 26(2)*, 85-102.

McPhie-Lalmansingh, A. A., Tejada, L. D., Weaver, J. L. & Rissman, E. F. (2008). "Sex chromosome complement affects social interactions in mice." *Horm Behav, 54(4)*, 565-70.

Nordeen, E. J., Nordeen, K. W., Sengelaub D. R. & Arnold, A. P. (1985). "Androgens prevent normally occurring cell death in a sexually dimorphic spinal nucleus." *Science, 229(4714)*, 671-3.

Parker, K. L. & Schimmer, B. P. (1997). "Steroidogenic factor 1: a key determinant of endocrine development and function." *Endocr Rev, 18(3)*, 361-77.

Phoenix, C. H., Goy, R. W., Gerall, A. A. & Young, W. C. (1959). "Organizing action of prenatally administered testosterone propionate on the tissues mediating mating behavior in the female guinea pig." *Endocrinology, 65*, 369-82.

Quinn, J. J., Hitchcott, P. K., Umeda, E. A., Arnold, A. P. & Taylor, J. R. (2007). "Sex chromosome complement regulates habit formation." *Nat Neurosci, 10(11)*, 1398-400.

Reisert, I., Engele J. & Pilgrim, C. (1989). "Early sexual differentiation of diencephalic dopaminergic neurons of the rat in vitro." *Cell Tissue Res, 255(2),* 411-7.

Reisert, I. & Pilgrim, C. (1991). "Sexual differentiation of monoaminergic neurons--genetic or epigenetic?" *Trends Neurosci, 14(10)*, 468-73.

Roselli, C. E., Larkin, K., Resko, J. A., Stellflug J. N. & Stormshak, F. (2004). "The volume of a sexually dimorphic nucleus in the ovine medial preoptic area/anterior hypothalamus varies with sexual partner preference." *Endocrinology, 145(2)*, 478-83.

Roselli, C. E., Stadelman, H., Reeve, R., Bishop C. V. & Stormshak, F. (2007). "The ovine sexually dimorphic nucleus of the medial preoptic area is organized prenatally by testosterone." *Endocrinology, 148(9)*, 4450-7.

Schulz, K. M., Molenda-Figueira H. A., & Sisk, C. L. (2009). "Back to the future: The organizational-activational hypothesis adapted to puberty and adolescence." *Horm Behav, 55(5)*, 597-604.

Smith-Bouvier, D. L., Divekar, A. A., Sasidhar, M., Du, S., Tiwari-Woodruff, S. K., King, J. K., Arnold, A. P., Singh, R. R. & Voskuhl, R. R. (2008). "A role for sex chromosome complement in the female bias in autoimmune disease." *J Exp Med, 205(5)*, 1099-108.

Smith, C. A. (2007). "Sex determination in birds: HINTs from the W sex chromosome?" *Sex Dev, 1(5)*, 279-85.

Swaab, D. F., Gooren, L. J. & Hofman, M. A. (1992). "The human hypothalamus in relation to gender and sexual orientation." *Prog Brain Res, 93*, 205-17; discussion 217-9.

Swaab, D. F., Gooren L. J., Hofman, M. A. (1995). "Brain research, gender and sexual orientation." *J Homosex, 28(3-4)*, 283-301.

Vasey, P. L. & Pfaus, J. G. (2005). "A sexually dimorphic hypothalamic nucleus in a macaque species with frequent female-female mounting and same-sex sexual partner preference." *Behav Brain Res*, *157(2)*, 265-72.

Wagner, C. K., Xu, J., Pfau, J. L., Quadros, P. S., De Vries G. J. & Arnold, A. P. (2004). "Neonatal mice possessing an Sry transgene show a masculinized pattern of progesterone receptor expression in the brain independent of sex chromosome status." *Endocrinology, 145(3)*, 1046-9.

In: Neuroendocrinology Research Developments
Editor: N. S. Penkava and L.R. Haight, pp.105-117
ISBN: 978-1-60876-983-4
© 2010 Nova Science Publishers, Inc.

Chapter 6

DEVELOPMENTAL NEUROENDOCRINOLOGY OF POSTTRAUMATIC STRESS DISORDER: THE BIOLOGICAL EFFECTS OF CHILDHOOD STRESS AND TRAUMA

Panagiota Pervanidou*[*] *and George P. Chrousos
Developmental and Behavioral Pediatrics Unit, First Department of Pediatrics, Athens University Medical School, Aghia Sophia Children's Hospital, Athens Greece

ABSTRACT

The Hypothalamic-Pituitary-Adrenal (HPA) axis and the locus caeruleus / norepinephrine-sympathetic nervous system (LC/NE-SNS), are involved in the pathophysiology of Posttraumatic Stress Disorder (PTSD), a clustering of symptoms that develop after exposure to traumatic life events. However, diverse biological patterns of disease have been reported and this can be attributed mainly on comorbidity, biological vulverability (genetic and transgenerational effects) and previous stress history and the developmental stage of the individual.

In pediatric PTSD, elevated peripheral cortisol concentrations are noted in the majority of studies, while low cortisol is the most frequent finding in adult studies. Furthermore, in contrast to adult studies, initially elevated evening cortisol in the aftermath of a traumatic event, was predictive of later PTSD development in children. Longitudinal data on pediatric and adolescent PTSD biology have shown that progressive divergence of cortisol and noradrenaline concentrations over time may be responsible for PTSD maintenance and may explain the discrepancies between the child and adult PTSD phenotypes.

Psychobiological abnormalities, through chronically disturbed HPA and LC/NE-SNS activity, in vulnerable periods of development may have irreversible effects on behavioral maturation and may affect specific vulnerable brain areas, altering CNS development,

[*] Corresponding author: Phone: 0030 210 746 74 57 (office), fax: 0030 210 77 59 167, Cell phone: 0030 693 6833936, E-mail: ppervanid@med.uoa.gr

increasing both the biological risk for psychopathology as well as the cardiometabolic risk in later life.

I. Introduction

Since Posttraumatic Stress Disorder (PTSD) was recognized as an anxiety disorder of childhood (1), a number of studies investigated the biological factors underlying the clinical manifestations of the disorder. Additionally, several studies have also focused on neuroendocrine parameters in maltreated children, independently of a formal DSM-IV PTSD diagnosis. Diversity of findings among these studies may be due to differential clinical manifestations in maltreated children the time of the assessment. However, even in children with a clear PTSD diagnosis, several additional parameters seem to have an effect on the neuroendocrine profile of the disease.

Neuroendocrine research in PTSD has mainly focused on the two axis of the stress system, the hypothalamic-pituitary-adrenal (HPA) axis and the locus caeruleus / norepinephrine-sympathetic nervous system (LC/NE-SNS). Normally, activation of the two axes of the stress system leads to behavioral and physical adaptive changes that improve an organism's ability to survive. However, excessive and prolonged activation of the stress system can lead to long-term emotional and behavioural symptoms and disorders and physical complications (2,3).

II. Developmental Aspects of PTSD Diagnosis

Diagnostic and Statistical Manual for Mental Disorders–IV (DSM-IV) provides diagnostic criteria for children older than 6 years, and adults with PTSD. Diagnosis include: a) Exposure to a traumatic life event that involved actual death, injury or a threat to the physical integrity of the individual or others and that evoked intense fear, helplessness, or horror (1). Traumatic events have been recognized most often in children in cases of natural disasters, war, sexual or physical abuse and accidents (4), b) Re-experience of the initial trauma via intrusive memories and/or dreams about the event, feeling as if the trauma was continuing to occur, and intense distress on exposure to cues that recall the event. c) Avoidance of stimuli associated with the trauma and numbing of overall responsiveness. d) Symptoms of excessive arousal, including insomnia, angry outbursts, hyper-vigilance, an exaggerated startle response, and difficulty concentrating (1,4).

Later, a set of developmentally appropriate criteria for preschoolers was proposed by Sheringa et al. (5,6). In fact, in young age groups, assessment of PTSD is frequently based on behaviours observed, since children of this age group are not able to describe their internal psychologic status and express their feelings. Infants or toddlers may become very aggressive or distressed at exposure to cues related to the trauma. Posttraumatic play, repeatedly mimicking the trauma, is also frequent in young children. A significant number of preschool and school age children are reported by their parents or teachers as being involved in repetitive play or drawings involving themes related to the trauma. Regression to earlier developmental stages is not rare in this age group. Children may also exhibit nightmares and significant sleep disruption. In school age kids aggression, withdrawal or avoidance and antisocial behaviour, at home and at school, may prevail. (5-7).

III. Hypothalamic Pituitary Adrenal Axis Dysregulation

Neuroendocrine studies in adults with PTSD have shown altered activity of the HPA axis, as evidenced by elevated basal cerebrospinal fluid (CSF) CRH concentrations (8) and differing results from peripheral cortisol measurements (9). In the majority of adult studies, low 24h excretion of urinary free cortisol (10-12), low or normal circulating plasma cortisol levels (11,13), or, more rarely high plasma cortisol levels (14,15) have been reported. The direction of HPA activity, as evidenced by peripheral cortisol measures, differs between studies whereas several factors, such as the type and chronicity of the trauma and the time since the stressful event occurred, as well as presence co-morbid disorders that may influence PTSD biology.

In accordance with adult studies, neuroendocrine research in pediatric PTSD has demonstrated lower or higher (16,17) cortisol levels in children with PTSD or a history of maltreatment. Childhood maltreatment, defined as physical or sexual abuse or neglect, represents the most widely studied chronic stressor in childhood. Though PTSD is the most common trauma-related disorder, occurred in 40-90% of children exposed in sexual abuse and in 11-50% among physically abused children, a great majority of studies in maltreated children have not clearly examined biological factors related to PTSD *per se*, but neuroendocrine parameters in children with a history of maltreatment exhibiting a variety of symptoms or disorders (18-21).

One of the first neuroendocrine studies, in sexually abused girls with histories of depression and suicidal behavior, revealed that these girls exhibited reduced evening basal and ovine CRH-stimulated plasma ACTH concentrations compared to matched non-abused girls (20). On the other hand, plasma cortisol responses to CRH stimulation did not differ between the two groups. This combined ACTH cortisol response to CRH was reminiscent of that observed in melancholic depression. Another study (17), investigated cortisol secretion in maltreated children, in the context of a day camp research program. Significant variation in cortisol secretion patterns were found, based on the subtypes of maltreatment the children had experienced. Furthermore, the type of symptoms was an additional determinant of the neuroendocrine profile of those children. In this study in the day camp, maltreated children who had both been physically and sexually abused, as well as neglected and/or emotionally abused, exhibited substantial elevations in morning cortisol levels. In contrast to the multiple abuse group, the subgroup of only physically abused children showed a trend toward lower morning cortisol relatively to non-maltreated children, and a smaller decrease in cortisol levels from morning to afternoon.

More recently (22), a study investigated morning cortisol levels in preschool aged foster children in relation to differential types of maltreatment. Foster children were subjected to a range of early adverse experiences, including neglect, abuse, and multiple caregiver disruptions. The study revealed that the foster children were significantly more likely to have low morning cortisol levels compared to the non-maltreated and low-income children. Furthermore, the type of the maltreatment was significantly associated with the foster children's morning cortisol levels: foster children with low morning cortisol levels had experienced more severe physical neglect than the other foster children. In contrast, foster children with high morning cortisol levels had experienced more severe emotional maltreatment. These findings are in accordance with the previous study and suggest that the type of early adverse experiences have differential effects on the functioning of the hypothalamic-pituitary-adrenal system.

The long-term effects of childhood stress and trauma in hypothalamic-pituitary axis have also been studied in adults with a history of child maltreatment. In a recent study (23), basal cortisol secretion, as measured with four saliva samples, was investigated in adults adopted as children. In this study, morning cortisol was lower in adoptees whose adoptive parents had reported severe neglect or abuse than in non-neglected or non-abused participants. Participants who had experienced severe childhood neglect, also had a flatter diurnal gradient in cortisol secretion compared to non-neglected adoptees. In contrast, adoptees whose parents reported moderately severe abuse had higher cortisol levels and a steep cortisol diurnal gradient relatively to non-abused participants. This study indicates that, early trauma is associated with cortisol levels and diurnal cortisol variation, even if children are raised in another environment after their early adverse experience.

Further to these findings, the effects of childhood emotional abuse on cortisol responsivity in adulthood was examined in a very recent study (24) using the dexamethasone/corticotropin releasing hormone (Dex/CRH) test. This test has been proposed as a potential tool for identifying endophenotypes relevant to mood disorders. The investigators examined cortisol secretion profiles in phenotypically healthy adults without psychiatric disorders, and revealed that a history of childhood emotional abuse significantly diminished cortisol response. This effect was amplified with advancing age of the individuals and was independent of the effects of other types of childhood maltreatment, lifetime diagnoses, and symptom scores. Researchers concluded that dampened cortisol reactivity in these individuals might be a consequence of childhood emotional abuse that is cumulative over time.

Further to neuroendocrine research on child maltreatment, fewer studies have also focused on the biology of childhood PTSD after an acute stressor. In a study after the 1988 Armenian earthquake, adolescents who lived close to the epicenter had more severe PTSD and lower baseline mean salivary cortisol levels and greater afternoon suppression of cortisol by dexamethasone than adolescents who lived 20 miles from the epicentre (25). Another study, found that high initial urinary cortisol immediately following an accident, were significantly correlated with subsequent PTSD symptoms, especially in boys (26).

Their study (27,28) examined prospectively and longitudinally the development of PTSD one and six months after a motor vehicle accident, in relation to neuroendocrine factors, in hospitalised children and adolescents for motor vehicle accidents (MVAs). Children's K-SADS (29) semi-structured interview was used for PTSD diagnosis and the PTSD-RI (30) questionnaire to assess symptoms severity one and six months after the accident. Serum cortisol and interleukin-6 and plasma catecholamine concentrations were measured, while salivary cortisol was measured 5 times a day to examine circadian variation, in all three assessments. In the cross sectional analysis, at month 1, salivary afternoon (6.00 pm) and evening (9.00) cortisol concentrations were higher in the PTSD than the non-PTSD and the control groups. No such differences were detected in month 6. In the longitudinal analysis, initially elevated evening salivary cortisol in the PTSD group gradually normalized at month

6. In the same study, biologic factors measured within 24hours after the accident were examined in relation to later PTSD development. We found that initially high evening salivary cortisol and high morning serum IL-6 concentrations were predictive of later PTSD diagnosis at month 6.

Another recent study, examined the impact of September 11, 2001 terror attacks in New York City, in bereaved children compared with children selected from the community. In this study, morning (am) and 4.00 pm baseline cortisol was significantly higher in bereaved than nonbereaved children. However, bereaved children with PTSD had significantly lower 4.00 pm baseline cortisol and significantly greater 4.00 pm cortisol suppression compared with bereaved children without psychopathology (31).

IV. The Sympathetic Nervous System

The locus caeruleus / norepinephrine-sympathetic nervous system is also involved in the pathophysiology of PTSD. The majority of adult and child neuroendocrine studies in PTSD show increased LC/NE-SNS activity. Indeed, increased 24h urinary catecholamine excretion or plasma norepinephrine concentrations (26,27,32-34) are reported in PTSD patients compared to control subjects. In clinical practice, increased blood pressure, heart rate, skin conductance and an exaggerated startle response have been reported in adults suffering from PTSD, reflecting increased noradrenergic activity (35). Norepinephrine plays important physiologic roles in arousal, attention, and memory and dysregulation of the LC/NE-SNS neurons may be involved in the hyperarousal and re-experience symptoms of PTSD (35,36). Stressful stimuli may enhance memory encoding in PTSD individuals, causing defective consolidation for the stressful event, leading to the development of intrusive thoughts, images, flashbacks, and repetitive nightmares (35,36).

In children, one of the first neuroendocrine studies revealed that sexually abused girls with histories of depression and suicidal behavior exhibited significantly greater 24-hour urinary concentrations of catecholamines and their metabolites than matched controls (21). Another study in child trauma victims (26), examined urinary cortisol and catecholamine concentrations collected soon after the trauma, and correlated them to the subsequent development of PTSD and depressive symptomatology six weeks later. High initial urinary cortisol and epinephrine levels were significantly correlated to the development of PTSD six months later. The findings suggested that high initial urinary cortisol and epinephrine levels immediately following a traumatic event may be associated with increased risk for the development of subsequent PTSD symptoms. Their longitudinal study in children after motor vehicle accidents, in accordance with the current literature, demonstrated significantly elevated plasma noradrenaline concentrations in children with PTSD, at both months 1 and 6 after the accident compared to the non-PTSD and control groups (27,28). Furthermore, a gradual increase in norepinephrine levels was noted within both the PTSD and the non-PTSD groups through time. Differences within the PTSD group, between month one and month six, were statistically significant. Interestingly, the non-PTSD group (those having experienced trauma but not fulfilled PTSD diagnosis) exhibited a similar pattern of norepinephrine increase through time. However, in their study, examining the predictive value of biomarkers in the aftermath of the trauma, unlike evening salivary cortisol and morning plasma IL-6, plasma epinephrine and norepinephrine concentrations were not predictive of later PTSD development.

V. Interactions between HPA Axis and the LC/NE-SNS

A minority of studies has examined interactions between the two axes of the stress system in pediatric PTSD and child maltreatment. Neuroendocrine measures in maltreated youth have shown an asymmetry between salivary alpha amylase (sAA), an indicator of the sympathetic nervous system, and cortisol reactivity to a social stressor: the researchers concluded that the maltreatment status moderated the relation between sAA and cortisol responses, in contrast to the comparison group, that showed significant correlations between the sAA and cortisol responses (37). A second study in girls with previous history of child maltreatment, showed that during the reactivity phase of the Trier Social Stress Test (TSST), the maltreated group exhibited an attenuated cortisol response, whereas the control group showed the increase and the gradual flattening over time (38). This blunted reactivity was independent of current symptoms of PTSD or depression. During the resting phase of the TSST, both groups exhibited a similar decline in cortisol levels. There were no group differences in resting and reactivity levels of heart rate, a clinical measure of SNS activity.

Their study examined longitudinally the interactions between cortisol and norepinephrine in PTSD development and maintenance in children and adolescents after motor vehicle accidents. Results from the longitudinal analysis revealed that children with continuous PTSD demonstrated a progressive divergence of cortisol and norepinephrine, with plasma norepinephrine gradually increasing and evening salivary cortisol decreasing over time. Interestingly, higher norepinephrine concentrations at month 6, relatively to month 1, were related to PTSD maintenance rather than PTSD severity as measured by the PTSD reaction index questionnaire. Findings from this study reveal a natural history of pediatric PTSD, after the impact of a single stressor, showing the continuous interrelations of the two axes of the stress system, as evidenced by peripheral measures of cortisol and catecholamine concentrations (27,28,39).

VI. Neuroendocrine Endophenotypes in PTSD: Investigating Diversity

In contrast to diverse patterns of cortisol secretion, as a peripheral marker of HPA axis function in PTSD, peripheral biomarkers of sympathetic nervous system activity are more consistent. However, the hypoactive HPA with the hyperactive LC/NE-SNS is the most prevalent finding among adults with chronic PTSD. Indeed, it has been suggested that exaggerated catecholamine secretion without the concurrent regulatory effect of accompanying cortisol elevations during stress, could result in defective consolidation of traumatic memories in the brain and subsequent PTSD symptomatology (40). As depicted in figure 1, the following parameters seem to contribute to diversity of PTSD neuroendocrine phenotypes among studies:

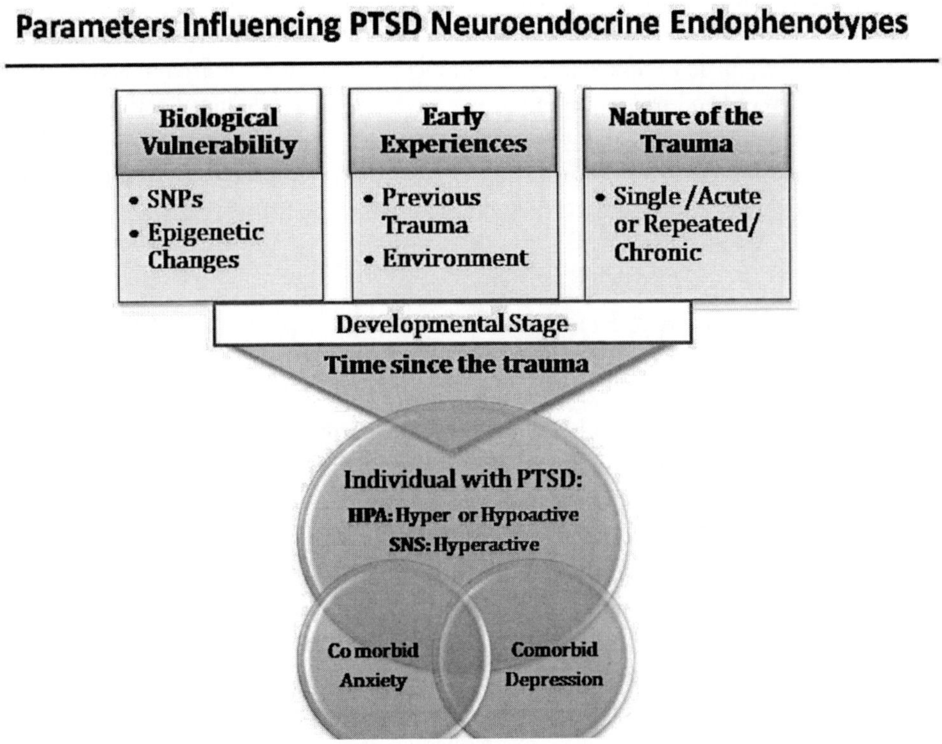

Figure 1. Parameters influencing Hypothalamic-Pituitary-Adrenal Axis Dysregulation (Hypet-or Hypo activation) in PTSD

A. Genetic Vulnerability

Family and twin studies have investigated the contribution of genetic variants, especially in combination with environmental factors, in the development, maintenance and resilience of PTSD. Genes associated with basic biochemical, endocrine, neuroanatomical, cognitive and psychiatric characteristics of the disorder, include the serotonin transporter (5-HTT), the dopamine transporter (DAT), the glucocorticoid receptor (GR), the glucocorticoid regulating genes (FKBP5), the GABA (A) receptor, the apolipoprotein E (APOE), the brain-derived neurotrophic factor (BDNF) and the neuropeptide Y (NPY) (41,42). Recently, the cannabinoid receptor gene (CNR1) was also associated with Attention Deficit Hyperactivity Disorder (ADHD) and PTSD (43).

B. Epigenetic Changes

Stress in utero, through fetal programming of the HPA axis, may also contribute to PTSD development in the offspring. In mothers exposed to the 11th September attacks during pregnancy, maternal PTSD was associated with awakening and bedtime salivary cortisol in their babies. Furthermore, lower cortisol values were noted in infants of PTSD mothers than those of exposed but non-PTSD affected ones (44). These data suggest that epigenetic mechanisms are also involved in biological susceptibility to PTSD. There is also evidence supporting that stress during pregnancy, through elevations of glucocorticoid levels, influence fetal brain development and programming of the HPA axis (45). Reduced activity of placental 11 beta-hydroxycorticosteroid dehydrogenase type 2, the enzyme that catalyses the conversion of maternal cortisol to cortisone, results in an increased exposure of the fetus to glucocorticoids and may contribute to HPA axis programming (45).

C. Developmental History: Previous Trauma and Time since the Trauma Occurred

Prior trauma exposure is a well known risk factor predisposing to development of PTSD. From a neuroendocrine percpective, exposure to previous trauma may contribute to altered HPA axis responses to a new stressor, and the low cortisol levels observed in adults with chronic PTSD (46, 47). This view hypothesizes that after an initial normal increase in cortisol levels, HPA axis functioning may be altered to a state of low basal cortisol levels, as time passes from the traumatic event. Indeed, a recent study in children (47) found that cortisol and PTSD symptoms were significantly positively correlated in children having recently experienced trauma, but negatively in children with distal trauma.

Thus, low cortisol levels found shortly after the trauma in adult studies, may be the impact of previous trauma exposure, which represents a preexisting vulnerability factor, rather than a biologic factor responsible *per se* for the subsequent development of PTSD (46,47). Children are, in general, less likely to have experienced a great majority of prior traumas, compared to adults, and less likely to exhibit comorbid disorders or alcohol or drug abuse. This might be the explanation of high cortisol levels reported more frequently in pediatric than in adult PTSD studies

D. Type of Stressor/Trauma (Acute vs. Chronic)

Acute and chronic trauma represent different types of stressors. Child maltreatment, defined as physical and/or sexual abuse or neglect is a chronic and complex stressor. Physical and/or sexual abuse most often co-exist with other psychosocial risk factors, such as low socioeconomic status, unemployment, parental psychopathology, drug and alcohol abuse. Furthermore, parental psychopathology in chronically maltreated children, may represent an additional innate biological risk factor for PTSD development. In contrast, accidents, or physical disasters are single traumas, potentially producing different clinical manifestations and neuroendocrine alterations. Terr differentiated single from repeated traumas and suggested that greater dissociation was related to repeated trauma (48).

E. Co-Morbid Disorders

PTSD is often comorbid with other disorders, such as major depressive disorder (MDD) and generalized anxiety disorder (GAD), as well as with a number of psychopathologic manifestations, such as somatic complaints, depressive symptoms or symptoms of dissociation (49). A study in adolescents revealed that depression was the most common comorbid diagnosis of PTSD, being reported in around one third of the PTSD population, while GAD was prevalent in 27%. Overlap of all three diagnoses may occur in 14% of the patients (49). The impact of comorbidity on neuroendocrine factors is highlighted in studies examining maltreated children. In a study in a day camp, mentioned before (17), maltreated children with internalizing problems demonstrated higher morning, afternoon and average daily cortisol levels, while non-maltreated boys with externalizing problems were more likely not to show the expected diurnal decrease in cortisol. This study, was one of the first to clarify the diversity of neuroendocrine patterns, depending on the type of maltreatment and the concurrent psychopathology in childhood.

VII. Conclusions and Effects of PTSD in the Developing Organism

In conclusion, PTSD in children and adolescents is associated with elevated norepinephrine and variable cortisol levels, depending on the time point of the assessment after the traumatic event. Genetic and epigenetic background, type and chronicity of the stressor, previous trauma and comorbidity are additional parameters related to neuroencocrine patterns of disease. High cortisol levels, reported in the majority of pediatric studies, and, in contrast to most of adult studies, may represent an initial alteration of the HPA axis in response to the traumatic experience.

Early trauma and childhood PTSD can cause alterations in the functioning of neuroendocrine structures and networks in the central nervous system (50). Childhood trauma may alter CNS development: early severe stress results in elevated levels of CRH and glucocorticoids affecting specific, vulnerable brain areas (50,51). A recent longitudinal study in children with PTSD demonstrated that PTSD symptoms and cortisol levels at baseline, predicted a reduction in hippocampal volume 12 to 18 months later. This study is in accordance with adult studies showing smaller hippocampal volumes in PTSD patients (52). In the same study, higher hyperarousal symptoms were related to smaller hippocampal volumes, whereas, in previous research, hyperarousal symptoms were related to cognitive difficulties in individuals with PTSD. In addition to stress-related brain changes, endocrine systems, which are crucial for growth and puberty, including the gonadal, growth hormone and thyroid axes, are influenced by chronic stress. Chronic changes in these systems during critical periods of development could have irreversible effects on growth and development (53).

In conclusion, the impact of childhood stress and trauma, in addition to concurrent symptoms and disorders, may "program" the developing organism of some individuals to be more susceptible to future stressors and thus, more vulnerable to develop mental and physical disorders. This is compatible with a kindling effect of stress mediators, such as CRH, on certain brain substrates resulting in hypersensitivity of these substrates to ensuing insults (2).

References

[1] American Psychiatric Association 1994 *Diagnostic and statistical manual of mental disorders-DSM-IV*, 4TH ed. Washington DC: American Psychiatric Press.

[2] Chrousos, GP; Gold, PW. The Concepts of Stress and Stress System Disorders. *JAMA* 1992, 267, 1244-1252.

[3] Chrousos, GP. Stress and disorders of the stress system. *Nat Rev Endocrinol.* 2009 Jul, 5(7), 374-81.

[4] Yule, W. Posttraumatic stress disorder in the general population and in children. *J Clin Psychiatry* 2001, 62 Suppl 17, 23-28.

[5] Scheeringa, MS; Zeanah, CH; Myers, L; Putnam, FW. New findings on alternative criteria for PTSD in preschool children. *J Am Acad Child Adolesc Psychiatry.* 2003 May, 42(5), 561-70.

[6] Scheeringa, MS. Developmental considerations for diagnosing PTSD and acute stress disorder in preschool and school-age children. *Am J Psychiatry.* 2008 Oct, 165(10), 1237-9.

[7] Pervanidou, P; Kolaitis, G; Chrousos, GP. Bio-behavioral consequences of traumatic stress in childhood and adolescence: The effects of war on children' s mental health, growth and development. In: Sher L, Vilens A (editors). War and Suicide. Hauppauge, New York: Nova Science Publishers, in press.

[8] Baker, DG; West, SA; Nicholson, WE; Ekhator, NN; Kasckow, JW; Hill, KK; Bruce, AB; Orth, DN; Geracioti, TD Jr. Serial CSF corticotropin-releasing hormone levels and adrenocortical activity in combat veterans with posttraumatic stress disorder. *Am J Psychiatry* 1999, 156(4), 585-8. Erratum in: *Am J Psychiatry* 1999, 156(6), 986

[9] Rasmusson, AM; Vythilingam, M; Morgan, CA. 3rd. The neuroendocrinology of posttraumatic stress disorder: new directions. *CNS Spectr.* 2003, 8(9), 651-656, 665-667.

[10] Yehuda, R; Giller, EL; Southwick, SM; Lowy, MT; Mason, JW. Hypothalamic-pituitary-adrenal dysfunction in posttraumatic stress disorder. *Biol Psychiatry* 1991, 30(10), 1031-1048.

[11] Yehuda, R. Biology of posttraumatic stress disorder. *J Clin Psychiatry* 2001, 62 (17), 41-46.

[12] Yehuda, R; Kahana, B; Binder-Brynes, K; Southwick, SM; Mason, JW; Giller, EL. Low urinary cortisol excretion in Holocaust survivors with posttraumatic stress disorder. *Am. Journal of Psychiatry* 1995, 152, 982-986.

[13] Boscarino, JA. Posttraumatic stress disorder, exposure to combat, and lower plasma cortisol among Vietnam veterans-findings and clinical implications. *J Consult Clin Psychol* 1996, 64, 191-201.

[14] Lemieux, AM; Coe, CL. Abuse related posttraumatic stress disorder: evidence for chronic neuroendocrine activation in women. *Psychosom. Med* 1995, 57, 105-115.

[15] Maes, M; Lin, A; Bonaccorso, S; van Hunsel, F; Van Gastel, A; Delmeire, L; Biondi, M; Bosmans, E; Kenis, G; Scharpe, S. Increased 24-hour urinary cortisol excretion in patients with post-traumatic stress disorder and patients with major depression, but not in patients with fibromyalgia. *Acta Psychiatr Scand*, 1998, 98(4), 328-335.

[16] De Bellis, MD; Thomas, LA. Biological findings of posttraumatic stress disorder and child maltreatment. *Curr Psychiatry Rep*, 2003 5(2), 108-117.

[17] Ciccheti, D; Rogosch, FA. Diverse patterns of neuroendocrine activity in maltreated children. *Dev Psychopathol*, 2001, 13(3), 677-693.

[18] *Children of Trauma: Stressful Life Events and their Effects on Children and Adolescents* / edited by Thomas Miller, 1998, International Universities Press, Inc.

[19] Kiser, LJ; Heston, J; Millsap, PA; Pruitt, DB. Physical and sexual abuse in childhood: relationship with post-traumatic stress disorder. *J Am Acad Child Adolesc Psychiatry.* 1991 Sep, 30(5), 776-8375

[20] De Bellis, MD; Chrousos, GP; Dorn, LD; Burke, L; Helmers, K; Kling, MA; Trickett, PK; Putnam, FW. Hypothalamic-pituitary-adrenal axis dysregulation in sexually abused girls. *JCEM* 1994, 78, 249-255.

[21] De Bellis, MD; Lefter, L; Trickett, PK; Putnam FW, Jr. Urinary catecholamine excretion in sexually abused girls. *J Am Acad Child Adolesc Psychiatry.* 1994, Mar-Apr, 33(3), 320-7.

[22] Bruce, J; Fisher, PA; Pears, KC; Levine, S. *Dev Psychobiol.* Morning cortisol Levels in preschool-aged foster children: differential effects of maltreatment type. 2009 Jan, 51(1), 14-23.

[23] van der Vegt, EJ; van der Ende, J; Kirschbaum, C; Verhulst, FC; Tiemeier, H. Early neglect and abuse predict diurnal cortisol patterns in adults A study of international adoptees. *Psychoneuroendocrinology*. 2009 Jun, 34(5), 660-9.

[24] Carpenter, LL; Tyrka, AR; Ross, NS; Khoury, L; Anderson, GM; Price, LH. Effect of childhood emotional abuse and age on cortisol responsivity in adulthood. *Biol Psychiatry*. 2009 Jul 1, 66(1), 69-75.

[25] Goenjian, AK; Yehuda, R; Pynoos, RS; Steinberg, AM; Tashjian, M; Yang, RK; Najarian, LM; Fairbanks, LA. Basal cortisol, dexamethasone suppression of cortisol, and MHPG in adolescents after the 1988 earthquake in Armenia. *Am J Psychiatry*, 1996 153(7), 929-934.

[26] Delahanty, DL; Nugent, NR; Christopher, NC; Walsh, M. Initial urinary epinephrine and cortisol levels predict acute PTSD symptoms in child trauma victims. *Psychoneuroendocrinology*. 2005 Feb, 30(2), 121-8.

[27] Pervanidou, P; Kolaitis, G; Charitaki, S; Lazaropoulou, Ch; Hindmarsh, P; Bakoula, Ch; Papassotiriou, I; Tsiantis, J; Ghrousos, GP. The natural history of neuroendocrine changes in pediatric posttraumatic stress disorder after motor vehicle accidents: progressive divergence of noradrenaline and cortisol concentrations over time. *Biol Psychiatry*, 2007 15, 62(10), 1095-1102.

[28] Pervanidou, P; Kolaitis, G; Charitaki, S; Margeli, A; Lazaropoulou, C; Papassotiriou, I; Ferentinos, S; Bakoula, C; Tsiantis, J; Chrousos, GP. Elevated morning serum IL-6 or evening salivary cortisol predict PTSD in children and adolescents 6 months after motor vehicle accidents. *Psychoneuroendocrinology*, 2007 32(8-10), 991-992.

[29] Kaufman, J; Birmaher, B; Brent, D; Rao, U; Flynn, C; Moreci, P; Williamson, D; Ryan, N. Schedule for Affective Disorders and Schizophrenia for School-Age

Children-Present and Lifetime Version (K-SADS-PL): initial reliability and validity data. *J Am Acad Child Adolesc Psychiatry*, 1997, 36(7), 980-988.

[30] Rodriguez, N; Steinberg, A; Pynoos, RS. UCLA Post Traumatic Stress Disorder Reaction Index for DSM-IV, Child, *Adolescent, and Parent Versions*, 1998 (available from the authors).

[31] Pfeffer, CR; Altemus, M; Heo, M; Jiang, H. Salivary cortisol and psychopathology in children bereaved by the september 11, 2001 terror attacks. *Biol Psychiatry*. 2007 Apr 15, 61(8), 957-65.

[32] Yehuda, R; Southwick, S; Giller, EL; Ma, X; Mason, JW. Urinary catecholamine excretion and severity of PTSD symptoms in Vietnam combat veterans. *J Nerv Ment Dis*, 1992, 180(5), 321-325.

[33] Southwick, SM; Paige, S; Morgan, CA 3rd; Bremner, JD; Krystal, JH; Charney, DS. Neurotransmitter alterations in PTSD: catecholamines and serotonin. *Semin Clin Neuropsychiatry*, 1999, 4(4), 242-248.

[34] Pitman, R; Orr, S. Twenty –four urinary cortisol and catecholamine excretion in combat–related posttraumatic stress disorder. *Biol Psychiatry*, 1990, 27, 245-247.

[35] O Donnell, TO; Hegadoren, KM; Coupland, NC. Noradrenergic mechanisms in the pathophysiology of post-traumatic stress disorder. *Neuropsychobiology*, 2004, 50, 273-283.

[36] Southwick, SM; Bremner, JD; Rasmusson, A; Morgan, CA 3rd; Arnsten, A; Charney, DS. Role of norepinephrine in the pathophysiology and treatment of posttraumatic stress disorder. *Biol Psychiatry*, 1999, 46(9), 1192-1204.

[37] Gordis, EB; Granger, DA; Susman, EJ; Trickett, PK. Salivary alpha amylase-cortisol asymmetry in maltreated youth. *Horm Behav.*, 2008 Jan, 53(1), 96-103.

[38] MacMillan, HL; Georgiades, K; Duku, EK; Shea, A; Steiner, M; Niec, A; Tanaka, M; Gensey, S; Spree, S; Vella, E; Walsh, CA; De Bellis, MD; Van der Meulen, J; Boyle, MH; Schmidt, LA. Cortisol response to stress in female youths exposed to childhood maltreatment: results of the youth mood project. *Biol Psychiatry.*, 2009 Jul 1, 66(1), 62-8.

[39] Pervanidou, P. Biology of Posttraumatic Stress Disorder in childhood and adolescence *J. Neuroendocrinol.*, 2008 May, 20(5), 632-638.

[40] Pitman, RK; Orr, SP; Shalev, AY. Once bitten, twice shy: beyond the conditioning model of PTSD. *Biol Psychiatry*, 33, 145-146.

[41] Broekman, FFP. Olff M, Boer F, The genetic background of PTSD. *Neuroscience and Behavioral Reviews.*, 2007. 31, 348-362

[42] Amstadter, AB; Nugent, NR; Koenen, KC. Genetics of PTSD: Fear Conditioning as a Model for Future Research. *Psychiatr Ann.*, 2009 Jun 1, 39(6), 358-367.

[43] Lu, AT; Ogdie, MN; Järvelin, MR; Moilanen, IK; Loo, SK; McCracken, JT; McGough, JJ; Yang, MH; Peltonen, L; Nelson, SF; Cantor, RM; Smalley, SL. Association of the cannabinoid receptor gene (CNR1) with ADHD and post-traumatic stress disorder. *Am J Med Genet B Neuropsychiatr Genet.*, 2008 Dec 5, 147B(8), 1488-94.

[44] Yehuda, R; Engel, SM; Brand, SR; Seckl, J; Marcus, SM; Berkowitz, GS. Transgenerational effects of posttraumatic stress disorder in babies of mothers exposed to the World Trade Center attacks during pregnancy. *JCEM*, 2005, 90(7), 4115-4118.

[45] Seckl, JR. Prenatal glucocorticoids and long-term programming. *Eur J Endocrinol*, 2004 151(Suppl 3), U49–U62

[46] Resnick, HS; Yehuda, R; Pitman, RK; Foy, DW. Effect of previous trauma on acute plasma cortisol level following rape. *Am J Psychiatry*, 1995, 152, 1675-1677.

[47] Weems, CF; Carrión, VG. Brief report: diurnal salivary cortisol in youth--clarifying the nature of posttraumatic stress dysregulation. *J Pediatr Psychol.*, 2009 May, 34(4), 389-95.

[48] Pervanidou, P; Chrousos, GP. Post-traumatic Stress Disorder in children and adolescents: from Sigmund Freud's "trauma" to psychopathology and the (Dys)metabolic syndrome. *Horm Metab Res.*, 2007 Jun, 39(6), 413-9.

[49] Kar, N; Bastia, BK. Post-traumatic stress disorder, depression and generalised anxiety disorder in adolescents after a natural disaster: a study of comorbidity. *Clin Pract Epidemol Ment Health*, 2006, 2, 17.

[50] De Bellis, MD; Baum, AS; Birmaher, B; Keshavan, MS; Eccard, CH; Boring, AM; Jenkins, FJ; Ryan, ND. A. E. Bennett Research Award. Developmental traumatology. Part I: Biological stress systems. *Biol Psychiatry,* 1999, 45(10), 1259-1270

[51] Teicher, MH; Andersen, SL; Polcari, A; Anderson, CM; Navalta, CP. Developmental neurobiology of childhood stress and trauma. *Psychiatr Clin North Am*, 2002, 25(2), 397-426.

[52] Carrion, VG; Weems, CF; Reiss, AL. Stress predicts brain changes in children: a pilot longitudinal study on youth stress, posttraumatic stress disorder, and the hippocampus. *Pediatrics.*, 2007

[53] Charmandari, E; Kino, T; Souvatzoglou, E; Chrousos, GP. Pediatric stress: hormonal mediators and human development. *Horm Res.*, 2003, 59(4), 161-79.

In: Neuroendocrinology Research Developments
Editor: N. S. Penkava and L.R. Haight, pp.119-131
ISBN: 978-1-60876-983-4
© 2010 Nova Science Publishers, Inc.

Chapter 7

GENETIC ASPECTS OF STRESS NEUROENDOCRINOLOGY

E. V. Daev*

Dept. Genetics & Breeding, Faculty of Biology and Soil Sciences, Saint-Petersburg State University, Saint-Petersburg, Russia, 199034

ABSTRACT

It is well established that response to stress is one of the fundamental reactions of highly developed organisms. In spite of the fact that more than 70 years have passed since Selye began to study this phenomenon, even now many issues in this particular area of scientific research remain unclear. Therefore there is a good reason to discuss some basic questions which seem important for the future perspectives.

During the last half century new methodologies have allowed scientists to obtain much new data about different aspects of stress reaction. However inadequate expansion of the meaning of the term "stress" has made the concept of stress a bit ambiguous. For that reason it is important to study the fine mechanisms of the interconnections between features of stress at the levels of the genome, the single cell, the organism (neuroendocrine reactions and other "classic" effects) and the population level. Meanwhile, it seems that the current value of some prospective research areas has been underestimated. This applies particularly to the studies of stress that influences genomic integrity in somatic and germ cells of animals.

In this paper I endeavor to mark some prospective research areas connecting the physiology, neuroendocrinology and genetics to study common mechanisms of stress reaction more effectively and try to better interpret its evolutionary significance.

* Corresponding author: E-mail: mouse_gene@mail.ru

INTRODUCTION

The widely used term "stress" describes one of the basic reactions of highly developed organisms. Despite the fact that more than 70 years have passed since Selye began to study this phenomenon, even now many things remain unclear in this area of scientific research. Therefore there is a good reason to discuss some questions which seem important for the future perspectives.

Claude Bernard's (1878) and Walter Cannon's (1932; 1935) ideas about homeostasis were developed further in Selye's research on unspecific adaptive response of the mammalian organism (Selye, 1936, 1946, 1950, 1973). In response to the action of some factors, mammals demonstrate a nonspecific set of reactions in their attempts to adapt. The resulting strain inside the organism appears as a very real and quite typical negative change in morphologic and functional features especially in different tissues and organs under control of the anterior lobe of the hypophysis (Selye, 1950). This phenomenon was described and defined by Selye as a subject for detailed study in the future.

For the last half century new methods have allowed scientists to obtain considerable new data about the different sides of a stress reaction. But it is necessary to note not only positive, but also negative moments. Among the latter is an inadequate expansion and content of the term "stress". As a result the concept has become too loose. It is very important to emphasize here that the subject to this study needs to be well defined.

In his later publications Selye himself declared that stress means life and *vice versa* (Selye, 1974) and started to subdivide stress into two parts. One he called "distress" (real stress) and the other "eustress" (Selye, 1979). Therefore, when he began to include in content of the term "stress" all normal reactions of the organism he perhaps made a huge step back. Since then, to study stress means to study whole life. It looks as though his later overgeneralization diminished the scientific value of his earlier discoveries. It seems much better for scientific research to restrict the basic meaning of the term "stress". There is no doubt that numerous surrounding factors may be bad or good in themselves but both may or may not evoke the stress state. And only if they do evoke stress, are they known as stressors. That is the area to study. As for "stresses" (which Selye had called "eustresses") that resulted in pleasurable or satisfying experience (Selye, 1979; Rice, 1987), it is likely that they are not a stresses at all. Or ... it is possible also that we simply do not notice long-term and sometimes too weak negative consequences of such "stirring" events. The last suggestion seems more probable.

As Selye made a "slip of a tongue" using "stress" instead of "strain" (Selye, 1975) even now in the scientific literature there is often not a clear difference between "stress" and "stressor". In many papers we can see at the same time quite different definitions, for example, such as ... "*Stress* is a broad term that implies a threat to which the body needs to adjust" and a few lines below "*Stress* is defined as a condition in an animal that results from the action of one or more stressors" (von Borell, 2001). Undoubtedly, the upper definition describes stressor.

Stress is not synonymous with an acting force or factor. It is a response to a stressor action. Sometimes lack of any influences (or habitual environmental factors) can be a strong stressor inducing a state of stress. Thus, this can be a source of some misunderstanding.

Another problem is in applicability of the term "stress" to the organisms with very simple nervous system or even to plants and unicellular organisms but those are completely different stories. Certainly, even single cells have nonspecific mechanisms for response external stimuli (heat, UV light, trace metals, and xenobiotics). And different cells may nevertheless often use the same mechanisms (for example, heat-shock response) to protect themselves from damages. There are many stress proteins which protect and repair injuries inside a cell when an organism is environmentally stressed. Cellular stress responses result in inactivation or down-regulations of many genes, including many housekeeping genes, while up-regulating stress genes perform orchestrated induction of key stress proteins. Several stress protein families, including hsp90, hsp70, chaperonin60, hsp40, the low molecular weight stress proteins, and ubiquitin, are expressed in cells of diverse phyla. It has been shown that genetic differences in stress proteins' pattern correlate with the organism resistance, suggesting that they help organisms adapt to acute environmental factors. So, the "cellular stress" response can be defined as a reaction of evolutionarily highly conserved intracellular mechanism to the threat of cell damage that could follow sudden environmental changes (Kültz, 2003; Macario A., Macario E., 2005).

In spite of the fact that the cellular stress response has been widely studied, knowledge of it is still fragmentary and "unifying concept explaining its universality for many different species and types of stress is lacking" (Kültz, 2003). Identifying the key players within the stress response network as well as whole stress proteome is an important task for future investigations.

Most of the stress researches focus on key proteins and their role inside the cell. But during the last few decades it is likely to find relatively new term "genomic stress" (Parsons, 1992). Genomic stress is defined as genome dysfunction which leads to disruption of its stability by fostering chromosome damages or single gene mutations. So, it is definitely a certain state of the cell' genome, but is not an "influence", as anybody probably could find on some Internet sites. Does exploring stress mean to analyze temperature, moisture or other stressors themselves?

Subject to study and success depends on the correct definition. It seems, more useful to define stress as a definite state of a living organism responding nonspecifically and rather negatively to some different external factor or factors.

Hans Selye's definition of stress applied to higher animals at the level of the whole organism. Therefore it included changes in axis hypothalamic-hypophyseal-adrenal-gonadal axis. But of course all following morphological and other changes are impossible without coarse rearrangements and disturbances of intracellular and genetic processes in target cells of target organs and tissues. And it seems there is a gap in research connecting the neuroendocrine with other mechanisms of the stress reaction at the genomic, cellular and organismal levels in spite of all that stress-responses are links of the same chain.

Here I will use stress mainly in its "primary" meaning accordingly early Selye works (Selye, 1936; 1946) with reference to higher animals and will try to talk more about stress' genetics.

Genes Are Necessary to Form a Stress Response

Response to any influence in higher organisms, for example, mammals includes few common steps such as:

1. reception of a signal by a receptor cell;
2. signal transformation and transduction to CNS;
3. processing of the information by CNS;
4. formation of a composite integral response.

This all depends on well the coordinated work of many receptor proteins, enzymes, and early and late stage genes, of all participating cells inside the recipient organism. This is we call normal life. And adaptation to the most of the acting factors is a result of organism response (Figure 1). But often the factors function is too strong or too long or they are very new, and organism cannot adapt to them with usual mechanisms. Activation of additional unspecific defense forces such as heat shock proteins etc. may be needed. The organism and its nervous system begin to work in force-majeure mode. That is a stress (Figure 1). Sometimes it looks like stress is nothing more than problem with neurotransmitter supplies (Teuchert-Noodt, 1992).

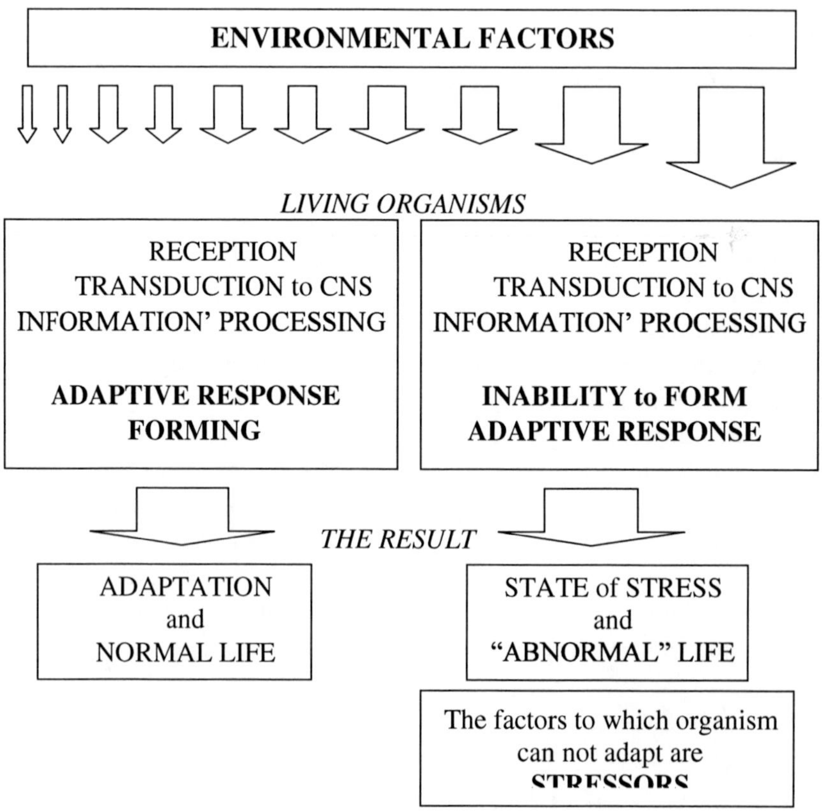

Figure 1. Difference between normal life and the stress.

Genes' activity is changed during any response occurring in all participating cells of the organism. Because stress is characterized by some common features (Figure 2) there is the network of genes whose activity in target cells changes drastically in response to the stressors action. It results in various organs hypertrophy or suppression (for example, involution of thymus or adrenals hypertrophy etc.). It is necessary to notice that just because of a genes abnormal activity and even genome partial disintegration in cells of target organs (hypothalamus, hypophysis, adrenals, thymus, gonads and others) we have stress consequences such as inhibition of immunity and deterioration of reproduction, long-term changes in central nervous system activity and animal behavior, reduction of general fitness and viability (Lee, McDonald, 1985).

Stress at the level of whole organism is directly connected with the target cells stress. And, in turn, cellular stress directly linked with genomic stress. So, it looks like the perspective direction in current neuroscience development seems to be revealing the interconnections between stress neuroendocrine characteristics, regulatory genetic changes and genomic instability in cells of different brain' regions as well as other affected organs. It will help to fill the gap in their knowledge about cross-talking mechanisms of stress at the level of single cell and stress of the whole organism.

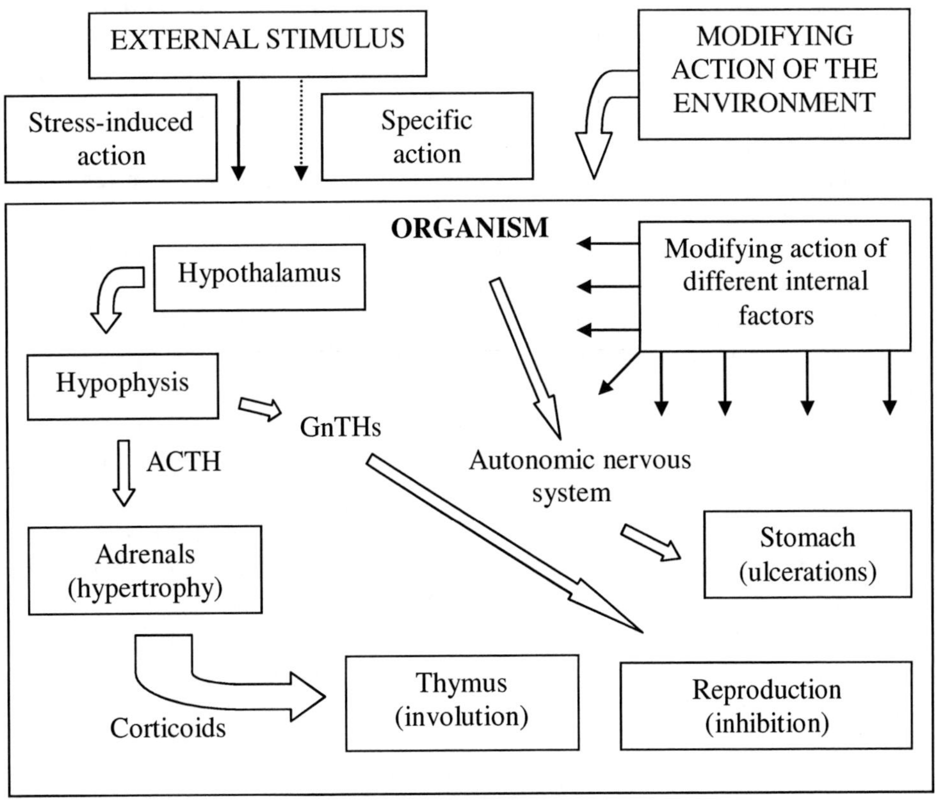

Figure 2. Main pathways of the animal organism response to stressors' action (after Selye, 1979). GnTHs – gonadotpopins; ACTH – adrenocorticotropin.

In some researches scientists investigate tissue specific expression patterns of genes which control such unspecific inducible mechanisms as lipids' peroxidation, heat shock proteins' activation, expression of receptor-proteins of different hormones and neurotransmitters under stress conditions. They study how intraspecific genetic differences between organisms determine their individual stress resistance and stress reactivity. There are data obtained on model organisms that shows the existence of common genetic mechanism controlling different links of stress-reaction (Rauschenbach et al., 2000). But, it seems, there are not so many works about organism's stress influences on genetic processes and stability of genetic machinery in different cells. In reality regulatory and other changes in genome functioning lead to further substantial long term biochemical, physiologic, morphologic and behavioral modifications. Therefore it seems necessary to mention some effects of organism' stress at the genetic level.

Stress is Necessary to Form Genetic Changes

There are few papers about an organism's stress influencing genetic processes. Accordingly academician D.K. Belyaev concept (Belyaev, 1979) stress state during domestication unveils hidden genetic heterogeneity in animal populations and seems to be an important factor in the evolutionary process. But he discussed mainly the problem of displaying already existing genetic variability. Only in few researches investigators have directly demonstrated newly acquired heterogeneity by increasing of recombination frequency in 1st and 2nd chromosomes of germ cells in mice after immobilization (Borodin, Belyaev, 1980; 1986).

Earlier the problem of neuroendocrine influence on genetic information realization had been discussed, at least, in Russian literature (Lopatina et al., 1975; Ponomarenko, 1976; Tsapigina, 1972). Later it was shown also that stress initiated by electric stimuli could induce chromosomal aberration frequency in mouse bone marrow cells. An interesting point was that tranquillizers significantly decreased the mutagenic effect of electric stimulation (Seredenin, Durnev, 1980). It has been shown also that olfactory induced stress in mice increased chromosomal aberration level in germ and somatic cells of mouse males (Daev, 1982; Tsapygina et al., 1979). This indicates that neuroendocrine changes that occur under stress conditions modify the structural stability of the genome in target cells. All these data confirmed the old hypothesis of Yu.Ya.Kerkis (1940) and M.E.Lobashev (1947) regarding the physiological nature of mutational process. This all suggests that stress can serve as a "tool" to study interconnections between genetic processes in single cells (genetic and cellular level) of some target tissues and neuroendocrine status of the whole organism.

Laboratory mice are a very suitable model to study the problem of organismal stress and its influence on intracellular genetic processes. For example, it is possible to show an interconnections among varying stresses at different levels with the following experiments.

There are no doubts that some mouse pheromones can act as stressors (Daev, 1983; 1994; 2007). Thus they can modify neuroendocrine status of the recipient mouse organism. Specifically, stress reaction changes appear in behavior of the recipient animals (Aron, 1979; Cavaggioni et al., 1999). It has been shown that pheromones induce adrenal hypertrophy (Archer, 1969; Wuensch, 1979), inhibit gonadal development (Lawton, Whitsett, 1979), and modify releasing-factors and pituitary hormones level (Dlusen et al., 1981; Dudley et al., 1996; Maruniak et al., 1978; Singer et al., 1988). Pheromonal cues change also immune response (Cocke et al., 1993; Moynihan et al., 1994). They can also disturb maturation and reproductive function in treated animals (Jemiolo, Novotny, 1994; Koyama, 2004). So, as typical stressors, some of them induce strain in the "hypothalamic –hypophyseal – adrenal – gonad" axis which results in changes described by Selye. These of course, do not negate the possibility of positive (non-stressor) action of some other pheromones on the recipient organism (Rekwot et al., 2001).

Sometimes it is possible to identify and dose olfactory stressor. There are also methods to estimate any cytogenetic changes in dividing cells of different tissues and organs that characterize stability of genetic machinery. Thus, cytogenetic analysis of chromosomal aberrations allows estimating negative consequences of stress reaction in target cells. At the same time such analysis demonstrates an existence of certain genetic link in the chain of stress response events.

There are reports about changes of sensitivity to odors in humans and animals depending on stage of estrous cycle and combination of estrogen-progesterone (Doty, 1986; Jechura, Lee, 2004; Havlicek, Roberts, 2009). We evaluated the ability of the 2,5-dimethylpyrazine (DMP) to induce *de novo* chromosomal aberrations in bone marrow cells of house mouse females with respect to their estrous cycle stage. Female testers sniffed the pheromone for 24 hrs, resulting in induction of mitotic disturbances. It was shown that females in pro-estrous – estrous were less sensitive to DMP action (Daev et al., 2007). These results indicate the existence of neuroendocrine mechanism of pheromone induced mutagenesis.

In a second experiment we allowed an experimental group of mouse males to sniff a pheromone-stressor for 24 hrs and after that checked the chromosome aberration level in dividing bone marrow cells. The frequency was significantly higher than in control group (Figure 3). This would indicate that part of bone marrow cells has many of genetic disturbances and at least part of them will incur the risk of lethality. As bone marrow is a very important organ of immune and hemopoietic system, death or mitotic disturbance in part of its cells marks a fitness decrease in the stressed animals. Possibly, the phenomenon of eosinopenia in mice (Southwick, 1959) could be explained by such a mechanism.

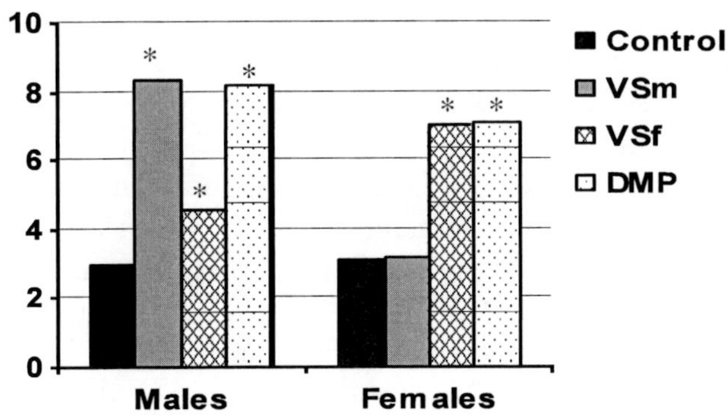

Figure 3. Total frequency of spontaneous and pheromone-induced cytogenetic abnormalities (%) in bone marrow cells of laboratory mice after sniffing VS_m or VS_f (volatile substances, which are contained in the protein fraction of dialyzed urine pooled from 10 single mouse males or females, correspondingly) or DMP - mouse female pheromone 2,5-dimethylpyrazine (0,01% water solution). Control – distilled water; *- significant differences from control group animals ($P<0.05$).

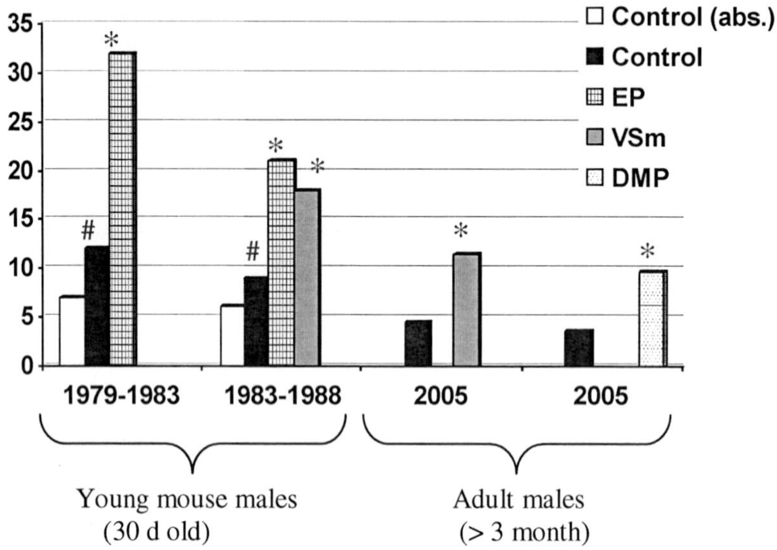

Figure 4. Total frequency of meiotic disturbances in spermatocytes I (%) of recipient mouse males after different influences. Control (abs.) – intact animals (absolute control); Control – influence of transferring animals into new cage with "clean bedding" (handling) or (after 1988) putting inside their own cage special capsule with distilled water; EP – influence of transferring animals into new cage with "soiled bedding" (bedding mixture with excretory products from 10 single adult males); VS_m and DMP-influence of putting into cage with recipient males special capsule with water solution of MUPs (main urinary proteins) pooled from 10 adult single male donors or with 0,01% water solution of female mouse pheromone 2,5-dimethylpyrazine. * - significant differences between treated group of males and Control I (P<0,05); # - significant differences between Control and Control I (handling-effect).

It is of interest that noradrenalin concentration drops to the zero level in nerve endings of mucous epithelium of the nose and in the testes tunica within 1hr after short-term exposure with 2,5-dimethylpyrazine. Only minute amounts of the hormone appear 24 hrs after the exposure with the pheromone (Daev et al., 2000). Also, sex specific influence of volatiles from donor urine indirectly supports hypothesis about the neuroendocrine connection to cytogenetic disturbances observed here. At the same time some "special" pheromones (DMP) act nonspecifically (Jemiolo, Novotny, 1994). In spite of all these data the impact of individual hormones into destabilizing of target cells genome remains unknown.

Similar results were obtained with germ cells of mouse males (Figure 4). Young males sniffed "soiled bedding" or volatiles from main urinary protein fraction of mature male dialyzed urine. Later we used DMP as stress-factor also. After sniffing stressor pheromones the frequency of meiotic abnormalities in recipient males was higher than in control (Daev, 1983; 1994; Daev, Dukelskaya, 2005).

It is necessary to note that the cytogenetic effect of adult male mouse pheromones depends on individual main urinary protein content. Absence of some protein fractions leads to changes of conjugated volatiles effectiveness (Daev, Sverdlova, 2002).

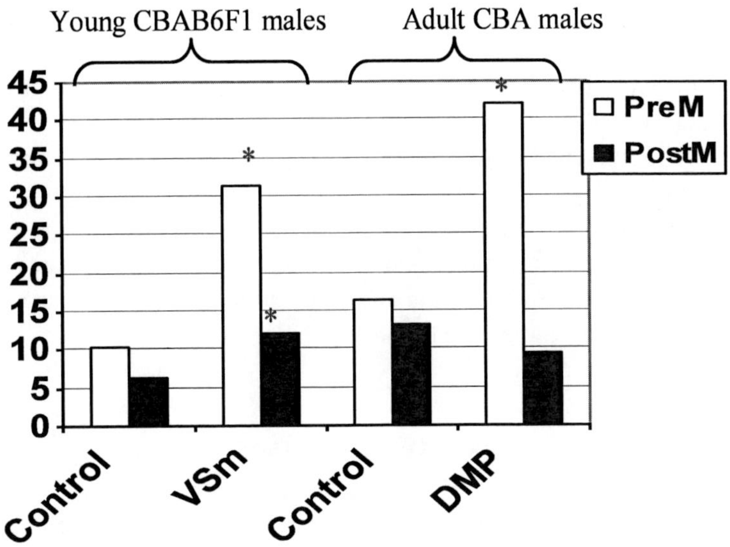

Figure 5. Pre- and post-implantation mortality (%) after short-term exposure of the young CBAB6F1 males with pheromones from excretory products of the adult CBA males (VS_m) or exposure (for 6-d) of the adult CBA males with 2,5 dimethylpyrazine (DMP).

PreM and PostM – pre- and post-implantation mortality, correspondingly. Mating of young males was conducted during 6th week after pheromones sniffing. Mating of adult males was conducted during 18-22 d after beginning of DMP sniffing (Daev et al., 1988; Daev, Dukelskaya, 2003). * - significant differences between treated animals and corresponding control (P<0,05).

At 17 days the level of abnormal sperm heads was increased (Arief'ev et al, 1986; Daev, Dukelskaya, 2003). The high level of dominant lethals was observed at pre- and post-implantation stages when males stressed by pheromones were mated with intact females. These males were also less successful in mating (Daev, 1983; 2003; Daev et al., 1988). The last result is similar to the well known pheromonal Bruce effect (Bruce, 1959), but with one big difference. In their experiments stressed males (not females) demonstrate a high mortality among their progeny after mating with undisturbed females (Figure 5). The frequency of dominant lethals (Ehling et al., 1978) induced by pheromones was 35% in the progeny of CBAB6F1 stressed males and 29% in the progeny of CBA males.

Animals after exposure with pheromones have also mating effectiveness in 1,3-1,4 times lower than in control males. This may possibly be explained by reduced fertilizing ability of sperm and abnormal sex behavior after action of pheromonal stressors.

Conclusion

Taken together, these data permit the proposal of a mechanism of pheromone action through neuroendocrine changes → stress state → genome destabilization in germ cells → decrease in sperm quality → inhibition of reproductive function of mouse males (Daev, 1983; 1994; 2007). In the case of immune system we have the similar situation. It is possible to consider such genetic destabilization under stress conditions as a part of self-regulation mechanism, which controls population density and changes microevolution rate by modifying the level of genetic diversity in germ cells (Daev, 1994, 2007). It seems that here we have an example of connection between cell's stress, organism's stress and stress at the population level. It may also be assumed that any stressor might lead to similar results in higher organisms with well developed cross-talking between neuro-immuno-endocrine system and genome of their cells.

It is my hope that this paper helps to initiate some perspective research in areas connecting the physiology, neuroendorinology and genetics to study more effectively the common mechanisms of the stress reaction and its evolutionary significance at the level of a single cell, tissue and organ, whole organism and population.

ACKNOWLEDGMENTS

I would like to thank Dr. Sam Rhine (IN, USA) and Alexander Pryor (Cambridge, UK) for correction of the manuscript. The research in the Animal Genetics laboratory of the Department of Genetics & Breeding was supported in part by RFBR grant N 09-04-00693.

REFERENCES

[1] Archer J. E. (1969). Adrenocortical response to olfactory stimuli in male mice. *J. Mammal., V.50,* 836-841 (in Rus.).

[2] Arief'ev, A. A., Daev, E. V., Kaidanov, L. Z., Lopatina, N. G. & Novikov, S. N. (1986). Anomalous spermatogenesis in laboratory mice after the influence of compounds contained in urine of sexually mature males. *Academiia nauk SSSR. Doklady Biological Sciences, V.291*, 1257-1259.

[3] Aron, C. (1979). Mechanisms of control of the reproductive function by olfactory stimuli in female mammals. *Physiol. Reviews, V.59,* 229-284.

[4] Bernard, C. (1878). *Les phe´nome`nes de la vie.* vol. 1. p 879. Librairie J. B. Baillie`re et Fils, Paris, France.

[5] Belyaev, D. K. (1979). Destabilizing selection as factor in domestication. *Journal of Heredity, V.70 (5)*, 301-308.

[6] Borodin, P. M. & Belyaev, D. K. (1980). Influence of stress on the frequency of crossing-over in the second chromosome of the house mouse. *Academiia nauk SSSR. Doklady Biological Sciences. 253 (1-6)*, 322-323.

[7] Borodin, P. M. & Belyaev, D. K. (1986). Influence of emotional stress on the frequency of crossing-over in the first chromosome of the house mouse. *Academiia nauk SSSR. Doklady Biological Sciences, V.286, (3).* 726-728.

[8] Bruce, H. M. (1959). An exteroceptive block to pregnancy in the mouse. *Nature, V. 184,* 105.

[9] Cannon, W. B. (1932). In: *The Wisdom of the Body.* p 24. W. W. Norton, New York.

[10] Cannon, W. (1935). Stresses and strains of homeostasis. *Am.J.Med.Sci., V.89,* 1-14.

[11] Cavaggioni, A., Mucignat, C. & Tirindelli, R. (1999). Pheromone signalling in the mouse: role of urinary proteins and vomeronasal organ. *Archives Italiennes de Biologie, V.137,* 193-200.

[12] Cocke, R., Moynihan, J. A., Cohen, N., Grota, L. J. & Ader, R. (1993). Exposure to conspecific alarm chemosignals alters immune responses in BALB/c mice. *Brain Behav. Immun. V.7.* 36-46.

[13] Daev, E. V. (1994). Pheromonal regulation of genetic processes: research on the house mouse (*Mus musculus* L.). *Russian Journal of Genetics, Vol. 30, N. 8,* 964 - 970.

[14] Daev, E. V. (2007). Stress, Chemocommunication, and the Physiological Hypothesis of Mutation. *Russian Journal of Genetics, Vol. 43, No. 10,* 1082–1092.

[15] Daev, E. V. (1982). Meiotic abnormalities in young males of the house mouse (*Mus musculus* L.) under the effect of exogenous metabolites of sexually mature animals . *Zool. Journal. [Zoologicheskii` journal], V. 61, N 8,* 1269-1271 (russ).

[16] Daev, E. V. (1983). *Action of exogenous metabolites on cytogenetic characteristics of spermatogenesis and reproductive function of immature males of house mouse.* Ph.D. thesis, Leningrad: VIR, 1-16 (in Rus.).

[17] Daev, E. V. (2003). Induction of Dominant Lethals in Progeny of CBA Male Mice after Pheromonal Action. *Russian Journal of Genetics, V. 39, N. 10,* 1347-1352.

[18] Daev, E. V., Dukelskaya, A. V. (2003). The Female Pheromone 2,5-Dimethylpyrazine Induces Sperm-Head Abnormalities in Male CBA Mice. *Russian Journal of Genetics, V. 39, N. 7,* 969-974.

[19] Daev, E. V., Dukelskaya, A. V. (2005). Induction of meiotic disturbances in spermatocytes I by pheromones as an inhibiting mechanism of male reproductive function in house mice. *Tsitologiia, V. 47 (6),* 505-509 (russ).

[20] Daev, E. V., Sverdlova, O. L. (2002). Analysis for Pheromone-Induced Cytogenetic Disturbances Depending on Major Urinary Proteins of Laboratory Mouse Males. *Russian Journal of Genetics, 38 (2),* 132-137.

[21] Daev, E. V., Tsapigina, R. I. & Lopatina, N. G. (1988). Frequency of dominant lethals in progeny of young house mouse (Mus musculus L.) after exposure to excretory products of adult males of the same species. *Russian Journal of Genetics, 24,* 2015-2021.

[22] Daev, E. V., Vorob'ev, K. V., Shustova, T. I., Zimina, S. A. & Samotokin, M. B. (2000). Genotype-specific changes in functional parameters of immunocompetent cells in laboratory male mice under conditions of pheromonal stress. *Russian Journal of Genetics, V.36 (8),* 872-876.

[23] Daev, E. V., Dukel'skaya, A. V., Kazarova, V. E. & Filkina, Ya. A. (2007). Effect of the estrus cycle stage on sensitivity to pheromone 2,5-dimethylpyrazine in the house mouse Mus musculus. *Journal of Evolutionary Biochemistry and Physiology, 43 (6),* 573-578.

[24] Dlusen, D. E., Ramirez, V. D., Carter, C. S. & Getz L. L. (1981). Male vole urine changes luteinizing hormone releasing hormone and norepinephrine in female olfactory bulb. *Science, V.212,* 573-575.

[25] Doty R. L. (1986). Reproductive endocrine influences upon olfactory perception: A Current Perspective. *Journal of Chemical Ecology, Vol. 12, No.2,* 497-511.

[26] Dudley, C. A., Rajendren, G. & Moss, R. L. (1996). Signal processing in the vomeronasal system: modulation of sexual behavior in the female rat. *Crit. Rev. Neurobiol., V.10,* 265-290.

[27] Ehling, U. Я., Machemer, L., Busselmaier, W. et al. (1978). Standard protocol for the dominant lethal test on male mice. *Arch. Toxicol., V. 39,* 173-185.

[28] Havlicek, J. & Roberts, S. C. (2009). MHC-correlated mate choice in humans: A review. *Psychoneuroendocrinology, V.34 (4),* 497-512.

[29] Jechura, T. J. & Lee, T. M.. (2004). Ovarian hormones influence olfactory cue effects on reentrainment in the diurnal rodent, Octodon degus. *Hormones and Behavior, 46 (3),* 349-355.

[30] Jemiolo B. & Novotny M. (1994). Inhibition of sexual maturation in juvenile female and male mice by chemosignal of female origin. *Physiol. & Behav., V.55,* 519-522.

[31] Kerkis Yu.Ya. (1940). Physiologic changes inside cell as a reason of mutation process [Physiologicheskie izmeneniya v kletke kak prichina mutatzionnogo processa]. *Successes of modern biology [Uspehi sovremennoi` biologii], N 1,* 344-350 (in Rus.).

[32] Koyama S. (2004). Primer effects by conspecific odors in house mice: A new perspective in the study of primer effects on reproductive activities. *Hormones and Behavior, 46 (3),* 303-310.

[33] Lawton, A. D. & Whitsett, J. M. (1979). Inhibition of sexual maturation by a urinary pheromone in male prairie deer mice. *Horm. Behav., V.13,* 128-138.

[34] Lee, A. K. & McDonald, I. R. (1985). Stress and population regulation in small mammals. *Oxford Rev. Reprod. Biol., V.7,* 261-304.

[35] Lobashev, M. E. (1947). Physiological (Paranecrotic) Hypothesis of the Mutation Process. *Bulletin of Leningrad State University* [*Vestnik Leningradskogo universiteta*], *№8,* 10-29 (in Rus.).

[36] Lopatina, N. G., Ponomarenko, V. V. & Smirnova, G. P. (1975). Hypothesis of nerve regulation of hereditary information realizing process . In: *Problems of higher nerve activity and neurophysiology.* Leningrad: Nauka, 107-121 (in Rus.).

[37] Macario, A. J. L. & Macario, E. C. (2005). Sick Chaperones, Cellular Stress, and Disease. *N. Engl. J. Med. V.353,* 1489-501.

[38] Maruniak, J., Coquelin, A. & Bronson, F. H. (1978). The release of LH in male mice in response to female urinary odors: characteristics of the response in young males. *Biol. Reprod., V.18,* 251-255.

[39] Moynihan, J. A., Karp, J. D., Cohen, N. & Cocke, R. (1994). Alterations in interleukin-4 and antibody production following pheromone exposure: role of glucocorticoids. *J. Neuroimmunol. V.54.* 51-58.

[40] Parsons, P. A. (1992). Fluctuating asymmetry: a biological monitor of environmental and genomic stress. *Heredity, 68,* Pt 4/-

[41] Ponomarenko, V. V. (1976). Genetics of behavior. In: *Physiological genetics.* Leningrad: Medicine. 350-382 (in Rus.).

[42] Rekwot, P. I., Ogwub, D., Oyedipe E. O. & Sekoni, V. O. (2001). The role of pheromones and biostimulation in animal reproduction. *Animal Reproduction Science. 65.* 157–170.

[43] Rice, P. L. (1987). *Stress And Health: Principles And Practice For Coping And Wellness.* Pacific Grove, CA: Brooks/Cole Publishing Company, 18-19.

[44] Selye, H. (1936). A syndrome produced by diverse nocuous agents. *Nature (USA), 138,* 32.

[45] Selye, H. (1946). The general adaptation syndrome and the diseases of adaptation. *J. Clin. Endocrinol., 6,* 117–230.

[46] Selye, H. (1950). *The physiology and pathology of exposure to stress.* Montreal: Acta Med. Publ. 203.

[47] Selye, H. (1973). The evolution of the stress concept. *Am. Sci., V.61(6),* 692-699

[48] Selye H. (1974). *Stress without Distress.* New American Library: New York.

[49] Seredenin, S. B., Durnev, A. D. & Vedernikov, A. A. (1980). Effect of emotional stress on the frequency of chromosome aberrations in the bone marrow cells of mice. *Bulletin of Experimental Biology and Medicine* [*Byulleten Eksperimentalnoi Biologii i Meditsiny*], *V.89(7),* 91-92.

[50] Selye, H. (1979). The stress concept and some of its implications. In: *Human Stress and Cognition: An Information Processing Approach.* V. Hamilton and D. M. Warburton (ed.).Wiley, New York.

[51] Singer, A. G., Clancy, A. N., Macrides, F., Agosta, W. C. & Bronson, F. H. (1988). Chemical properties of a female mouse pheromone that stimulates gonadotropin secretion in males. *Biol. Reprod., V.38,* 193-199.

[52] Southwick, C. H. (1959). Eosinophil response of C57Br mice to behavioral disturbance. *Ecology, V.40,* 156-157.

[53] Tsapigina, R. I. (1972). *Studying of role of central nerve system in cytogenetic processes regulation by method of conditioned reflex.* Ph.D. thesis. Leningrad, 1-16 (in Rus.).

[54] Tsapigina, R. I., Daev, E. V. & Novikov, S. N. (1979). Action of exogenous metabolites on cell division process in germ tissue of laboratory animals. In: *Study of biological action of anthropogenic factors, which polluted lakes.* Irkutsk, 157-162 (in Rus.).

[55] von Borell, E. H. (2001). The biology of stress and its application to livestock housing and transportation assessment. *J. Anim. Sci., 79(E. Suppl.),* E260–E267.

[56] Teuchert-Noodt, G. (1992). Stress-induced alterations in both peripheral and central nerve system: environmental stress and the mesoprefrontal dopamine projection. *Bielefelder Ökologische Beiträge, Band 6,* 69-70.

[57] Rauschenbach, I. Yu., Khlebodarova, T. M., Sukhanova, M. G. et. al. (2000). There is uniform genetic control of different stress-reaction links. In: *Modern concepts of evolutionary genetics.* V.Shumny and A. L. Markel (ed.). Novosibirsk:IC&G, 86-94 (in Rus.).

[58] Wuensch, K. L. (1979). Adrenal hypertrophy in mice following exposure to crowded males odors. *Behav. Neural Biol., V.27(2),* 222-226.

In: Neuroendocrinology Research Developments
Editor: N. S. Penkava and L.R. Haight, pp.133-142
ISBN: 978-1-60876-983-4
© 2010 Nova Science Publishers, Inc.

Chapter 8

THE STATE OF ART ON THE IMMUNE AND NEUROENDOCRINE FUNCTIONS OF CORTICOTROPHIN-RELEASING HORMONE AND UROCORTIN IN INVERTEBRATES

Enzo Ottaviani and Davide Malagoli
Department of Animal Biology, University of Modena and Reggio Emilia,
Via Campi, 213/D, 41100 Modena, Italy

ABSTRACT

Corticotrophin-releasing hormone (CRH) and urocortin (UCN) are well-known peptides whose functions, in mammals, include different aspects of stress-response, such as the activation of the hypothalamus-hypophysis-adrenal gland axis and the reduction of the appetite, respectively. Expecially in vertebrates, numerous sequences are now available for CRH, UCN and their paralogs that are collectively dubbed as CRH-family members. Together with a better understanding of their functions, the increased availability of CRH-family member sequences allowed sequence comparison and the consequent flourishing of evolutive hypotheses. Even if problems and conundrums still persist about the origin and the diversification of the CRH-family components, there is growing evidence that this family of peptides, the related receptors and their binding proteins evolved before the split of deuterostomian and protostomian lineages. In invertebrates, CRH-like molecules have been isolated and described mainly in insects whereas no sequence information have so far been derived from other models, such as molluscs or annelids. In insects, the molecules considered as the most probable paralogs of vertebrate CRH-family members are usually ascribed to the group of diuretic hormones. However, in numerous invertebrate taxa, morphological, functional and molecular data indicate the presence of CRH and/or UCN orthologs in circulating and immune-related cell types, that we refer to as immunocytes. Here we review the evidence connecting the presence of invertebrate CRH- and UCN-like peptides to the immune and neuroendocrine system, suggesting that their involvement with the stress response is probably one of their most primitive characteristic, despite the different anatomical scenario within which the stress response occurs in divergent metazoan taxa.

Keywords: CRH; UCN; evolution; HPA-axis; invertebrate stress response

INTRODUCTION

Since its discovery in 1981 (Vale et al.,1981), corticotrophin-releasing hormone (CRH) has been subjected to extensive studies that demonstrated its involvement in the adjustment of stress-related behaviours (Silberstein et al., 2009) and immunity (Bamberger and Bamberger, 2000). More precisely, in vertebrates CRH is well-known as the activator of hypothalamus-hypophysis-adrenal glands (HPA) axis (Chrousos, 1995), but several evidence suggested a possible role for CRH in other fundamental functions. Beside the central nervous system (CNS), the CRH can be retrieved in the human placenta, the ovary, the endometrium, in peripheral nerves and in inflammated tissues (Bamberger and Bamberger, 2000). CRH is the first example of a protein family that, in mammals, include also urocortin (UCN), UCN2 and UCN3. In bony fish, the paralogue of UCN is considered urotensin I (Vaughan et al., 1995; Lovejoy and Jahan, 2006), whereas in the frog *Phyllomedusa sauvagei* the still enigmatic peptide, sauvagine, has been retrieved (Montecucchi et al., 1980).

CRH and UCN are molecules that frequently appear related to both neural and immune response (Bamberger and Bamberger, 2000), representing one of the most clear example of the overlap existing between the mediators shared by neuroendocrine and immune systems. By interpreting these findings from an evolutive perspective, one of the Author of the present chapter advanced the hypothesis that immune and neuroendocrine system may have a common evolutive root, that's to say that in the ancestors of complex pluricellular organisms the edge between immune and neuroendocrine components was quite blurred, if not indistinguishable (Ottaviani and Franceschi, 1996). This hypothesis found support in experiments performed on molluscan circulating and phagocytic cells (immunocytes), in which the mediators of HPA axis seem to be all present and act in the same order observed in mammals (Ottaviani and Franceschi, 1997).

Interestingly, genetic data indicate that in insects are present only CRH paralogs, known as diuretic hormones (DHs) and essentially connected to water and salt balancing. This has led to the hypothesis that CRH have become connected to the HPA axis only in vertebrates and after the evolution of HPA axis (Lovejoy and Jahan, 2006). This second hypothesis still awaits for genetic and functional evidence in molluscs and annelids, collectively labelled as lophotrocozoan invertebrates (Adoutte et al., 2000), and presents some important drawbacks in the highly different organization of CRH and DH genes and the small molecular size of the mature peptides (Huising and Flick, 2005). However, it is almost established that the CRH system evolved before the split of deuterostomian and protostomian lineages of metazoan (Huising and Flick, 2005; Lovejoy and Jahan, 2006). This conclusion is confirmed by several morphological, functional and genetic evidence relating also to CRH receptors (CRH-R) and the regulating factor, CRH binding protein (CRH-BP).

Within this intriguing and somehow contradictory context, the present reviews aims to summarize morphological and functional data concerning CRH- and UCN-like molecules in invertebrate models, with a special focus on molluscs and annelids, that represent less investigated taxa, from a genetic perspective.

Presence of CRH- and UCN-like Molecules in Invertebrates: Morphological and Genetic Observations

In invertebrates, immunoreactive CRH molecules were found in the CNS of the annelid *Dendrobaena subrubicunda* (Rémy et al., 1982), the insect *Periplaneta americana* (Verhaert et al., 1984), the mollusc *Planorbarius corneus* (Sonetti et al., 1986) and the annelid *Lumbricus terrestris* (Lubics et al., 2003). The presence of these molecules were found not only in the brain but also in other non-nervous tissue. In the pulmonate molluscs *P. corneus* and *Viviparus ater* we detected CRH-like material in the immunocytes and the hemolymph by immunocytochemistry and radio-immuno assay (RIA), respectively (Ottaviani et al., 1990, 1994a). *In situ* hybridization experiments revealed, that immunocytes of *Mytilus galloprovincialis* contain mRNA encoding for CRH-R1 and CRH-R2 (Malagoli et al., 2000). Moreover, a proCRH ortholog was cloned and characterized in the cabbage moth *Mamestra brassicae* (Mb-proCRH) starting from extracts of the hemocyte cell line IZD-MB-0503 (Malagoli et al., 2002).

In insects, a wide family of neuropeptides, defined as DHs, plays an important neuroendocrine role on the excretory system allowing the control of water balance. DHs, found at least in nine species from five insect orders, are considered usually as the paralogs of CRH and UCN, together with urotensin I and sauvagine (Coast, 1998; Furuya et al., 2000). However, several variants of DHs have been identified and it is complex to establish evolutionary relationships (Lovejoy and Jahan, 2006). These peptides are considered CRH paralogs, being relatively similar in terms of sequence and structure to mature vertebrate CRH. Various insect DHs have been described, including *Manduca* -DH, *Locusta*-DH, *Periplaneta*-DH, *Acheta*-DH (see for review, Coast, 1996; Lovejoy and Jahan, 2006). Using antibodies specific for *Locusta*-DH, DH-like molecules were found in the neurons of CNS, in neurohemal sites of *corpus cardiacum*, abdominal nerves, hindgut and endocrine-like cells of the midgut of the blood-feeding bug *Rhodnius prolixus* (Te Brugge et al., 1999). Even if DHs, despite the differences in sequence similarity, are frequently described as the obvious correspondent of vertebrate CRH (Lovejoy and Jahan, 2006), the Mb-proCRH we have cloned (GenBank accession no. AY079100) present a higher degree of sequence similarity with vertebrate CRH than with lepidopteran DH (Figure 1), and should therefore considered as a good CRH ortholog candidate. A BLAST search (Zhang et al., 2000) performed on July, 30 2009, in nr database (i.e., all GenBank+EMBL+DDBJ+PDB sequences, but no EST, STS, GSS, environmental samples or phase 0, 1 or 2 HTGS sequences) using Mb-proCRH as template and standard research parameters, finds *Astatotilapia burtoni* CRH (GenBank accession no. EF363131.1) and *Tilapia mossambica* proCRH (GenBank accession no. AJ011835.1) as first hits, followed by CRH sequences of several primates, including human (GenBank accession no. BT007453.1). When the BLAST search is performed after aligning Mb-proCRH and the silkworm *Bombyx mori* DH (GenBank accession no. BAAB01018830.1) (Lovejoy and Jahan, 2006) a "No significant similarity found" outcome is obtained. Also when the BLAST search was limited to insect database, no DH was found to be similar to Mb-proCRH. However, despite this absence of sequence similarity, the gene encoding for Mb-proCRH appears to be organized as that of insect DHs, i.e., four exons and three introns (Malagoli et al., 2002; Lovejoy and Jahan, 2006) and not as that of vertebrate CRH (2 exons and 1 intron) (Lovejoy and Jahan, 2006). The discrepancy between the observations on DH and that on Mb-CRH might be attributed to a different approach in sequence comparison. DHs are usually compared to the mature form of mammalian CRH (41 aminoacids) (Lovejoy and Jahan, 2006), while Mb-proCRH is always compared to vertebrate CRH precursor (Malagoli et al., 2002). The first approach is more strictly focalized on the active component of the mammalian molecule, but it has to be underlined that also the precursor proCRH has been demonstrated to have biological activity in *in vitro* and *in vivo* model of vertebrates (Castrol et al., 1995; Morrison et al., 1995; Malagoli et al., 2004).

With regards the presence and distribution of UCN, scanty data are available in invertebrates. UCN-like material was evidenced in the ventral ganglia of the annelid *L. terrestris* (Lubics et al., 2003), in the cerebral ganglia of the gastropod *Aplysia californica* (Gonzalez et al., 1991, 1992) and in the neurons of pedal ganglia, microglial cells and immunocytes of the bivalve mollusc *M. galloprovincialis* (Malagoli et al., 2007).

Immune and Neuroendocrine Functions of CRH- and UCN-Like Molecules in Invertebrates

The fact that CRH-like and, to a lesser extent, UCN-like molecules are present in different tissues of various invertebrate species, suggests that these two molecules have been conserved during evolution, at least in terms of structure. In mammals, the presence of CRH in lymphocytes turned out to be due to cross-reactivity of anti-CRH antibody with UCN (Bamberger et al., 1998). However, it is interesting to note that no co-localization of UCN- and CRH-like material was found in the neural cells of *L. terrestris* (Lubics et al., 2003) and *M. gallloprovincialis* (Malagoli et al., 2007). If we admit the existence of both CRH and UCN in invertebrates, a question arises relatively to their function. It is well known that in vertebrates CRH and UCN are involved in important immune and neuroendocrine responses. More precisely, it has been suggested that UCN plays a redundant role in activating the HPA-axis, and its role would become evident only as a consequence of a reduced availability of CRH (Bamberger and Bamberger, 2000). In periphery, even though UCN may reduce perfusion pressure in inflammated sites (Torpy et al., 1999), CRH and UCN are usually considered as pro-inflammatory molecules (Zhang and Li, 2009). A similar involvement of CRH- and UCN-like molecules in stress and immunity does occur also in invertebrates?

As mentioned above, the CRH paralogs, DHs, are involved in insect diuresis and are of peculiar importance in hematophagous insects, in which a very rapid diuresis finalized to the elimination of exceeding water and salts after the ingestion of big amount of blood is necessary (Coast, 1996). Coast (2009) reports that in bugs of the genus *Rhodnius* and in mosquitoes, the neurohormones acting on the Malpighian tubules have a dominant role in the control of ionic homeostasis. A different frame is detected in vertebrates where the role of CRH in controlling the body fluid balance remains unclear. In this context, a relationship between CRH secretion and the stimulation of the lateral parabrachial nucleus in controlling thirst and sodium appetite has been reported in rats (De Castro e Silva et al., 2006).

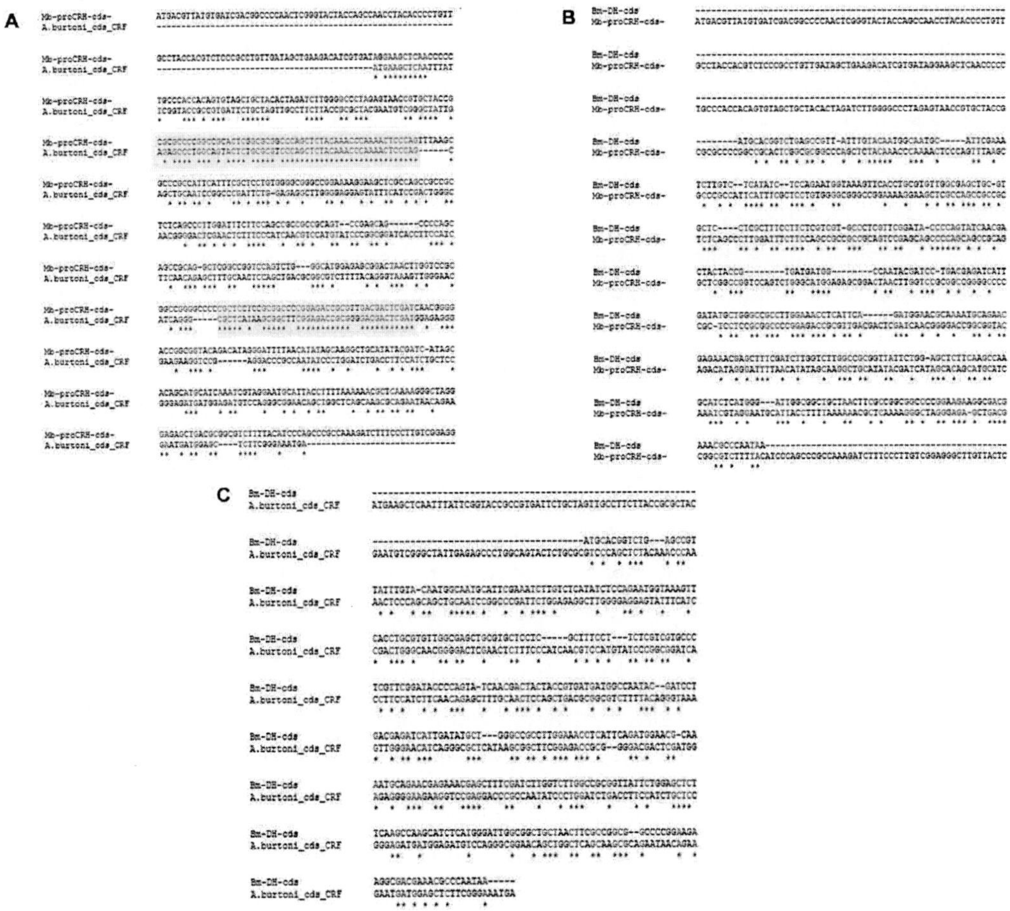

Figure 1. Comparison through Clustal W algorithm (Thomposn et al., 1994) of the coding sequences of Mb-proCRH (GenBank accession no. AY079100) (Mb-proCRH-cds), *A. burtoni* CRH (GenBank accession no. EF363131.1) (A.burtoni_cds_CRF) and *B. mori* DH 31 (GenBank accession no. NM_001130907) (Bm-DH-cds). (A) The high degree of similarity between *M. brassicae* and *A. burtoni* proCRH coding sequences is demonstrated by the highlighted stretches (minimal length 40 nucleotides; similarity between 82 and 90%). These highly similar regions were not found neither by comparing (B) Mb-proCRH with *B. mori* DH 31 nor by comparing (C) *A. burtoni* CRH with *B. mori* DH 31.

While in insects DHs are connected to water balancing, in other invertebrate models, CRH- and UCN-like molecules have been related to the immune and neuroendocrine responses. In molluscs, CRH-like molecules have been demonstrated to be involved in immune-related functions such as chemotaxis and phagocytosis (Genedani et al., 1994; Ottaviani et al., 1994) as well as in stress response (see for review Ottaviani and Franceschi, 1996). Chemotaxis, a nonrandom-type locomotion that allows the cells to move toward a recognized chemoattractant, was stimulated by human CRH in molluscan immunocytes (Genedani et al., 1994). CRH has been reported to inhibit human granulocyte and *Mytilus edulis* immunocyte motility in a stereospecific manner (Stefano et al., 1993), whereas it can also stimulate human monocyte locomotion (Genedani et al., 1992). When the chemoattractant is a particulate substance, such as bacteria, chemotaxis may be followed by engulfment and phagocytosis. The incubation of the molluscan immunocytes with bacteria showed that the cells were able to engulf bacteria and the phagocytic activity was increased in the presence of human CRH (Ottaviani et al., 1994b). As far as the role of CRH-like molecules during the neuroendocrine response of invertebrates, it should be remarked here that several data suggest that, beside CRH, also other molecular mediators of stress response have been conserved during evolution (Ottaviani et al., 2007). In vertebrates, CRH intervenes in stress response allowing the body to cope with a variety of agents threatening life. This fundamental defense mechanism responsible of the soma integrity appears to have been maintained during evolution, remaining remarkably similar in vertebrates and invertebrates. In particular, we have found in molluscs the main factors involved also in vertebrate stress response, including CRH (see for review Ottaviani and Franceschi, 1996). Human CRH is able to induce the release of biogenic amines as well as the release of adrenocortocotropic hormone (ACTH)-like molecules from molluscan immunocytes (Ottaviani et al., 1992; 1993). On the whole, these findings depict an ancestral type of stress response, similar to the vertebrate CRH-ACTH-biogenic amines axis. However, while in vertebrates this molecular axis is anatomically distributed within the HPA-axis, in molluscs the whole cascade seem to be represented within the immunocytes. This concentration of mediators in a single cell type should not appear heterodox, because also human lymphocytes have already been described as immune-neuroendocrine cells (Blalock and Smith, 1985).

With regards the involvement of UCN-like molecules in invertebrate stress response, we have found in *M. galloprovincialis* that high salinity induced a significant increase of the UCN immunoreactivity in immunocytes, but not in neurons (Malagoli et al., 2007). It is interesting to underline that microglial cells, that contain UCN-like material in control animals, were not found after application of high-salinity stress, suggesting that those cells leave the ganglia as a reaction to the stressful experimental condition.

CONCLUSION

Despite CRH has been isolated almost 30 years ago, and several CRH-family members have now been described in vertebrates and invertebrates, several questions persist on the distribution, structure and function of these molecules outside mammals. The existence of CRH-like molecules in metazoans before the split of deuterostomian and protostomian lineage is now unquestioned. It is interesting to observe that by one side functional, morphological and some molecular data, collected primarily in molluscs, point towards the involvement of CRH- and UCN-like molecules in invertebrate stress-response. On the other side, genetic and *in silico* predictions, link invertebrate CRH paralogs (i.e., insect DHs) to water and saline balance (Figure 2). Genetic divergence of CRH-family genes and the absence of reliable molecular databases from annelids and molluscs make impossible to draw a definitive conclusion, at present. Stress response is reasonably as ancient as diuretic balance, therefore further functional and genetic evidence is eagerly awaited in order to clarify the still elusive history of one of the most important and ancient family of metazoan peptides.

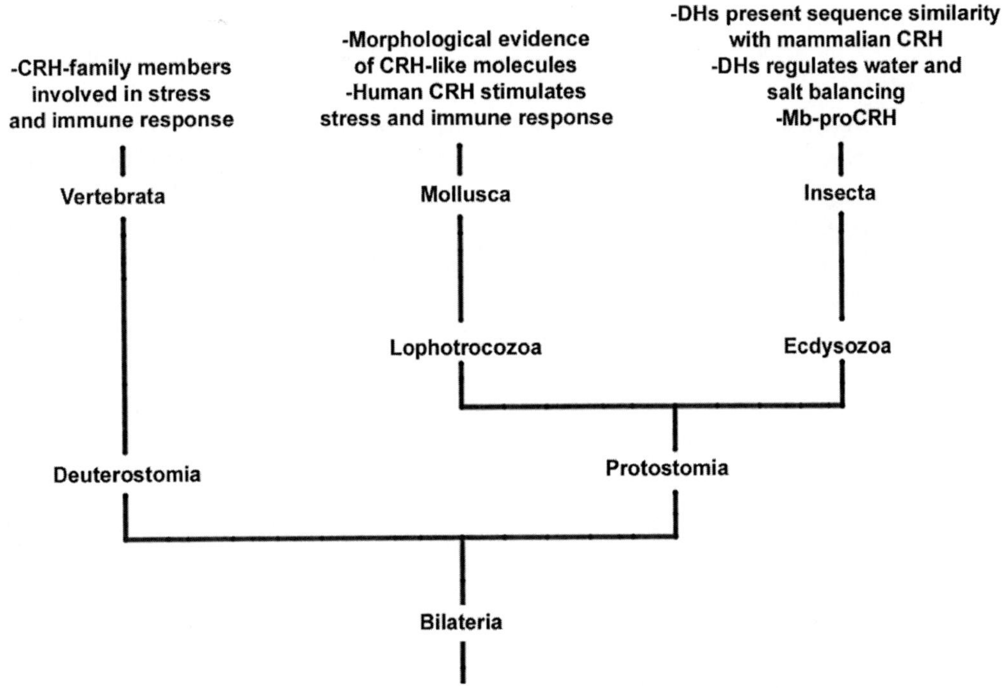

Figure 2 Schematic representation of bilaterian metazoan phylogeny evidencing the principal characteristics and functions of CRH-family members in the three fundamental clades, Deuterostomia, Lophotrcozoa and Ecdysozoa. The numerous other taxa included in the three clades but not discussed in the present review have been excluded on purpose. Annelids are included, together with molluscs, among lophotrocozoans (Adoutte et al., 2000).

REFERENCES

Adoutte, A; Balavoine, G; Lartillot, N; Lespinet, O; Prud'homme, B; de Rosa, R. The new animal phylogeny: reliability and implications. *Proc. Natl. Acad. Sci. U. S. A.*, 2000, 97, 4453–4456.

Bamberger, CM; Bamberger, AM. The peripheral CRH/urocortin system. *Ann. N. Y. Acad. Sci.*, 2000, 917, 290-296.

Bamberger, CM; Wald, M; Bamberger, AM; Ergün, S; Beil, FU; Schulte, HM. Human lymphocytes produce urocortin, but not corticotropin-releasing hormone. *J. Clin. Endocrinol. Metab.* 1998, 83, 708-711.

Castrol, MG; Tomasec, P; Morrison, E; Murray, CA; Hodge, P; Blanning, P; Linton, E; Lowry, PJ; Lowenstein, PR. Mitogenic effects and nuclear localisation of procorticotrophin-releasing hormone expressed within stably transfected fibroblast cells (CHO-K1). *Mol. Cell. Endocrinol.*, 1995, 107, 17-27.

Coast, GM. Neuropeptides implicated in the control of diuresis in insects. *Peptides*, 1996, 17, 327-336.

Coast, GM. The influence of neuropeptides on Malpighian tubule writhing and its significance for excretion. *Peptides*, 1998, 19, 469-480.

Coast, GM. Neuroendocrine control of ionic homeostasis in blood-sucking insects. *J. Exp. Biol.*, 2009, 212 (Pt 3): 378-386.

Chrousos, GP. The hypothalamic-pituitary-adrenal axis and immune-mediated inflammation. *N. Engl. J. Med.*, 1995, 332, 1351–1362.

De Castro e Silva, E; Fregoneze, JB; Johnson, AK. Corticotropin-releasing hormone in the lateral parabrachial nucleus inhibits sodium appetite in rats. *Am. J. Physiol. Regul. Integr. Comp. Physiol.*, 2006, 290, R1136-1141.

Furuya, K; Harper, MA; Schegg, KM; Schooley DA. Isolation and characterization of CRF-related diuretic hormones from the whitelined sphinx moth *Hyles lineata. Insect Biochem. Mol. Biol.*, 2000, 30, 127-133.

Genedani, S; Bernardi, M; Baldini, MG; Bertolini, A. Influence of CRF and alpha-MSH on the migration of human monocytes in vitro. *Neuropeptides*, 1992, 23, 99-102.

Genedani, S; Bernardi, M; Ottaviani, E; Franceschi, C; Leung, MK; Stefano, GB. Differential modulation of invertebrate hemocyte motility by CRF, ACTH, and its fragments. *Peptides*, 1994, 15, 203-206.

Gonzalez, GC; Martinez-Padron, M; Ko, D; Lukowiak, K; Lederis, K. Urotensin I-like immunoreactivity in the central nervous system of *Aplysia californica*. Peptides 1991, 12, 787-793.

González, GC; Martinez-Padrón, M; Lederis, K; Lukowiak, K. Distribution and coexistence of urotensin I and urotensin II peptides in the cerebral ganglia of *Aplysia californica. Peptides*, 1992, 13, 695-703.

Huising, MO; Flik, G. The remarkable conservation of corticotropin-releasing hormone (CRH)-binding protein in the honeybee (*Apis mellifera*) dates the CRH system to a common ancestor of insects and vertebrates. *Endocrinology*, 2005, 146, 2165-2170.

Lovejoy, DA; Jahan, S. Phylogeny of the corticotropin-releasing factor family of peptides in the metazoa. *Gen. Comp. Endocrinol.*, 2006, 146, 1-8.

Lubics, A; Reglodi, D; Szelier, M; Lengvári, I; Kozicz, T. Comparative distribution of urocortin- and CRF-like immunoreactivities in the nervous system of the earthworm *Lumbricus terrestris. Peptides*, 2003, 24, 205-213.

Malagoli, D; Di Paolo, I; Ottaviani, E. Presence of and stress-related changes in urocortin-like molecules in neurons and immune cells from the mussel *Mytilus galloprovincialis. Peptides*, 2007, 28, 1545-1552.

Malagoli, D; Franchini, A; Ottaviani, E. Synergistic role of cAMP and IP(3) in corticotropin-releasing hormone-induced cell shape changes in invertebrate immunocytes. *Peptides*, 2000, 21, 175-182.

Malagoli, D; Mandrioli, M; Ottaviani, E. Cloning and characterisation of a procorticotrophin-releasing hormone in the IZD-MB-0503 immunocyte line from the insect *Mamestra brassicae. Peptides*, 2002, 23, 1829-1836.

Malagoli, D; Mandrioli, M; Ottaviani, E. ProCRH in the teleost *Ameiurus nebulosus*: gene cloning and role in LPS-induced stress response. *Brain Behav. Immun.*, 2004, 18, 451-457.

Montecucchi, PC; Anastasi, A; de Castiglione, R, Erspamer, V. Isolation and amino acid composition of sauvagine. An active polypeptide from methanol extracts of the skin of the South American frog *Phyllomedusa sauvagei. Int. J. Pept. Protein Res.*, 1980, 16, 191-199.

Morrison, E; Tomasec, P; Linton, EA; Lowry, PJ; Lowenstein, PR; Castro, MG. Expression of biologically active procorticotrophin-releasing hormone (proCRH) in stably transfected CHO-K1 cells: characterization of nuclear proCRH. *J. Neuroendocrinol.*, 1995, 7, 263-272.

Ottaviani, E; Caselgrandi, E; Franchini, A; Franceschi, C. CRF provokes the release of norepinephrine by hemocytes of *Viviparus ater* (Gastropoda, Prosobranchia): further evidence in favour of the evolutionary hypothesis of the mobile immune-brain. *Biochem. Biophys. Res. Commun.*, 1993, 193, 446-452

Ottaviani, E; Caselgrandi, E; Petraglia, F; Franceschi, C. Stress response in the freshwater snail *Planorbarius corneus* (L.) (Gastropoda, Pulmonata): interaction between CRF, ACTH, and biogenic amines. *Gen. Comp. Endocrinol.*, 1992, 87, 354-360.

Ottaviani, E; Franceschi, C. The neuroimmunology of stress from invertebrates to man. *Prog. Neurobiol.*, 1996, 48, 421-440.

Ottaviani, E; Franceschi, C. The invertebrate phagocytic immunocyte: clues to a common evolution of immune and neuroendocrine systems. *Immunol. Today*, 1997, 18, 169-174.

Ottaviani, E; Franchini, A; Caselgrandi, E; Cossarizza, A; Franceschi, C. Relationship between corticotropin-releasing factor and interleukin-2: evolutionary evidence. *FEBS Lett.*, 1994a, 351, 19-21.

Ottaviani, E; Franchini, A; Fontanili, P. The effect of Corticotropin-releasing factor and pro-opiomelanocortin-derived peptides on the phagocytosis of molluscan hemocytes. *Experientia*, 1994b, 50, 857-859.

Ottaviani, E; Malagoli, D; Franceschi, C. Common evolutionary origin of the immune and neuroendocrine systems: from morphological and functional evidence to *in silico* approaches. *Trends Immunol.*, 2007, 28, 497-502.

Ottaviani, E; Petraglia, F; Montagnani, G; Cossarizza, A; Monti, D; Franceschi, C. Presence of ACTH and beta-endorphin immunoreactive molecules in the freshwater snail *Planorbarius corneus* (L.) (Gastropoda, Pulmonata) and their possible role in phagocytosis. *Regul Pept.*, 1990, 27, 1-9.

Rémy, C; Tramu, G; Dubois MP. Immunohistological demonstration of a CRF-like material in the central nervous system of the annelid *Dendrobaena. Cell Tissue Res.*, 1982, 227, 569-575.

Silberstein, S; Vogl, AM; Bonfiglio, JJ; Wurst, W; Holsboer, F; Arzt, E; Deussing, JM; Refojo, D. Immunology, signal transduction, and behavior in hypothalamic-pituitary-adrenal axis-related genetic mouse models. *Ann. N. Y. Acad. Sci.*, 2009, 1153, 120-130.

Sonetti, D; Vacirca, F; Fasolo, A. Localization of Substance P (SP)-, Neuropeptide Y (NPY)-, and Corticotropin Releasing Factor (CRF)-like immunoreactive cells in the CNS of the freshwater *Planorbis corneus. Neurosci. Lett. Suppl.*, 1986, 26, 322.

Stefano, GB; Smith, EM; Cadet, P; Hughes, TK Jr. HIV gp120 alteration of DAMA and IL-1 alpha induced chemotaxic responses in human and invertebrate immunocytes. *J. Neuroimmunol.*, 1993, 43, 177-184.

Te Brugge, VA; Miksys, SM; Coast, GM; Schooley, DA; Orchard, I. The distribution of a CRF-like diuretic peptide in the blood-feeding bug *Rhodnius prolixus. J. Exp. Biol.*, 1999, 202 (Pt 15), 2017-2027.

Thompson, JD; Higgins, DG; Gibson, TJ. CLUSTAL W: improving the sensitivity of progressive multiple sequence alignment through sequence weighting, position-specific gap penalties and weight matrix choice. *Nucleic Acids Res.*, 1994, 22, 4673-4680.

Torpy, DJ; Webster, EL; Zachman, EK; Aguilera, G; Chrousos, GP. Urocortin and inflammation: confounding effects of hypotension on measures of inflammation. *Neuroimmunomodulation*, 1999, 6, 182-186.

Vale, W; Spiess J; Rivier, C; Rivier, J. Characterization of a 41-residue ovine hypothalamic–peptide that stimulates secretion of corticotropin and betaendorphin. *Science*, 1981, 213, 1394–1397.

Vaughan, J; Donaldson, C; Bittencourt, J; Perrin, MH; Lewis, K; Sutton, S; Chan, R; Turnbull, AV; Lovejoy, D; Rivier, C; Rivier, J; Sawchenko, PE; Vale, W. Urocortin, a mammalian neuropeptide related to fish urotensin I and to corticotropin-releasing factor. *Nature*, 1995, 378, 287-292.

Verhaert, P; Marivoet, S; Vandesande, F; De Loof, A. Localization of CRF immunoreactivity in the central nervous system of three vertebrate and one insect species. *Cell Tissue Res.* 1984, 238, 49-53.

Zhang, R; Li, S (2009). COX-2 as a novel target of CRF family peptides' participating in inflammation. *Biochem. Biophys. Res. Commun.*, 382, 483-485.

Zhang, Z; Schwartz, S; Wagner, L; Miller, W. A greedy algorithm for aligning DNA sequences. *J. Comput. Biol.*, 2000, 7, 203-214.

In: Neuroendocrinology Research Developments
Editor: N. S. Penkava and L.R. Haight, pp.143-150
ISBN: 978-1-60876-983-4
© 2010 Nova Science Publishers, Inc.

Chapter 9

NEONATAL LEPTIN SURGE

Takashi Higuchi*
Department of Integrative Physiology, Faculty of Biomedical Sciences, University of Fukui, Eiheij-cho, Matsuoka, Fukui 910-1193, Japan

ABSTRACT

An under- or over-nutritional intrauterine environment and over-nutrition in early postnatal period is associated with long-term metabolic consequences, including obesity, insulin resistance, and type 2 diabetes in adulthood. At least in rodents, leptin surge in neonatal pups may be involved in mediating this programming. Fetal under-nutrition results in reduced or premature leptin surge and maternal obesity induces exaggerated or premature leptin surge. Administration of leptin to neonatal pups to induce premature or supraphysiologicalleptin surge may cause hypothalamic programming that brings about metabolic abnormality in adulthood. Although there are many problems to be clarified, neonatal leptin surge may be involved in establishing hypothalamic neuronal system that controls food intake and energy expenditure.

INTRODUCTION

Obesity and related metabolic disorders are a major health problem in modern society. Converging lines of evidence from epidemiological and animal model studies indicate that the origins of obesity and related metabolic disorders lie not only in the interaction between genes and traditional adult risk factors, such as unbalanced diet and physical inactivity, but also in the interplay between genes and the embryonic, fetal and early postnatal environment (Taylor and Poston, 2007).An adverse intrauterine environment is associated with long-term metabolic consequences, including obesity, insulin resistance, and type 2 diabetes(Hales and Baker, 1992; Hales and Baker, 2001; Gluckman and Hanson, 2004). On the other hand, intrauterine over-nutrition because of maternal obesity has been linked childhood obesity.

* Phone; 81-776-61-8309, Fax; 81-776-61-8134, E-mail; higuchit@u-fukui.ac.jp

There is apparent association between excessive weight gain in pregnancy and the BMI of the adolescent child (Lowlor et at., 2007; Oken et al., 2009). It is unknown what is the mechanism for the maternal over- or under-nutrition and/or neonatal over-nutrition predisposes offspring to become obese in adults.

The adipose hormone leptin is an important regulator of energy balance. Leptin signal nutritional status and energy storage levels to feeding center in the arcuate nucleus (ARC) of the hypothalamus, through its action on the orexigenic neurons which produce neuropeptide Y (NPY) and agouti related protein (AGRP), and anorexigenic neurons that produce pro-opiomelanocortin (POMC) and cocaine- and amphetamine-regulated transcript (CART), resulting in suppression of food intake and increasing energy expenditure (Schwartz et al., 2000; Morton et al., 2006). Leptin does not play a role to regulate appetite and body weight but a neurotrophic role during the development of the hypothalamus during neonatal critical period (Bouret et al., 2004).

This review highlights the role of leptin as a mediator for metabolic problems in adults programmed by nutritional imbalance in utero and early postnatal life.

Maternal under- or over-Nutrition

The epidemiological association between an adverse intrauterine environment and the later onset of adult metabolic and cardiovascular disorders led to the concept of fetal programming and the fetal origins hypothesis. This hypothesis proposes that unfavorable prenatal environment is thought to trigger adaptations that improve fetal survival or prepare the fetus in expectation of a particular range of postnatal environments. However, these adaptations may later prove to be a disadvantage when the prenatal and postnatal environments are widely discrepant with an over abundance of nutrients (Hales and Baker, 1992; Hales and Baker, 2001; Gluckman and Hanson, 2004). Regardless of whether the maladaptaion theory is correct or not (Speakman, 2007), fetal under-nutrition induces impaired neuroendocrine regulation in which hyperleptinemia, hyperinsulinemia, and insulin and leptin resistance may lead to hyperphagia and obesity during adult life. The animal models closely resemble the clinical and metabolic abnormalities seen in humans with low birth weight have been extensively investigated(Vickers et al., 2000; Yura et al., 2005).

Maternal obesity and/or gestational diabetes in humans may predispose offspring to alftered energy balance and increased adiposity in adulthood (Lowlor et at., 2007; Oken et al., 2009). The pups born to obese mothers have an enhanced risk of becoming obese and developing metabolic syndrome (Guo and Jen, 1995; Levin &Govek, 1998).Maternal over-nutrition exerts an adverse influence on offspring in programming brain appetite and fuel-sensing regulators, which lead to early-onset obesity with metabolic disorders in rats(Chen et al., 2008; Kirk et al., 2009).

Leptin Levels in Neonate

There is a surge plasma levels of leptin during the 2nd postnatal week without correlation with body fat mass in rats (Rayner et al., 1997; Delahaye et al., 2008)and mice (Ahima et al.,

1998). The high level of leptin during the neonatal period is surprising, because this is an important growth phase and it seems counterintuitive to have such a high satiety signal.

With intra uterine under-nutrition, when fed a high-fat diet, develop pronounced weight gain and adiposity. exhibited a premature onset of neonatal leptin surge compared to offspring with intrauterine normal nutrition (Yura et al., 2005). In rats maternal under-nutrition drastically reduces the postnatal surge of plasma leptin(Delahaya et al., 2008). On the other hand, offspring of obese rats display an amplified and prolonged neonatal leptin surge (Kirsh et al., 2009). These results suggest that nutritional environment in the uterus may inversely influence the leptin concentrations in neonatal animals; over-nutrition induces reduced leptin surge and under-nutrition induces exaggerated or premature leptin surge.

The relationship between nutritional status in the uterus and blood leptin levels in neonate is different from humans. There is a strong correlation between leptin levels and neonatal birth weight exist which can be a reflection of the correlation of body fat mass in determining leptin levels in neonate as well (Alexe at al, 2006). The difference may come from the difference in adiposity, because in the human embryo, leptin mainly sourced from developing fat cells (Bajoria et al., 2002). However, adipose tissue is hardly detectable even in newborn pups from obese rat dams (Delahaya et al., 2008).Leptin may come from mother's milk in rats (Walker et al., 2004). Anyhow, the intrauterine nutritional states must be informed to the origin of leptin secretion to modulate leptin surge in neonates.

Exogenous Leptin Treatment in Neonate

Leptin treatment from day 3-13 resulted in normalized caloric intake, locomotor activity, body weight, fat mass and fasting plasma glucose, insulin, and leptin concentrations in programmed offspring in adult life of undernourished mothers who developed all these features on a high-fat diet (Vickers et al., 2005). The sameleptin treatment had no demonstrable effects on the adult female offspring of normally fed mothers (Vickers et al., 2005) but resulted in diet-induced weight gain and related metabolic disorders, including hypreleptinemia and increased total body adiposity (Vickers et at., 2008). Leptin's effect may be modulated by gender as well as by prenatal and postnatal nutritional status.

Neonatal leptin treatment for the first 10 days in rat pups born to normal mothers, programmeshyperleptinemia, hyperinsulinemia, hyprephagia and obesity in adulthood (de Oliveia et al, 2002; Toste et al., 2006). Similar treatment with leptin for the last 10 days also induced similar results (de Oliveira et al., 2002). These results suggest that supraphysiologicalleptin surge or delayed leptin surge also determine the occurrence of long-term metabolic squeal.

Both offspring with intrauterine under-nutrition and neonatallyleptin-treated offspring with intrauterine normal nutrition exhibited an impaired response to leptin administrations and accelerated weight gain with high-fat diet (Yura et al., 2005). They further demonstrated that on a high-fat diet, the body weight of the ob/ob with undernutrition in utero paralleled that of the ob/ob offspring exposed to normal intrauterine nutrition. In contrast early exposure to leptin in the ob/ob offspring exposed normal nutrition in utero reproduced the development of pronounced obesity on a high-fat diet in adulthood (Yura et al., 2008).

Although it is not clear whether the timing or the amplitude of leptin surge is critical for the neonatal programming, these experimental results suggest that abnormal leptin surge plays an essential role in the developmental origins of obesity as a programming signal during the early neonatal period.

Leptin Effect on the Hypothalamus in Neonates

Both offspring with intrauterine undernutrition and neonatallyleptin-treated offspring with intrauterine normal nutrition exhibited an increased density of nerve terminals containing NPY or CART in the paraventricular nucleus (PVN) that receives the downstream leptin signaling from theARC (Yura et al., 2005).

Maternal obesity was linked to reduced hypothalamic NPY and increased POMC mRNA expression. Postnatal over-nutrition of offspring from obese dams amplified these hypothalamic changes (Chen et al., 2008).At weaning, the suppressed orexigenic signals in offspring from obese dams were normalized after overnight fasting, although anorexigenic signaling appeared impaired in these animals. This may contribute to their hyperphagia and faster growth (Chen et al., 2009).

The marked decrease of plasma leptin levels in neonates induced by maternal under-nutrition precedes the diminution of POMC mRNA in the ARC of developing rats (Delahaya et al., 2008). This result is in part in line with the observations indicating that in the ob/ob mutant mice, the absence of endogenous leptin markedly affects both NPY/AgRP and POMC pathways (Bouret et al., 2004). Although they did not observe any detectable modification of NPY, POMC nerve fibers projecting to the PVN is drastically reduced, indicating maternal perinatal under-nutrition seems to preferentially affect the POMC anorexigenic pathway in the rats (Delahaya et al., 2008).

These results suggest that intrauterine under-nutrition and postnatal over-nutrition may affect the organization of the neuron system that produces orexigenic or anorexigenic peptides in the ARC. However, it is not clear whether these changes are a consequence of changes in the offspring's body weight and adiposity-related hormones or they reflect developmental changes in utero or in neonatal period that persist over the long time. Chang et al. has reported that the offspring of dams on a high-fat diet from embryonic day 6 to postnatal day 15 show increased expression of orexigenic peptides, galanin, enkephalin and dynorphin, in the PVN and orexin and melanin-concentrating hormone in the perifornical lateral hypothalamus, without any changes in peptide production in the ARC (Chang et al., 2008). The increased density of these peptide-expressing neurons, evident in newborn offspring as well as postnatal day 15 offspring cross-fostered to dams on the normal chow. They speculate the markedly increased lipids in the blood of the offspring from obese mother may be responsible for the long-term (Chang et al., 2008).

Development of leptin-sensitive projection pathways

While leptin seems to have little effect on food intake during early postnatal period, it affects neuronal activity in the ARC during this phase. Acute peripheral leptin treatment at postnatal day 10 (P10) increased mRNA expression of suppressor of cytokine signaling 3 (a marker of leptin receptor activity), POMC mRNA levels, but decreased NPY mRNA levels in the ARC (Proulx et al., 2002).

Using axonal tracer Dil to label axons of the ARC in mice at various postnatal ages, the ontogeny of projections from the ARC was visualized (Bouret and Simerly, 2004). The neurons of the ARC do not extend axons to the majority of their target nuclei the 2nd week of postnatal life. Arcuate projections extend through the periventricular zone of the hypothalamus to provide inputs to the dorsomedial hypothalamus (DMH) by P6, followed by inputs to the PVN between P8 and P10. Projections from the ARC to the lateral hypothalamic area (LHA) appeared on P12. The pattern of arcuate projections does not achieve their adult-like distribution until P18 (Bouret and Simerly, 2004).

As the postnatal surge in letpin levels coincides with the development of ARC projection, the surge acts as a signal promoting the development of ARC connections to the targets nuclei that are involved in the control of appetite and energy expenditure. Leptin deficiency in ob/ob mice causes a severe, permanent reduction and significant delay in the formation of ARC projections to each target nucleus (Bouret et al., 2004). By comparing projection pathways from the ARC in leptin-deficient (ob/ob) and wild-type mouse pups, leptin deficiency was shown to cause a dramatic reduction in the density of axons emanating from the ARC and innervating the DMH, PVN and LHA (Bouret et al., 2004). Both NPY/AgRP and POMC projections are affected. Leptin treatment in adult ob/ob mice is largely ineffective in reversing innervations pathways, whereas supplementation during the neonatal period fully restores the density of arcuate project to that found wild-type mice (Bouret et al., 2004).

It is tempting to speculate abnormal leptin surge may induce aberrant neuronal organization resulting in metabolic disorder in adulthood, but there is a report that must regarded with caveat. Leptin deficient (ob/ob) mice differ form wild-type mice in the numbers of excitatory and inhibitory synapses and postsynsptic currents onto NPY and POMC neurons. When leptin is delivered systemically to ob/ob mice, the synaptic density rapidly normalizes, and effect detectable within 6 hours, suggesting that structural alterations in the ob/ob hypothalamus do not result from leptin deficiency during development (Pint et al., 2004).

Problems to Be Clarified

There are some problems to be determined in order toestablish the role of neonatal leptin surge in programming the regulation system of metabolism.

1. From where does theleptin surge in rodents come from?
2. How is the nutritional state in the uterus reflected to the neonatal leptin surge?
3. How does leptin surge organize the hypothalamic neurons that are responsible for regulation of food intake and energy expenditure?
4. How does both under- and over-nutritional conditions bring about similar metabolic maladaptation?

If the programming theory by neonatal leptin surge is established and similar leptin surge exists in humans, a new strategy to prevent obesity can be developed.

CONCLUSION

Leptin surge in neonatal rodent pups may reflect nutritional status in the uterus and together with over-nutrition in early postnatal period programmes the regulation system of metabolism resulting in obesity in adults.

REFERENCES

Ahima, R. S., Prabakaran, D., & Flier, J. S. (1998). Postnatal leptin surge and regulation of circadian rhythm of leptin by feeding.Implications for energy homeostasis and neuroendocrine function. *J Clin Invest*, *101*, 1020-1027.

Alexe, D. M., Syridou, G., & Petridou, E. T. (2006).Determinants of early life leptin levels and later life degenerative outcomes.*Clin Med Res*, *4*, 326-335.

Bajoria, R., Sooranna, S. R., Ward, B. S., & Chatterjee, R. (2002). Prospective function of placental leptin at maternal-fetal interface. *Placenta*, *23*, 103-115.

Bouret, S. G., Draper, S. J., & Simerly, R. B. (2004). Trophic action of leptin on hypothalamic neurons that regulate feeding. *Science*, *304*, 108-110.

Bouret, S. G., & Simerly, R. B. (2004). Minireview: Leptin and development of hypothalamic feeding circuits. *Endocrinology*, *145*, 2621-2626.

Chen, H., Simar, D., Lambert, K., Mercier, J., & Morris, M. J. (2008). Maternal and postnatal overnutrition differentially impact appetite regulators and fuel metabolism. *Endocrinology*, *149*, 5348-5356.

Chen, H., Simar, D., & Morris, M. J. (2009). Hypothalamic neuroendocrine circuitry is programmed by maternal obesity: interaction with postnatal nutritional environment. *PLoS One* 4, e6259.

de Oliveira Cravo, C., Teixeira, C. V., Passos, M. C., Dutra, S. C., de Moura, E. G., & Ramos, C. (2002). Leptin treatment during the neonatal period is associated with higher food intake and adult body weight in rats. *HormMetab Res*, *34*, 400-405.

Delahaye, F., Breton, C., Risold, P. Y., Enache, M., Dutriez-Casteloot, I., Laborie, C., Lesage, J., & Vieau, D. (2008). Maternal perinatalundernutrition drastically reduces postnatal leptin surge and affects the development of arcuate nucleus proopiomelanocortin neurons in neonatal male rat pups. *Endocrinology*, *149*, 470-475.

Gluckman, P. D., & Hanson, M. A. (2004). Living with the past: evolution, development, and patterns of disease. *Science*, *305*, 1733-1736.

Guo, F., & Jen, K. L. (1995). High-fat feeding during pregnancy and lactation affects offspring metabolism in rats. *PhysiolBehav*, *57*, 681-686.

Hales, C. N., & Barker, D. J. (1992). Type 2 (non-insulin-dependent) diabetes mellitus: the thrifty phenotype hypothesis. *Diabetologia*, *35*, 595-601.

Hales, C. N., & Barker, D. J. (2001). The thrifty phenotype hypothesis. *Br Med Bull*, *60*, 5-20.

Kirk, S. L., Samuelsson, A. M., Argenton, M., Dhonye, H., Kalamatianos, T., Poston, L., Taylor, P. D., & Coen, C. W. (2009). Maternal obesity induced by diet in rats permanently influences central processes regulating food intake in offspring. *PLoS One*, *4*, e5870.

Lawlor, D. A., Smith, G. D., O'Callaghan, M., Alati, R., Mamun, A. A., Williams, G. M., & Najman, J. M. (2007). Epidemiologic evidence for the fetal overnutrition hypothesis: findings from the mater-university study of pregnancy and its outcomes. *Am J Epidemiol*, *165*, 418-424.

Morton, G. J., Cummings, D. E., Baskin, D. G., Barsh, G. S., & Schwartz, M. W. (2006). Central nervous system control of food intake and body weight. *Nature*, *443*, 289-295.

Oken, E. (2009). Excess gestational weight gain amplifies risks among obese mothers. *Epidemiology*, *20*, 82-83.

Pinto, S., Roseberry, A. G., Liu, H., Diano, S., Shanabrough, M., Cai, X., Friedman, J. M., & Horvath, T. L. (2004). Rapid rewiring of arcuate nucleus feeding circuits by leptin. *Science*, *304*, 110-115.

Proulx, K., Richard, D., & Walker, C. D. (2002). Leptin regulates appetite-related neuropeptides in the hypothalamus of developing rats without affecting food intake. *Endocrinology*, *143*, 4683-4692.

Rayner, D. V., Dalgliesh, G. D., Duncan, J. S., Hardie, L. J., Hoggard, N., & Trayhurn, P. (1997). Postnatal development of the ob gene system: elevated leptin levels in suckling fa/fa rats. *Am J Physiol*, *273*, R446-50.

Schwartz, M. W., Woods, S. C., Porte, D. J., Seeley, R. J., & Baskin, D. G. (2000). Central nervous system control of food intake. *Nature*, *404*, 661-671.

Speakman, J. R. (2007). A nonadaptive scenario explaining the genetic predisposition to obesity: the "predation release" hypothesis. *Cell Metab*, *6*, 5-12.

Taylor, P. D., & Poston, L. (2007). Developmental programming of obesity in mammals. *Exp Physiol*, *92*, 287-298.

Toste, F. P., de Moura, E. G., Lisboa, P. C., Fagundes, A. T., de Oliveira, E., & Passos, M. C. (2006). Neonatal leptin treatment programmesleptin hypothalamic resistance and intermediary metabolic parameters in adult rats. *Br J Nutr*, *95*, 830-837.

Vickers, M. H., Breier, B. H., Cutfield, W. S., Hofman, P. L., & Gluckman, P. D. (2000). Fetal origins of hyperphagia, obesity, and hypertension and postnatal amplification by hypercaloric nutrition. *Am J PhysiolEndocrinolMetab*, *279*, E83-7.

Vickers, M. H., Gluckman, P. D., Coveny, A. H., Hofman, P. L., Cutfield, W. S., Gertler, A., Breier, B. H., & Harris, M. (2005). Neonatal leptin treatment reverses developmental programming. *Endocrinology*, *146*, 4211-4216.

Vickers, M. H., Gluckman, P. D., Coveny, A. H., Hofman, P. L., Cutfield, W. S., Gertler, A., Breier, B. H., & Harris, M. (2008). The effect of neonatal leptin treatment on postnatal weight gain in male rats is dependent on maternal nutritional status during pregnancy. *Endocrinology*, *149*, 1906-1913.

Walker, C. D., Deschamps, S., Proulx, K., Tu, M., Salzman, C., Woodside, B., Lupien, S., Gallo-Payet, N., & Richard, D. (2004).Mother to infant or infant to mother?Reciprocal regulation of responsiveness to stress in rodents and the implications for humans. *J Psychiatry Neurosci*, *29*, 364-382.

Yura, S., Itoh, H., Sagawa, N., Yamamoto, H., Masuzaki, H., Nakao, K., Kawamura, M., Mogami, H., Ogawa, Y., & Fujii, S. (2008). Neonatal exposure to leptin augments diet-induced obesity in leptin-deficient Ob/Ob mice. *Obesity (Silver Spring)*, *16*, 1289-1295.

Yura, S., Itoh, H., Sagawa, N., Yamamoto, H., Masuzaki, H., Nakao, K., Kawamura, M., Takemura, M., Kakui, K., Ogawa, Y., & Fujii, S. (2005). Role of premature leptin surge in obesity resulting from intrauterine undernutrition. *Cell Metab*, *1*, 371-378.

In: Neuroendocrinology Research Developments
Editor: N. S. Penkava and L.R. Haight, pp.151-191

ISBN: 978-1-60876-983-4
© 2010 Nova Science Publishers, Inc.

Chapter 10

THE NEUROENDOCRINOLOGY OF TESTOSTERONE – SOCIOSEXUAL BEHAVIOR RELATIONS

George T. Taylor**, Joshua Dearborn and Susan Fortenbury
Behavioral Neuroscience, Univ. of Missouri, St. Louis, MO 63121 USA

ABSTRACT

Steroids produced in the periphery have long been of interest to reproductive biologists. The emergence of neuroendocrinology as a dominant subfield of behavioral studies appeared to demote steroids to a lesser status than the exciting neuropeptides that clearly interacted with many regions of the brain. Seminal findings in recent years, however, have propelled the study of steroids back onto center stage. In this chapter we identify the seminal findings and describe why they are revolutionary. These new findings have demonstrated steroids have the capacity to modify the structure and function of brain regions both related to and unrelated to reproduction. The consequences on behavior are likely to be profound. This chapter focuses on one steroid, testosterone, because it occupies a strategic position in the metabolic cascade of the sex steroids. It is a position that can influence the actions of androgens and estrogens, as well as the adrenal precursors of testosterone and the recently identified neurosteroids, on the brain and behavior. We believe future research will reveal testosterone to have behavioral effects extending well beyond those related to reproduction. Still, the massive literature on testosterone – sociosexual behavior provides a solid background on which to begin that work.

* Correspondence concerning this article should be addressed to George T. Taylor, Ph. D. Professor of Psychology & Director of Behavioral Neuroscience, University of Missouri - St. Louis, One University Blvd. St. Louis, MO 63121 U. S. A. Tel: (314) 516-5475; Fax: (314) 516-5392; E-mail: geot@UMSL. edu.

SECTION I. INTRODUCTION

Reproductive function, most notably sexual behavior, has been the meat and potatoes of behavioral endocrinology for over a century. Androgens, and especially testosterone (TS), have been front and center for much of the century.

The first experimental manipulation of the endocrine system often cited in textbooks is of a demonstration of castrated roosters being implanted with testes. The treatment restored the color and size of their combs, as well as fully restored crowing, fighting and sexual behaviors. Later, an aging researcher reported rejuvenation of sexual prowess with an implant of an aqueous solution from crushed testes of experimental animals injected into his own abdominal cavity (Wilson 2000). Few can watch today's television commercials on topical TS without smiling and thinking how little times have changed.

These early studies point to four important features that defined much of the research in endocrinology for the next decades. First, there was a clear focus on practical therapeutic application to humans. Understanding the basic biology of sex hormones was only of secondary interest. Second, the studies demonstrated a fundamental research paradigm of endocrinology – ablation and hormone replacement as the experimental manipulation with functional restoration as the outcome measure. Third, the studies focused on the relation of a hormone to function and dysfunction of systems related to reproduction. A special focus was on sociosexual behaviors, defined as behaviors related to successful reproduction. Finally, the hormones on which most attention was placed were the sex steroids. It was TS and males in the early days, but today there has been at least equal focus on estrogens and progesterone in females.

Later still came the recognition that a non-sex steroid, corticosteroid, was intimately involved in the response to stressors. The bind that tied corticosteroids to sex steroids were the findings that stress could suppress reproductive physiology and function. Without doubt, steroids were firmly entrenched into the field of behavioral endocrinology (Beach 1981).

Behavioral neuroendocrinology emerged as the dominant subfield with a handful of seminal findings in recent decades These results have made it clear that steroids do more than simply maintain peripheral structures and reflexively activate subcortical brain regions to initiate regulatory behaviors. The seminal findings suggest sex steroids do more, much more.

One of the more satisfying outcomes is to give contemporary legitimacy to a behavioral biologist with interest in the steroids. The new findings also allowed researchers to move beyond the simple correlational studies of circulating TS and behavior. We now can understand better puzzling findings from the earliest days in behavioral endocrinology. More important, the seminal findings have thrust the brain into a central position in the study of steroids.

Their goal in this chapter will be to address the current status of TS and behavior in relation to the recent findings. We will use reproductive behaviors as the exemplary literature because that is surely the most complete. There are already excellent reviews of endocrine - sociosexual behavior relations (Archer 1994, Baum 2002, Meisel and Sachs 1994, Meston, 2000). Rather than presenting another similar review, we have organized topics to emphasize the changes in thinking induced by the seminal findings as they have impacted the study of TS. We characterize these findings as "revolutionary" for several reasons. 1) The findings were more or less unexpected. 2) They introduced a level of complexity for the study of steroid - behavior interactions that few would have envisioned in the early days of endocrinology. 3) They provided a searchlight to guide their study of the fundamental mechanisms in the brain responsible for the steroid – behavior correlations.

It is their hope that the reader who persists to the end of this chapter will better appreciate the neuroendocrine complexities researchers have encountered in the study of a seemingly simple hormone – behavior interaction. Emphasis will be primarily on male animal models and men, although the emerging role of TS on female behaviors will be discussed where appropriate. Finally, the chapter may also prove helpful to students and researchers in behavioral neuroendocrinology because similar complexities likely apply to other hormone – behavior relations.

I.1. Sexual Behaviors Can Be Separated into Motivation and Performance Behaviors

A first step in digesting the large literature on sexual behavior is to distinguish its two separate components, motivation and performance. Sexual motivation refers to measures of the male's interest to engage in sexual activity, sometimes referred to as sexual arousal or libido. Sexual performance is the effectiveness of the male to initiate and complete a copulatory bout. The two components of sexual behavior involve distinct, quantifiable behaviors.

Successful reproduction requires the male to be sufficiently motivated to find a receptive female. Clever methods have been adopted to quantify intensity of sexual motivation in laboratory animals. One example is a small treadmill on which a male mouse must continue to run to stay nearby the stationary female (Craigen and Bronson 1982). More commonly, the measure of motivation is latency to initiate a mount of the female (Meisel and Sachs 1994) or time spent near an inaccessible estrous female (Taylor, *et al* 1991). Sexual motivation in females can be assessed also by time spent near a reproductive male or by recording solicitations, a species-specific set of behaviors used in the pre-copulatory phase (Taylor, *et al* 1989).

Copulation can be more easily observed than motivation in animal models. There are a number of distinct behaviors that can be independently measured, most notably latencies and frequencies of mounting, intromissions and ejaculations (Taylor and Weiss 1987). The single behavioral marker of receptivity in the female is lordosis, the bent-back positioning by the female, exposing her genitals and allowing the male to penetrate her.

In humans, the most common measures of both sexual interest and activity are self-reports, either from recall or a diary. There are a number of sophisticated recording instruments available to researchers, but they are intrusive and have limited use. Self-reports remain most convenient and most popular.

I.2. Distinct Brain Pathways Have Evolved for Sexual Motivation and Performance in Males

The two components of sexual behavior also involve different underlying neural systems. An exemplary experiment (Everitt 1990) demonstrated the different neural systems underlying sexual motivation and performance. Male rats pressed a bar to deliver a receptive female rat into his chamber. After training, the medial preoptic area (MPOA) of the hypothalamus was lesioned in one group of males. The animals continued to bar press for the female but no longer would attempt to mount and copulate with her. Both amygdalae were lesioned in a second group. These males no longer bar pressed to produce the receptive female. If she was placed inside the chamber, however, the male readily copulated. The suggestion is clear that an intact MPOA is necessary for normal copulatory performance whereas the amygdala is intimately involved in sexual motivation.

That experiment, and many others before and afterwards (Pfaus 1996), have demonstrated that the CNS ultimately holds the key to understanding sexual function in both males and females. The structures in the brain most often cited as being directly related to the control of male sexual behavior are the olfactory tubercles, corticomedial nuclei of the amygdaloid complex, bed nucleus of the stria terminalis (BNST), and the hypothalamus, especially the medial preoptic area (Baum 2002, Cooke, *et al* 1999b, Dominguez and Hull 2005).

Circulating levels of TS and the other sex hormones readily cross the blood brain barrier and, joined by a host of neurotransmitters and neuropeptides involved in reproduction, exert profound influence on the activity of these structures (Hull, *et al* 1999, McEwen, *et al* 1995). The evidence is overwhelming that TS is critical for the organization and activation of sexual motivation and performance of males. We present in the next section five findings (highlighted in bold and listed as II. 1, II. 2 and so forth) that changed, indeed revolutionized, the study of steroid physiology and behavior.

Section II. Findings That Revolutionized the Study of Neuroendocrinology of Testosterone – Behavior Relations

II.1. Fetal Testosterone Organizes Male Brain Circuitry

The influence of TS on the brain begins early. Beginning in the prenatal phase and continuing as the brain and periphery develop in the neonate, TS or its absence determines sexual differentiation. Early exposure to TS permanently masculinizes the male for an array of behavioral and physiological functions. The fetal and postnatal periods of testicular activity have profound effects on male sexual differentiation, whereas in the female early sexual development occurs without influence of ovarian function. In the absence of circulating TS, the mammalian brain and urogenital systems are feminized and de-masculinized.

Other data confirm male perinatal physiology being more reactive than that of females to sex hormones. Testosterone is being released in the male fetus long before the hypothalamic –

pituitary - gonadal (HPG) axis has matured. Still, the HPG axis is fully functional in the male rat during the last days of gestation (Huhtaniemi 2000). In the first hours after birth, only the male experiences a burst of TS that increases circulating titers to near adult levels for a short period of time (Timiras and Cons 1982). This dramatic increase may or may not have consequences for later adult sociosexual behaviors (McGivern, *et al* 1998). By contrast, the fetal ovary is in a quiescent state, and its endocrine activity begins in earnest only with the first signs of puberty.

Sex steroidal influences lay relatively dormant in the postnatal animal until puberty. Then the same sex hormones, along with surges of gonadotropins and neuropeptides, activate the circuits organized during fetal development. This two phase influence of TS on behavior is the now classic organizational – activational model (Arnold and Gorski 1984, Phoenix, *et al* 1959). Fetal organization of sexually dimorphic brain morphology and circuitry can be observed in behaviors prior to puberty. Examples are the sexually dimorphic play and cognitive behaviors of prepubertal animals (Hodes and Shors 2005, Taylor 1980a). Clearer differences emerge with the activation of the circuitry by pubertal hormones. The results are gender-typical adult sociosexual behaviors, as well as influences on an array of non-reproductive behaviors.

The organizational – activational concept remains a powerful guide and is treated today as dogma by most neuroendocrinologists (Hall, *et al* 2004). However, there are several refinements of the original organizational – activational model that are based largely on the rodent brain (Ball and Balthazart 2006). For example, a key step suggested by rodent studies is that metabolism of TS to estradiol is necessary to induce a masculine organization of the brain. There is little evidence, however, to indicate that step is necessary in primates. Testosterone is likely directly responsible for the masculinization of the primate brain (Breedlove and Hampson 2002, Cooke, *et al* 1999a). Nonetheless, these findings point out the importance of the metabolic cascade for the synthesis of steroids for understanding the influence of TS on sociosexual behaviors.

II.2. Estradiol Is a Metabolite of Testosterone

The metabolic cascade of steroidal hormones is remarkably complex and details remain unclear (Ball and Balthazart 2006, Occhiato, *et al* 2004). One basic feature is that the two primary metabolites of TS are estradiol (E2) and dihydrotestosterone (DHT). Thus, TS may directly activate steroid-sensitive tissues or be metabolized to either E2 or DHT which in turn activates the tissue. Whether TS or its metabolites activate the target cell is dependent upon the presence or absence of specific enzymes. Aromatase is responsible for converting TS to E2 and 5alpha-reductase converts TS to DHT (Payne and Hales 2004).

In tissue containing aromatase, and that includes many brain regions, the result is that TS is a prohormone in adult males. The direct effect on function is after TS is metabolized to E2 and E2 binds the estrogen receptor (Adkins-Regan 1981, Cooke, *et al* 1998). Evidence comes from the many reports with experimental animals showing E2 alone could restore sexual behaviors of castrated adult males (Baum 2002). For example, castrated male rats were injected either with TS, E2 or DHT. Only DHT failed completely to restore the animals' sexual behaviors (Johnston and Davidson 1972).

More recent work has confirmed that it is the conversion of TS to estrogen that is the critical step (Ball and Balthazart 2006). Blocking aromatase activity or injecting an anti-estrogen into the MPOA blocked the activation of male-typical sexual behavior by TS. Administering an estrogen directly to the MPOA in castrated animals activated male-typical sexual behavior.

Not to be outdone, DHT had its own surprise. It turns out to be a more potent androgen than TS. Upon conversion of TS to DHT in many peripheral sites, DHT binds the androgen receptor with higher affinity (Martini, *et al* 1990).

DHT also can magnify the effects of TS, as exemplified with its role in maturation of the penis at puberty. During adulthood, DHT also has primary responsibility for maintaining normal function of many of the secondary sex characteristics, as well as pathological conditions. Benign prostatic hyperplasia, prostate cancer, acne, androgenic alopecia in men, and hirsutism in women are all related to DHT production (Occhiato, *et al* 2004).

Originally, it seemed that DHT and E2 had divided the androgenic labor (Bonsall, *et al* 1992, Martini, *et al* 1990). The idea was of DHT being the active metabolite in peripheral tissues and E2 being the metabolite in the brain. Thus, E2 was the steroid most responsible for behavior in males. Supporting data came from administering DHT to a castrated rat. When given peripherally, DHT was less effective than TS in activating sexual behavior in castrated male rats (Butera and Czaja 1989). Integrity of the penis was maintained, but DHT did little to restore sexual behavior. Administering E2 did the opposite for a castrated male. Penile morphology was disturbed, but sexual motivation was intact (Sachs, *et al* 1984).

Such parsimony is rare in endocrinology, and it was not to last long. In rodents, it appears TS influences sexual behaviors of the males after it is converted to E2 while, in the brains of primates, it is TS interacting directly with the AR that underlies male sexual behaviors (Michael, *et al* 1987). We now know also that DHT is found in abundance in the brain (Bonsall, *et al* 1985), along with concentrations of the 5alpha-reductase enzyme converting TS to DHT (Cooke, *et al* 2003). Clearly, DHT influences brain structure and function. The functional dichotomy for DHT and E2 was officially put to rest with findings that E2 plays a critical role in male peripheral structures and functions (Akingbemi 2005, Sharpe 1998).

II.2.1. There are two Metabolic Pathways for Synthesizing Testosterone

TS is the major androgenic steroid in circulation, with the Leydig cells of the testes as the principal source of the hormone in males. The adrenal glands supplement TS synthesis by secreting the hormone precursors androstenedione (ANDRO), dehydroepiandrosterone (DHEA) and its sulfate (DHEAS). Adrenal steroids are converted to TS in peripheral tissues, often in the skin or fat (Payne and Hales 2004).

The role of the adrenal precursors of TS, especially DHEA, in normal physiology is of considerable recent interest (Beck and Handa 2004). Development of a mature adrenal gland, known as adrenarche, typically begins in children between 6 and 8 years of age, i. e., well before the onset of puberty. One functional outcome is the appearance of pubic hair. Interestingly, the dramatic increase in levels of the adrenal precursors of TS occurs without corresponding increases in the other adrenal steroids, corticosteroids and mineralocorticoids. Peak levels of DHEA are found in adult humans during the 20s and 30s and decline progressively thereafter.

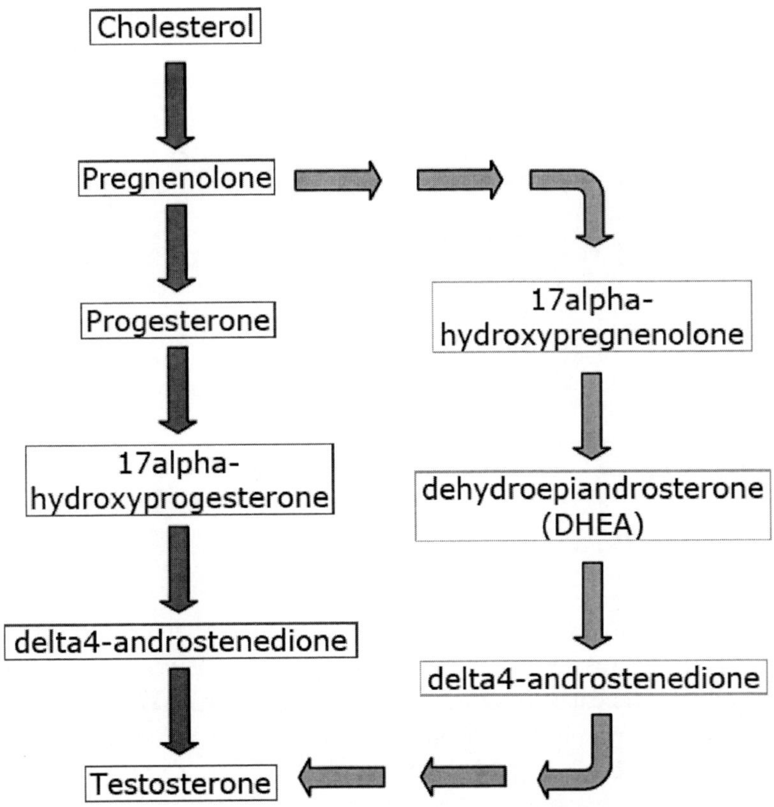

Figure 1. Metabolic cascade for the synthesis of testosterone and its potent metabolites, estradiol and dihydrotestosterone. The primary pathway is represented by the blue arrows.

Steroidogenesis of androgens, ovarian steroids and adrenal corticosteroids involves many of the same precursors. Two pathways are used for the synthesis of TS. The typical, preferred pathway is cholesterol –> pregnenolone –> progesterone –> 17alpha-hydroxyprogesterone –> ANDRO –> TS (Lieberman and Prasad 1990). A secondary route however is from pregnenolone –> DHEA –> ANDRO –> TS.

II.2.2. Supplements of the adrenal precursor androstenedione do not increase testosterone

A fundamental question about steroid metabolism is under what conditions is the secondary pathway used in place of the preferred pathway? We do not know. We do know, however, that there are surprising outcomes from manipulating precursor levels that may involve switching between the two pathways. For example, ANDRO supplements would seem to predict increased levels of TS by providing more precursor for increased production of TS. The enzyme responsible for converting ANDRO to TS, 17beta-hydroxysteroid dehydrogenase, is found in most body tissues. Androstenedione is also produced by some plants and has been marketed as a product for increasing blood TS concentrations, that is, as a natural alternative to anabolic steroid use. At least that was surely the thinking of baseball player Mark McGwire and other professional athletes who were self-administering ANDRO.

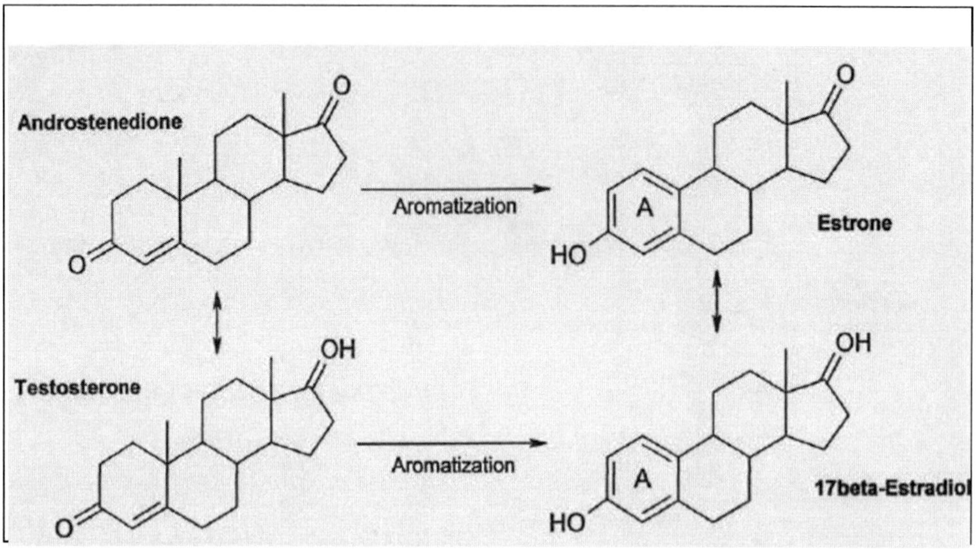

Figure 2. Metabolic cascade for the two possible pathways for the metabolism of androstenedione (ANDRO).

However, the interconversion of ANDRO and TS and metabolism to other bioactive steroids is complex. The results are often surprising. For example, supplements of a TS precursor may not have the expected effects on TS or its functions (Arlt, *et al* 1999, King, *et al* 1999). Oral ANDRO supplements revealed none of the expected increases in serum TS nor did it promote muscle strength (Birchard 1999). We also were surprised by their findings when castrated male rats were administered ANDRO. In TS restored castrates, concomitant ANDRO treatments suppressed androgen-sensitive behaviors (Taylor, *et al* 1994).

The key may be that in addition to serving as a precursor to TS, ANDRO is closely connected to estrogens (King, *et al* 1999). Androstenedione can be converted directly to an estrogen, specifically estrone, thereby completely bypassing testosterone (Labrie, *et al* 1998, Welt, *et al* 2006). Alternatively, because TS is also aromatized to E2, it also is possible that increased production of TS following ANDRO administration may result in increased aromatization, which would further attenuate any increase in the blood TS concentration (King, *et al* 1999). Sure enough, a study of young men with normal TS values confirmed the increased estrogen levels. The only steroids to increase with oral ANDRO supplements were serum E2 and estrone (King, *et al* 1999).

II.2.3. Female sexuality may be more sensitive to the adrenal precursor dhea

Androstenedione, however, has not received the research attention lavished on the other major TS precursor synthesized by the adrenal glands. DHEA appears to be a more potent precursor and perhaps serves both reproductive and non-reproductive functions.

DHEA and its sulphate DHEAS are easily detected in circulation of humans, although only with some difficulty in rodent models. DHEAS serves as reservoir for DHEA and the conversion is via cellular sulfatase. DHEA can then serve as a precursor for a number of other steroids, including ANDRO, TS, and E2 (Chen, *et al* 2005).

One set of findings that has focused attention on DHEA and DHEAS is that both show a progressive decline in adults with age that corresponds to physical aging. Circulating levels of DHEA and DHEAS are dramatically reduced in aged primates, including humans.

There has been considerable discussion recently over whether to consider DHEA a hormone. At this time, DHEA is more appropriately referred to as a steroid, a prohormone or an androgen precursor (Dhatariya 2005, Labrie, *et al* 2005). It is not an androgen nor is it a hormone. DHEA does not bind to either the estrogen or androgen receptor and, therefore, it has no direct androgenic activity. Unlike other major steroids, a receptor for DHEA or one of its metabolites has not been definitively isolated in the reproductive system or in the brains of animal models (Johannsson, *et al* 2002). Consequently, the problem of proponents of DHEA therapies is to identify a cellular mechanism of action for DHEA (Widstrom and Dillon 2004). One possibility is that DHEA exerts functional effects by neuromodulation and improvement in endothelial cell function (Piroli, *et al* 2002). Another is DHEA may act as a neurosteroid by binding a cell membrane-bound receptor in the brain. Unfortunately however, this potential receptor is yet to be isolated (Widstrom and Dillon 2004).

Still, the best evidence is that DHEA plays an important role in the periphery by its role as a precursor for the peripheral synthesis of TS, DHT, and E2. Levels of DHEA predict androgen and estrogen concentrations in peripheral tissues, although they have little effect on circulating levels of the sex hormones (Chen, *et al* 2005). Other possible influences on the periphery include enhancement of the immune system, antagonism of corticosteroids, and involvement in cellular pathology and even obesity. Williams (Williams 2000) has reviewed the literature on each of these possible functions as well as critiquing the mechanisms suggested for DHEA influences on the periphery.

More relevant here is to consider the role of DHEA in sociosexual behaviors. Interestingly, there has been more enthusiasm for a DHEA – sexuality relation in females than in males. This may reflect the notable paucity of findings supporting a clear role for DHEA in males. For example, a study of sexual behaviour in young healthy eugonadal men also assayed adrenal and testicular sex steroids. Serum DHT concentration was the only independent hormonal predictor of their sexuality (Mantzoros, *et al* 1995).

In an experiment with animals, we treated castrated rats daily for 4 wks with adrenal steroids in the presence or absence of restorative doses of TS (Taylor, *et al* 1994). DHEA, DHEAS, and ANDRO were administered as cyclodextrin complexes to mimic the pharmacodynamics of the endogenous products. DHEA supplements alone were unable to maintain integrity of sociosexual responses and androgen target tissues after castration (Beyer, *et al* 1973). More remarkable was that DHEA suppressed the normal restorative functions of TS therapy to the castrated animals.

The story is quite different in females, especially in postmenopausal women. That low levels of circulating DHEA have been demonstrated in women with diminished libido and other symptoms of sexual dysfunction has suggested the use of DHEA as a supplement to increase androgenic activity (Saltzman and Guay 2006). Acute DHEA exposure, however, induced no changes on subjective (self-report) or physiological (vaginal photoplethysmograph) sexual responses to erotic stimuli in premenopausal women (Meston and Heiman 2002). Chronic DHEA treatment was more successful in women with androgen deficiency due to hypopituitarism. Oral DHEA raised the serum levels of DHEAS to normal age-related reference ranges, but only slightly increased TS titers. Despite subnormal TS levels, the DHEA treated women increased their initiation of sexual activity (Johannsson, *et al* 2002).

II.2.4. Testosterone is important for sexual motivation in women

Testosterone appears to have been adopted by the female endocrine system for some aspects of successful reproduction. Aggression is possibly one behavioral example (Dabbs and Hargrave 1997), but sexual motivation is more likely. Although not without controversy, TS seems to play an important role in sexual interest exhibited by the female (Federman 2004).

Most of the supporting data comes from studies of women because it proves more difficult to assess initiation of a sexual encounter in animal models. One reason is that non-human females are solicitous of sex only when in estrus, which makes separating the effects of TS from other sex hormones difficult. Moreover, there are surprisingly few studies of animal models in which previously untreated adult females are treated with TS and behavior is measured. An exception is an experiment by Van de Poll and colleagues (VandePoll, *et al* 1988). Female rats treated for 14 days with exogenous TS spent more time near a male than untreated control females. Interestingly, urinary marking by the females increased immediately upon injection of TS.

The steroid metabolic cascade revealing that E2 is a metabolite of TS suggested two conclusions. Testosterone, the prototypical masculine hormone, is a requisite precursor for the estrogens found in females (Goldstein, *et al* 2004). And, that one may find detectable amounts of unmetabolized TS in circulation of females.

Subsequent assays of serum confirmed the existence of TS in females. Indeed, levels of TS were surprisingly high, higher even than circulating estrogens. Although at levels that are approximately 10% of the titers found in males, women typically have more absolute amounts of TS in circulation than E2 (Miller, *et al* 2001, Miller 2002). This is partly because E2 is synthesized at low rates. Androgens are quantitatively the predominant sex steroid in women, circulating in the micromolar and nanomolar concentration range, compared with picomolar levels of estrogens (Sarkola, *et al* 1999, Young, *et al* 2000).

In the male, the majority of TS production occurs in the testes. In the female, 25% of TS is produced in the adrenals, 25% in the ovaries, and 50% in the peripheral tissues from precursors released from the adrenals and ovaries (Bachmann 2002).

Serum levels of TS follow a pattern of increases and decreases across the menstrual cycle that somewhat mimic the rise and fall of estrogens (Dougherty, *et al* 1997, Miller, *et al* 2001). Peak levels are found at mid-cycle and remain detectable throughout the cycle.

The next question is whether TS activates brain processes underlying reproduction and non-reproduction function in females. The answer suggested is yes for both functions. For example, data from a recent study of ovariectomized rats were that hippocampal neurons responded to TS in a similar manner to the influence of E2 on dendritic morphology in the hippocampus, a brain region critical for learning and memory (Leranth, *et al* 2004a).

Other findings suggested an impact of circulating TS on female sexual behavior. A correlational study of premenopausal women with or without complaints of sexual dysfunction revealed lower adrenal precursors and TS of the latter group (Guay, *et al* 2004). Indeed, the predominant symptom of women with androgen deficiency is loss of sexual desire (Davis 1999). Low TS levels may accompany a variety of conditions in women of reproductive age, including hypothalamic amenorrhea, hypopituitarism, premature ovarian failure, and premenstrual syndrome, as well as glucocorticosteroid or oral estrogen therapies (Kalantaridou and Calis 2006). Consequences of androgen insufficiency include various peripheral changes such as increased vasomotor flushing, loss of bone and muscle mass and replacement of muscle with adipose tissue, as well as a pattern of declining sexual functioning. Along with decreased sexual motivation, there is a reduction of sexual fantasy and enjoyment; , diminished sexual arousability, and decreased vaginal vasocongestion in response to erotic stimuli (Bachmann 2002).

The more common cause of androgen decreases is simply aging. Serum androgen levels exhibit a progressive stepwise decline from 20 to 49 years of age (Guay, *et al* 2004). Women in their forties have approximately half the level of circulating total TS as that of women in their twenties (Dennerstein, *et al* 2002).

The best evidence for a TS – sexual motivation relation is the value of TS therapy on the sexual vitality of postmenopausal women (Shifren 2004, Somboonporn, *et al* 2005). Although the evidence for TS as fundamental to low sexual interest in younger women has proved more inconclusive (Guay, *et al* 2004, Nyunt, *et al* 2005), there is greater support from androgen treatments of postmenopausal women (Davis 1999).

For example, Sherwin et al. (Sherwin, *et al* 1985) assessed sexual functioning in menopausal women administered TS over a 3 months period. It was clear that exogenous androgen enhanced the intensity of sexual desire and arousal and the frequency of sexual fantasies. However, the results were limited to sexual motivation rather than sexual activity. This may be a reflection only that sexual activity involves non-endocrine factors such as marital status, partner interest and past experiences.

Postmenopausal women volunteers were administered either oral estrogens with or without concomitant androgen for eight weeks in a double-blind study. Sexual function was assessed with a questionnaire. Results were that sexual desire, satisfaction and frequency increased significantly more in the group receiving androgen than in women receiving by estrogen only or estrogen-progestin therapy (Sarrel, *et al* 1998). Finally, in a single-blind study TS was administered by implants for 2 years to postmenopausal women. Results indicated significantly greater scores for sexual activity, satisfaction, pleasure, and orgasm compared with controls (Davis, *et al* 1995).

An unanswered question is whether TS directly increases arousability in women or if it must be first converted to E2 (Bancroft 2005). In the latter case, it would suggest that estrogen therapy would have the same effect on sexual motivation. The studies cited above suggest that not to be the case. Sexuality of postmenopausal women was greater with a combination of TS and estrogen compared to women receiving estrogen alone (Davis, *et al* 1995, Dobs, *et al* 2002). More recently (Davis, *et al* 2006) there was a report that an aromatase inhibitor in combination with TS therapy had no significant effect on sexual restoration in women. The suggestion is that it is TS acting on the androgen receptor and that is the key to sexual motivation in women.

II.3. Androgen Receptors are Found in Structures Both Related and Unrelated to Reproduction

Molecular biology has allowed identification of receptors for steroidal hormones and for localizing concentrations of the receptors in tissues throughout the body. Estrogen receptors (ER) and androgen receptors (AR) were found in the periphery and brains of both genders of common laboratory animals. Surprisingly the receptors appear in brain regions responsible for reproduction as well as in brain regions with little relation to reproduction (Nyborg, 1994).

It came as a further surprise to many of us to learn that there is no specific TS receptor. The receptor is the more generic androgen receptor (AR). As already noted, TS serves both as an active hormone and as a prohormone. Genetic evidence indicates that TS and DHT work via a common intracellular receptor (Wilson, *et al* 2002). Testosterone has good affinity for the AR, but, interestingly, DHT has a notably higher affinity for the androgen receptor. Either directly or after conversion to E2 or DHT, TS interacts with sex steroid receptors to produce both peripheral and central activation that underlies sociosexual behaviors in the male.

In the periphery, steroid receptors are found in a remarkable variety of tissues, from muscle and bone to cranial motor nuclei to the cornea and retina of the eye (Wickham, *et al* 2000). Some of the influences of TS on these structures appear to require aromatization, bone for example, and others not, muscle for example (Bronwyn, *et al* 2003). The greatest concentration of AR, however, is where one would expect to find it, in the reproductive tract. Estrogen receptors are often found co-localized with the AR, for example in the testes (Carreau, *et al* 2003). The result is that TS and its metabolites are integral in maintaining the structure and function of peripheral structures involved in normal male sexual function (Goldstein, *et al* 2004). More specifically, TS directly impacts sexual behaviors by its effects on peripheral neurons that trigger and complete copulatory reflexes (Keast 1999). The influence on genital organ sensitivity plays an important role in sexual arousal and orgasm.

II.3.1. Distribution of androgen receptors in the brain

In the rodent brain, conversion of androgens into estrogens by aromatase is a key mechanism by which TS regulates many physiological and behavioral processes, including the activation of male sexual behavior, brain sexual differentiation and negative feedback effects of steroid hormones on gonadotropin secretion (Balthazart and Ball 1998). Therefore, cells that express steroid hormone receptors are integral to the action of gonadal hormones and represent essential components of the mechanism underlying masculinization of the brain.

Neurons with ARs in their nuclei are distributed widely in many regions of the brain including the preoptic area of the hypothalamus, septal area-bed nucleus, amygdala, and brain stem (Bonsall, *et al* 1985). ARs are also concentrated in areas of the brain that are not primarily involved in reproduction, such as the basal forebrain, hippocampus, caudate putamen, midbrain raphe and brainstem locus coeruleus (McEwen 2001).

The brain regions most closely related to male-specific sexual behaviors are located in various limbic structures and in the olfactory system. Most critical are the hypothalamus and amygdala. Testosterone and its metabolites interact with steroid receptors in hypothalamic limbic structures, where they elicit conscious perception and pleasurable reactions by influencing the release of specific neurotransmitters.

Although traditionally believed to be only in subcortical regions, ARs are also found in cortical and subcortical brain regions unrelated to reproduction, notably the hippocampus. AR immunoreactivity and binding are very similar in rat hippocampus as in the sexual behavior-dependent hypothalamus. ARs are concentrated in the CA1 region, an area that plays a major role in learning and memory (Xiao and Jordan 2002). That ARs are present also on axons and dendrites in cerebral cortex highlights the likelihood that androgens play an important and novel extra-nuclear role in neuronal function (DonCarlos, 2003}. This lays the groundwork for other surprises that have changed the way neuroendocrinologists think about sex steroids and behavior.

II.3.2. Gender differences in steroid receptors predict sexual behavior differences but not dimorphic non-reproductive behaviors

When neuroendocrinologists talk about "brain sex" or a brain being organized as masculine or feminine, it could mean many things. It could mean males and females having more neurons in certain brain areas, leaving those areas larger. It could mean having the same number of neurons but the neurons are connected differently leaving neurotransmitter pathways wired differently. It could also refer to the different numbers of steroid receptors in masculine and feminine brains with those receptors being distributed differently. Or it could refer to a brain region that metabolizes the same hormones differently. The net result of all these possibilities is that the same hormone, whether it be TS or estrogen or another hormone, delivered to the brain of an adult can lead to sexually dimorphic behaviors (Resko and Roselli 1997, Simerly 2002).

Still, much of the interest has centered on size differences and on receptor differences, likely because they are the easiest to quantify. Only a couple of size differences exist, most famously is the clearly larger size of the higher vocal center (or HVC) in male songbirds (Nottebohm and Arnold 1976). There are reports of subtle size differences in brain regions between men and women. The amygdala and hypothalamus appear to be larger in men. Both regions are also the same regions that contain high concentrations of steroid receptors (Hamann 2005).

It is notable that the both androgen and estrogen receptors are detected in the same brain regions in males and female animal models. ARs are found in neuroanatomical areas of both genders in the medial hypothalamic area, ventromedial and dorsomedial nucleus, preoptic area, arcuate nucleus, amygdala and regions of the hippocampus, arcuate-median eminence and BNST, with the greatest AR density reported in the preoptic and hypothalamic areas, septum and amygdala of these animals.

Receptor numbers differ in the expected direction in some brain regions. The two subtypes of estrogen receptor (ER), designated as ER-alpha and ER-beta, are distributed differently in male and female brains (Shughrue, *et al* 2000). Although ER-beta is found in the hippocampus of male and female rats, females have higher concentrations (Zhang, *et al* 2002).

Using 4 strains of male and female mice Lu (Lu, *et al* 1998) found sexually dimorphic receptor concentrations in various brain regions. Males had a higher absolute number of AR than females. Concentrations of AR were higher in males in brain regions associated with male-typical sexual behaviors, e. g., BNST and MPOA. AR decreased significantly with castration. Indeed, most differences in AR numbers between the sexes are detected in hypothalamic nuclei and other structures related to reproduction (Chen and Tu 1992, Lu, *et al* 1998).

In many non-reproductive structures, however, there are surprisingly few or no sex differences in distribution and concentrations of ERs and ARs (Michael, *et al* 1995, Scott, *et al* 2000). Moreover, where there may be sex differences, there is no clear functional logic for the existence of different receptor numbers. An example is the AR findings from autopsies of a small number of men and women between 20 years and 39 years (Fernandez-Guasti, *et al* 2000). Again, ARs were found in high numbers in both male and female hypothalamus. However, men had higher AR concentrations in the suprachiasmatic nucleus of the hypothalamus, a region generally agreed to be related to diurnal activity rather than sexual behavior.

The presence of large numbers of ER and AR in both sexes would seem to pose interpretation problems for relating dimorphic functions to the steroid receptor. High concentrations of ERs in males can be explained, however, by the metabolism of TS into E2 in brain tissues to interact with ERs. Notably, amounts of aromatase are higher in many brain regions of male animal models than of females (Lu, *et al* 1998, Roselli and Resko 1997). The presence of high concentrations of ARs in the brains of females is more puzzling (Xiao and Jordan 2002).

II.4. Steroids Act through Genomic AND Non-Genomic Mechanisms

Steroid hormones are unique endocrine products in the way they interact with nuclear DNA. This capacity allows for many of the distinctive features of steroids to induce the long-lasting changes that are observed, for example, the surge of TS with the oncoming breeding season in feral animals or the onset of puberty in humans.

In the past decade another mechanism for influences on brain and behavior has been identified. In addition to the well-established nuclear action of steroid receptors, membrane-associated receptors for gonadal steroid hormones have been discovered. This finding has revolutionized the way we think of steroids, recognizing rapid actions of steroids that could not be attributed to transcriptional regulation. Considerable evidence has now accumulated to support the existence of these nonnuclear receptors. Their ideas have now been broadened to recognize gonadal steroid receptor action via extranuclear sites.

II.4.1. The classic mechanism for steroidal influence is genomic and slow

It has been known for some time that TS and the other steroids have direct influence on DNA transcription in the nucleus of target cells. The result is that the genomic effects are slow because it requires time for the multiple steps to initiate DNA activation and subsequent protein synthesis to initiate functional changes. Genomic changes, consequently, are long-lasting.

Steroidal hormones belong to a ligand-activated nuclear receptor family. Members of this family have been defined by their ability to bind to specific DNA sequences in promoter regions of hormone responsive genes.

Unbound TS in circulation enters a cell and binds the androgen receptor (AR) to form a steroid ligand. Prior to confronting TS, the AR is loosely bound to a protein in the cellular cytoplasm or nucleus. Surprisingly, the exact location of the steroid-hormone receptor is not known. What is known is that TS diffuses into the cell and binds the receptor and the TS – AR complex then diffuses into the cell nucleus. The TS - AR complexes bind to specific sequences of DNA called steroid-response elements, as well as to nuclear-receptor coactivators or repressors (Gruber, *et al* 2002). Upon binding to these hormone response elements in the DNA, the receptors are capable of exerting powerful modulatory effects on transcription of specific genes.

The outcomes are prominent changes in neural morphology and function. Testosterone surges are linked to an increase in neuron somal size, neuritic growth, plasticity and synaptogenesis in both motoneurons of the spinal nucleus of the bulbocavernosus muscle in the reproductive system of males and several populations of pelvic autonomic neurons (Bialek, *et al* 2004). The genomic influences of TS are now known to extend beyond the reproductive system. Changes in lateralized function of the hemispheres and hippocampal activation are but two examples.

Castration of adult rats is reported to induce a decrease of dendritic spines in the CA1 region of the hippocampus (Leranth, *et al* 2004b). Castration also reduced numbers of acetylcholine neurons in some cortical areas, and 4 weeks of exogenous TS restored the cholinergic pathways in the adult rats. These data suggest that the presence or absence of TS profoundly influenced the cholinergic population in cortical and subcortical areas of the adult rat brain (Nakamura, *et al* 2002). These and other data have led to the speculation that TS is a neuroprotective agent (Frye and McCormick 2000).

One final word on androgen receptors and it has a familiar ring. There is more complexity than researchers had hoped. The concept of a single hormone activating a single receptor is being replaced by a more complex model (Vanderschueren and Bouillon 2000). The picture emerging is of the original hormonal signal undergoing transformation in the target tissue from processes such intracellular enzyme activities, receptor concentration and function, and post-receptor cross-talk. The result is modulation of the original signal and fine-tuning of the biological response.

II.4.2. A second mechanism for steroidal influence is non-genomic and fast

Steroids are usually identified as genomic regulators. Recently a body of evidence has accumulated demonstrating specific membrane effects more akin to neurotransmitter activities. That is, steroids can help coordinate neural firings by interacting with both membrane and intracellular receptors. The resulting rapid modulation of cellular activity is measured in seconds or minutes and suggests a non-genomic role for certain steroids. Rapid steroid synthesis and metabolism have been found to exist in the CNS, and downstream effects can be seen in both the central and peripheral nervous systems.

The mechanism for rapid, non-genomic action is suggested by the findings that ARs are present on axons and dendrites within the mammalian central nervous system. AR expression in axons was identified in the rat brain at the light microscopic level and details confirmed at the ultrastructural level. AR-immunoreactive axons were observed primarily in the cerebral cortex and were rare in regions where nuclear AR expression is abundant. This suggests that there are separate functional systems for the genomic and non-genomic influence of the sex steroids. The observation that ARs are present in axons and dendrites highlights the possibility that TS plays an important and novel extra-nuclear role in neuronal function (DonCarlos, *et al* 2003).

Current levels of circulating steroids can induce changes in neural morphology that would appear to be too fast to be genomic. The best example comes from estrogen and female rats. The rapid rise and fall of estrogen during the 4-day estrous cycle of f rats is accompanied by equally rapid increases and decreases in numbers of dendrites in certain hippocampal regions (Woolley 1998). Significantly, those are the same regions responsible for certain types of memory.

The implications that steroids have fast, membrane-mediated influences on the brain function are nothing short of revolutionary. That steroids can have acute, momentary actions opens a new avenue of thinking about the brain. The pharmaceutical industry has been among the first to recognize the potential of non-genomic steroidal actions. A prominent example is that sex steroids may contribution to brain plasticity.

II.4.3. Steroids play a role in brain plasticity

Neuroscientists use the word "plasticity" to refer to brain tissues that maintain the capacity for structural changes in mature animals. That TS and the other sex steroids could contribute to brain plasticity is a remarkable development for several reasons.

To set the scene, recall the original organizational - activational model. The suggestion is that organizational effects are structural and irreversible, whereas activational effects were functional and reversible. The thought was that once fetal development and its sensitive periods to TS had passed, the organized morphology of the brain would not change with changes in circulating adult hormones.

The activational component, on the other hand, was considered labile and modifiable, say by castration or hormone supplements. The hormonal influences that activated a function after puberty, sexual motivation for instance, were completed without changing integrity of the long-ago established structures. As long as those masculinized brain tissues have sufficient current levels of TS from the adult testes, we would see normal male sexual functioning. Remove the testes and TS and we would observe sexual behaviors beginning a downhill slide. Brain anatomy does not change with castration, but the behavior activated by TS does.

In general, the structural – functional distinction between organization – activation roles of the model have been largely upheld today. But, the line between function and structure has been blurred in the brain. Current research on the effects of gonadal steroids on the brain and spinal cord indicates that these agents can have profound trophic effects on many aspects of neuronal functioning. As example, TS induced structural remodeling of the neuromuscular junctions of the peripheral nervous system in the male rat reproductive tract (Gordon, *et al* 1990). Cranial nerves also show morphological sensitivity to androgens. Some of these effects may be genomic and some non-genomic. Regardless of the mechanism of action, the consequences are notable on cell survival, growth and metabolism, elaboration of processes, synaptogenesis, and neurotransmission (Jones, *et al* 1999).

Still, the best evidence that some structures in the brain maintain plasticity to hormones is the capacity of hormones to change the physical structure of the adult hippocampus. Specifically, features of hippocampal anatomy can be molded by current levels of ovarian hormone in cycling female rats. The initial findings were of neural morphology rapidly changing with fluctuations of endogenous sex hormones in adult female rats (Woolley, *et al* 1993). More recently, ovariectomized rats administered TS induced similar increases in dendritic spines (Leranth, *et al* 2004a). Male brains may or may not undergo similar changes.

These data highlight both the plasticity of the adult brain and the importance of hormone fluctuations on the brain during the activational phase (Breedlove and Jordan 2001).

There are good reasons, however, to believe that the male brain will show less plasticity than female brains, and that TS will be less likely to be as important of a player as ovarian hormones. A key difference between male and female brains is that only the females undergo dramatic endocrine fluctuations over days. It is probably accurate to suggest that even neuroendocrinologists have not fully appreciated the dramatic differences between a fluctuating endogenous hormonal stimulus experienced by females and a more or less constant one experienced by males (Taylor and Pitha 1988).

II.5. The Brain Synthesizes Its Own Steroids

We have known for decades that steroid hormones influence the brain. That is to say, a sex hormone released by the far-away gonads is pumped in the blood to the brain where it binds a steroid receptor. But, it has been recognized only in the past decade or so that the brain appears to be producing its own steroids. This has led, among other things, to a confusion of terms.

Terminology in the steroid hormone literature has not shown ideal consistency. The result is confusion about the definitions of steroids in the periphery and the CNS (Stoffel-Wagner 2001). We have already introduced one example, DHEA, which is referred to erroneously as an androgen or as a hormone.

"Biologically active steroids" are steroids that have the ability to bind to a steroid receptor in the periphery or the CNS. Examples are TS, E2, progesterone and corticosteroid. "Neuroactive steroids" are those substances that bind to a steroid receptor in the CNS. All the aforementioned steroids also meet the criterion for neuroactive steroids.

But the brain synthesizes its own steroids for local use in the brain. These became known as "neuroactive steroids" (Baulieu 1998), i. e., steroids used by the brain for both reproductive and non-reproductive functions. The most important feature is that neurosteroids are synthesized directly in the brain. The neuroactive steroids are not the familiar steroids, and include DHEA and progesterone metabolites such as allopregnanolone. Likely neurosteroids use non-genomic mechanisms to quickly modify brain activity and behavior (Rupprecht and Holsboer 1999). The terminology details may seem like splitting of hairs, but it is an important distinction because there are revolutionary implications in the concept of a neurosteroid.

One implication is that, rather than relying entirely on the peripheral endocrine organs for its hormones, the brain has evolved the capacity to synthesize its own steroids (Corpechot, *et al* 1981, Mellon 1994). This can be demonstrated by removing the peripheral organs, adrenals and gonads, and the amounts of neurosteroid in the brain do not change (Baulieu 1997). Economically, neurosteroids are synthesized mostly from the same precursors and enzymes as used for peripheral synthesis.

Another implication is perhaps more profound and has the potential to open a new chapter for steroidal influence on brain and behavior (Engel and Grant 2001). The mammalian brain has adapted both peptides and steroids used in reproduction for other neural functions. The ancient hormones synthesized in the periphery now have a new role. Rather than evolving completely new substances for complex behaviors such as memory or mood, steroids have been hijacked by the brain for other uses (Belelli and Lamber 2005, Birzniece, *et al* 2006).

SECTION III. CIRCULATING TESTOSTERONE AND SOCIOSEXUAL BEHAVIORS

III.1. Testosterone in Circulation Shows Wide between and within Individual Differences

A basic tenet of endocrinology is that endocrine products are released from glands to be carried by the bloodstream to target tissues some distance away. Sometimes this bloodstream is nearby and served by a specially evolved vascular source, a so-called portal system. The direct portal connection between hypothalamus and anterior pituitary is an important example. Much more commonly, the blood delivery system is general circulation, and that is almost always the source obtained for analyses of the steroids. There are myriads of methods to collect blood from experimental animals (Weiss, *et al* 2000), including the one familiar to human patients.

Once blood is drawn from men and assayed, the serum reveals only 2% found in the bloodstream is so-called unbound or free TS. That is, the portion of TS that is not bound to a protein, either albumin or sex hormone binding globulin (SHBG). The free fraction has traditionally been viewed as the source of biologically active TS that could enter cells and interact with a receptor. For example, aging men experience both reduced free TS and increased levels of SHBG (Swerdloff and Wang 2004). Much has been made of this observation. This includes a comparison of bound and free TS in patients with probable Alzheimer's disease with the conclusion that only free TS is significantly lower in male patients (Moffat, *et al* 2004).

Now it seems that albumin bound TS can be uptaken by cells and dissociated from the protein to interact with the receptor. Moreover, the bound form is a type of reservoir of TS that may actually facilitate the entry of hormone into the cell (Goldstein and Sites 2002). The result is that a considerable portion of the TS in circulation actually is in a readily bioactive form in males. The anxiety of researchers and clinicians over bound and free TS is probably unwarranted (Davidson, *et al* 1982). Serum TS levels and free TS are often highly correlated in healthy males (Stalenheim, *et al* 1998).

III.1.1. Within individual assays revealed that testosterone is released in pulses throughout the day and night

In the mid-1970s an important discovery was made about the way that gonads release their hormones into circulation. Release is not by slow leakage but in a series of episodic bursts throughout the day (Bartke and Dalterio 1975, Sodersten, *et al* 1983). Soon, the findings were extended to other endocrine glands, including those outside the HPG axis (Linkowski, *et al* 1985, Penny 1985, Samuels, *et al* 1990). This pattern became known as pulsatile release. The term continues to be used to distinguish circadian pulses from the gradual increases in hormone known as surges that occur, for example, in males of seasonal breeding species or with the advent of puberty in boys.

Recognition of the ubiquity of pulsatile release of endocrine products forced researchers to better control sampling protocols. Most prominent was to measure hormone levels at the same time of the day. With that control in place, however, it was possible to make comparisons among and within males.

Little TS is stored in the testes and newly synthesized TS is quickly released into the bloodstream in 6-10 pulses of different amplitudes per day in men. The pattern is variable both between males and over days in the same male. Still, in men there is a fairly reliable TS pulse early in the morning, around daybreak. The pulse-generator responsible for the pattern of pulsatile release of TS is unknown, but we do know it is more than simply the HPG axis. Specifically, neurons projecting from various subcortical brain regions influence the amplitude and frequency of hypothalamic gonadotropin releasing hormone (GnRH) released from the hypothalamus into the pituitary (Abbud, *et al* 1999, Scott, *et al* 1997).

One result of this pulsatile feature is that hormone sensitive tissue responds best to aperiodic stimulation. Indeed, a continuous stream of hormone can produce a paradoxical suppression of target tissue activity (Southworth, *et al* 1991). That feature has made its way into hormone therapies as GnRH agonists are used to suppress the downstream release of luteinizing hormone and, thus, TS (Matthews, *et al* 1998, Rosler and Witztum 1998).

III.1.2. Differences in endogenous testosterone between males do not explain differences in sexual behavior

Reports of within individual variability were quickly followed by findings of considerable variability between individual males. Testosterone values in healthy young males of many species, including humans, range over values that differ significantly. In men the lower limit for normative values is 300 ng/ dl but the values may range to 900 ng/ dl or more (Howell and Shalet 2001). Upon reflection, individual differences in TS were not surprising. Males within a social group differ, of course, along many physical and behavioral continua. Some of these differences are androgen dependent, including sexual behaviors. Yet, the surprise was that in normal adult males the wide individual variability in circulating TS levels did not seem to be linked in any meaningful way with individual differences in any aspects of sexual behavior (Meston and Frohlich 2000, Schiavi and White 1976).

Of course, a certain amount of TS is necessary for normal sexuality. Castrated animal models and men (Greenstein, *et al* 1995) typically experience dramatic decreases in all measures of interest and performance. In gonadally intact males, hypogonadism is also associated with low level of male sexual behavior (Gray, *et al* 1981, Sternbach 1998).

Yet repeatedly the findings from studies of intact laboratory animals and men are that individual differences in endogenous TS levels and measures of sexual behaviors are not significantly related (Damassa, *et al* 1977, Meston and Frohlich 2000). Phoenix and Chambers for instance have made an exhaustive study of the sexual behaviors of rhesus monkeys and laboratory rats. One dominant theme is their conclusion that circulating TS is not the key factor in individual differences in the sexual behaviors of intact young or old males (Chambers and Phoenix 1992). Even administering exogenous hormone to elevate TS titers of so-called sexually sluggish young male monkeys failed to improve their performance (Phoenix and Chambers 1986).

The same absence of a TS – sexual behavior relation appears to hold for non-traditional animal models. A study of male and female meerkats (Carlson, *et al* 2004) reported no rank-related differences in circulating levels of TS among males. Dominant, breeding males and females, however, did have significantly higher cortisol levels than the subordinates, non-breeding meerkats.

Similar conclusions have been reported for men (Brown, *et al* 1978, Schiavi and White 1976, Zitzmann and Nieschlag 2001). The former study employed collection of two samples taken a week apart from 101 young adult men. Serum TS concentrations in the two samples were highly correlated, indicating good reliability and consistency. However, there was no correlation with their self-reported frequencies of sexual behaviors. The conclusion was that differences among men in circulating TS concentration within the normal range do not account for differences in sexual interest or activity (Brown, *et al* 1978).

One finds data in the literature suggesting a positive correlation of TS and sexuality (Knussmann, *et al* 1986). However, the bulk of the data supports the original conclusions. There is little correlation between circulating levels of the hormone and performance measures.

There are many possible explanations for the absence of correlation between resting TS and sexual behavior. One possibility is differences in nocturnal hormone pulses that are not typically measured. After finding the usual absence of a correlation between TS levels and copulation in rhesus monkeys, the researchers measured nocturnal hormone titers (Michael, *et al* 1984). They found that the most sexually active males had less of a nadir of the circadian rhythm at night, thus maintaining a higher level of TS during sleep. The implication is that, considered over the entire day, the TS levels were higher in the more sexually active male.

Another possibility is that the relation is in the opposite direction, that is, sexual activity increases TS in males rather than TS increasing the behavior. Sure enough, sexually experienced male rats have larger testes and higher TS levels (Frankel 1984, Taylor, *et al* 1985) compared to virgin males. However, the increases of TS appear to be only observed with chronic sexual contact. Testosterone is not released with copulation. Measurement of various hormones in male rhesus monkeys following copulation revealed no acute increases in circulating TS (Phoenix, *et al* 1977). Only cortisol increased in the monkeys. Although it was with masturbation, the same result for TS was reported after orgasm in men. Only prolactin increased (Kruger, *et al* 2003).

Interestingly this same relation, or absence of a relation, may not hold for females. As noted in a previous section, it is likely that TS is responsible for libido in women. Although there are far fewer studies of women than men, resting levels of TS appear to be related to self-reports of sexual interest in women (Sherwin, *et al* 1985).

III.1.3. Rather than a dose-response model, a threshold model may be more accurate for the testosterone – behavior relations

These findings led to the conclusion that the relation of TS and sexual behavior, and likely all behaviors, were better described by a threshold hormone model than a dose-response model. Simply the idea is that, once a threshold is passed, increases in circulating TS will have no further effects on behavior (Buena, *et al* 1993, Ewing, *et al* 1979, Isidori, *et al* 2005).

One prediction from the threshold model is that TS restored castrates will show similar sexuality as before the surgery. That is, exogenous TS to a formerly sexually active castrated male will restore his sexual behavior, but only to his previous level. The data support that prediction (Phoenix and Chambers 1986).

Additional evidence for the threshold model is that when TS levels are manipulated to ensure high or low TS values within the normal male range, sexuality of the two groups are the same (Buena, *et al* 1993, Taylor, *et al* 1985). In the former study, two groups of healthy men were treated for 9 weeks with a GnRH agonist to slightly suppress or exogenous TS to slightly increase TS serum levels. Sexual function evaluated by daily dairies revealed no significant differences in overall scores or in subcategories of intensity of sexual feelings or sexual activity between the two groups. The authors' conclusion was that a minimal value of TS above threshold was sufficient to fully restore sexual behavior in men (Buena, *et al* 1993).

The threshold model remains a dominant concept today despite mounting evidence that some behaviors, including aspects of sexual behaviors, may show a dose-response relation to TS (Gray, *et al* 2005). The threshold vs. dose-response issue continues to define much of the research in this area, both basic research and applications to clinical populations. More recently the debate has included the effects of TS supplements to eugonadal men, defined as healthy males with normal endocrine functions (O'Connor, *et al* 2004). That controversy surrounds the consequences from use and abuse of anabolic steroids, as well as the value of supplement of TS to healthy men. Those issues will be addressed in the last sections of this chapter.

An important feature of the literature reviewed above is to emphasize that the typical paradigm is a study of baseline or steady-state hormone. Researchers refer to this as "current levels" or "prevailing levels" of hormone in serum. Better perhaps is "resting levels" because it focuses on the key concept that the values reported are the serum steroidal titers of a male in a normal, unstimulated condition. And the threshold model seems to most accurately describe current TS levels – sociosexual behavior relations in males.

III.2. Acute and Chronic Changes in TS Induce Behavioral Changes

The conclusion that resting TS levels of healthy males are seldom informative in explaining individual differences in behavior would seem to place a cloud on further research on TS – behavior relations. There is, however, another way to ask questions about the relation. Rather than resting levels, for instance, do changes in TS induce reliable changes in behavior? Given the proclivity of experimentalists and clinicians to manipulate, it is not surprising that the changing hormone literature is much larger, with more interesting outcomes, than the literature on resting hormone titers.

III.2.1. Momentary changes in testosterone can change sexual function

As discussed at length above, a basic principle of steroid endocrinology is that the primary pathway for influencing behavior is genomic. The result is that, in most situations, TS and the other steroids are unlikely to show a momentary relation to behaviors. Rather hormones help set the conditions that a behavior will occur in the presence of a specific stimulus (Wade 2006). This is because most steroid effects require some period of time to influence the genome.

There have been clever attempts to identify the time period. One example in humans was with women exposed to a dose of TS while watching pornographic films. Sublingual intake of exogenous TS was followed by a sharp increase in plasma TS levels within 15 minutes. The circulating levels declined gradually over the next 90 minutes to reach baseline values. Only 3 to 4 hours after reaching peak levels was there a significantly increased genital responsiveness (Tuiten, *et al* 2000). These data suggest behavioral changes can occur within a few hours, although the time period is likely longer for other steroid – behavior relations.

The time delays of the classic genomic activity of steroids raised the puzzle of how it was possible for sudden changes in TS to have an immediate effect on physiology and behavior (Sachs 1997). Such momentary changes have been demonstrated in a variety of experimental paradigms.

Males of many species experience a rapid increase in TS levels to the appearance of a receptive female, her odors or even an environment in which the male had previously copulated (Fukada, *et al* 1988, Huang, *et al* 1989, Taylor 1980b). Those males may also exhibit an immediate increase in sociosexual behaviors (Taylor, *et al* 1984). These results also point out the important concept of hormone – behavior relations being a two-way street. Environments and behavior can modify the endocrine milieu which, then, can influence the behavior sensitive to the hormone (Aluja and Torrubia 2004).

More recent studies have confirmed the influence of the environment, as well as providing additional neurophysiological evidence of a rapid activation of neural activity to receptive females. For example, using nuclear fos immunoreactivity as a marker of neuronal activation (Kelliher, *et al* 1999), male rats were exposed to the soiled bedding of the female. Those males showed significantly more neuronal fos immunoreactivity than clean-bedding control males in the nucleus accumbens, medial amygdala, BNST and MPOA. Even greater neuronal fos responses were detected in these brain regions in males allowed to mate.

Molecular changes in the brain with acute exposure to exogenous TS include an experiment in which androgen receptor concentrations were examined in castrated adult male rats and gonadally intact females (Xiao and Jordan 2002). Animals received an injection of either TS propionate or vehicle 2 hours prior to sacrifice. AR receptor numbers within the CA1 region of the hippocampus increased in both genders to the acute TS injection. Interestingly, the increases were greater in the left hippocampus than the right, but only in the males, suggesting a sex difference in laterality of AR in hippocampal structure and function.

Still, the most important conclusion for their discussion is that the rapid rise in AR numbers point to a non-genomic effect of steroids in the hippocampus. Additional evidence comes from findings that a single acutely stressful event quickly enhanced dendritic spine density in the male hippocampus but reduced density in the female hippocampus (Shors, *et al* 2001).

Rapid behavioral changes to acute changes in circulating steroids have been reported in other paradigms. These include increased aggression in male rats to acute increases in corticosteroids (Haller, *et al* 2000), and an immediate response by women to a recently formed metabolite of TS. This is in the form of attraction to the odors of androstenol from men that is found in the apocrine glands located in the axillae of the skin in the armpits and pubic region (Kohl, *et al* 2001).

A more titillating behavioral example is the so-called Coolidge effect (Dewsbury 1981). This refers to the reinstitution of copulation in sexually satiated males with the introduction of a new, unmated female. In this paradigm, a male is allowed to copulate to exhaustion, identified by the male refusing to attempt to initiate another copulation. However, removal of that female and replacement with a novel, receptive female is quickly followed by renewed, vigorous copulation. This procedure can be repeated several times with a new female and the same male, with the same result.

The implication is of a momentary rise in TS followed by an immediate behavioral change. The most likely explanation is for non-genomic activities of steroid hormones. We know now that steroids, including androgens, have the capacity for membrane-induced activation of neurotransmitter pathways underlying behavior (Frye 2001). Steroid receptors on the presynaptic and postsynaptic neurons can quickly influence neural activity and, thus, behavior.

Another mechanism for fast changes in sexual responsiveness of the male changes to momentary changes in TS is an indirect effects. We have demonstrated that female rats prefer a male with high TS levels. Intact females given a choice between inaccessible castrated males restored with different amounts of TS preferred to spend time near the higher TS male (Taylor, *et al* 1982). It is possible that the adaptive value of a sudden pulse of TS in the male is that the female will be more responsive to the male, thus increasing his sexual prowess.

III.2.2. Chronic changes in testosterone are likely to change sexual function

Most of the research on changing levels of hormone, however, has looked at long term TS exposure. This is in recognition that typically steroid hormonal changes slowly modify sexual behavior.

Chronic hormonal changes can be either from natural changes or experimentally induced changes. Most often the changes are to increase circulating hormone. Puberty or increases during a breeding season represent natural elevation of TS. Exogenous administration to castrated animals or hypogonadal men represent the most studied groups for behavioral changes accompanying chronic increases in TS titers. Natural declines with aging are a notable instance of decreases in circulating TS.

An interesting study group are men convicted of felonies for sexually deviant behaviors. Often they are pedophiles. Studies of surgical castration in a large study of 104 sex offenders found highly significant decreases in sexual arousal or performance in 90% of the men. Further studies of recidivism indicated a significant decrease in sex offenders following castration (Stone, *et al* 2000).

Still, it is notable that castrated males do not immediately lose sexual capacity (Baum, *et al* 1986). In male rats, the decline in copulatory performance takes a time course that is the reverse of the normal sequence of mounting without intromission, multiple intromissions followed by ejaculation. With castration of the rat, the first copulatory response to be lost is ejaculation and the last to be lost is mounting (Davidson 1966). Actually the very first sexual response, sexual motivation, is the last to be lost, and may never disappear entirely in castrated males, most notably men. The same is observed with a pharmacological agent that blocked the conversion of TS to E2 in the brains of male rats. All aspects of sexual behavior were eventually disrupted, but again the ordering of behavioral disruption was the sequence of ejaculation to sexual motivation (Bonsall, *et al* 1992).

The point is that a sudden and dramatic decrease in TS requires time to impact most androgen – sensitive structures and, especially, behaviors. In the following sections, we will consider paradigms that underline the importance of significant changes in circulating TS and the impact on sexual behaviors.

III.2.3. Aging represents a natural chronic decrease in testosterone and sexual function

In assessing the behavioral consequences of changes in circulating hormone levels and sexual behavior, a good place to start is with the aging male literature. Studies with non-human animals and humans have repeatedly confirmed the informal observations of many of us; aging is accompanied by a decrease in sexual behavior. Sexual performance declines earlier and more dramatically with aging than does sexual interest, but both performance and motivation show declines (Bancroft 2005, Taylor, *et al* 1996). There is also a progressive and systematic decrease in systemic TS in males (Lupo-DiPrisco and Dessi-Fulgheri 1980, Seidman 2003). Endocrine aging is less dramatic than the menopause of women, but aging exacts a toll on males and androgen-sensitive functions.

In a study of gonadally intact 22-24 months old male rats in good general health, we used multiple measures of sociosexual behavior and reproductive physiology to demonstrate that even healthy aging is accompanied by endocrine declines (Taylor, *et al* 1996). The untreated old animals showed clear decrements on all 13 measures of hypothalamic – pituitary – testicular function. This included reduced TS titers and decreased sexual activity.

The same is reported for a retrospective and prospective evaluation of sexual function and behavior in 77 healthy married men aged 45 to 74 years. There were significant age-related decreases in sexual desire, sexual arousal and activity, and increases in erectile problems. Aging also was negatively correlated with TS (Schiavi, *et al* 1991).

III.2.4. Hormone therapy to aged males increases sexual behaviors

There may or may not (Haren, *et al* 2002, Mazur, *et al* 2002) be a clearly identifiable causal relation between the two events, but a logical step for treatment of low sex hormone levels and reduced sexuality accompanying aging is hormone supplementation (Hayes 2000). There is understandable reluctance for clinicians to recommend TS therapy for aging men, given the well-known androgen sensitivity of the vulnerable prostate gland (Hijazi and Cunningham 2005). Nonetheless, given the success in experimental animals, TS supplementation for aging men remains an attractive therapy (Swerdloff and Wang 2004).

Clearly, androgen sensitive reproductive structures in older male animal models maintain sensitivity to additional TS (Chambers, *et al* 1991, Chubb and Desjardins 1984). The bulk of the data confirm benefits of TS to older males (Davidson, *et al* 1982, Schiavi, *et al* 1997). Treated males do not experience complete recovery to the behaviors of young males, but treated old males show more sexual interest and, to a lesser extent, increased copulatory capabilities.

Benefits of androgen therapy are accrued best in aged animal models and humans that are free of the diseases of old age (Wespes and Schulman 2002) and in aging males suffering the lowest TS levels (Corona, *et al* 2004). Not surprisingly, supplementation during middle age may be most effective. Testosterone supplements to 13 months old male rats, an ontogenetic period that models middle age in men, successfully increased most aspects of sexual behavior (Gray, *et al* 1981).

On rare occasion, experiments have been devised to increase endogenous circulating TS. In one experiment, we took advantage of the findings cited earlier that young males experience acute increases in TS to the presence of receptive females. We first asked if the same would be observed in old rats, and the results confirmed a significant rise in TS in old males (Taylor, *et al* 1996). Using the same receptive female exposure paradigm, we compared chronic endogenous and exogenous TS increases on two groups of healthy 22-24 months rats. Old male rats were administered either exogenous (ExT) supplementations daily for 6 weeks or were exposed to brief daily exposures to an inaccessible estrous female for additional episodes of endogenous (EnT) hormone over the same time period. Neither treatment restored their healthy old male rats to levels of sexual behavior approximating those of untreated young adults. Nonetheless, EnT males showed greater increases in sexual motivation and performance than ExT males. Their conclusions included that aged sexual behaviors of healthy old rats retain notable capacity, particularly, for endogenous TS activation of sociosexual behaviors (Taylor, *et al* 1996).

III.2.5. Testosterone to hypogonadal young males increases sexual behavior

Success is often reported with chronic TS supplementation in young hypogonadal men. Insufficient production of TS results in various sexual deficits affecting both sexual interest and sexual performance. Testosterone therapy commonly improves both significantly.

For example, men 25 – 40 yrs of age were diagnosed with severe hypogonadism by having a mean TS level of 35 ng/ dl, compared to the minimal level of 300 ng/ dl in eugonadal males (Burris, *et al* 1992). Patients were injected with 200 mg TS enanthate intramuscularly every 2 weeks for up to a year. Results were striking. Nocturnal erections in the hypogonadal men increased steadily during hormone replacement and were in the normal range with 6 to 12 months of treatment. The hypogonadal men also reported increases in several aspects of sexual activity, including sexual interest and the number of spontaneous erections.

It is interesting to highlight that this was clearly a genomic effect of the steroids. Serum TS concentration increased immediately and finally reached the upper range of normal levels. Yet, the behaviors only gradually changed with the immediate changes in circulating TS (Burris, *et al* 1992).

Other studies have reported similarly significant improvements in sexual function in hypogonadal young men treated with testosterone (Arver, *et al* 1996, Ashmed, *et al* 1988). A recent meta-analysis (Isidori, *et al* 2005) of men with TS levels below 300 ng/ dl receiving chronic TS therapy concluded that hormone treatment was moderately effective, likely because some were moderately hypogonadal. Even with this analysis, the men reported improvements in the number of nocturnal erections, sexual thoughts and motivation, number of successful intercourses, erectile function and overall sexual satisfaction.

Adolescent boys with delayed puberty also appear to benefit from TS supplementation, however, the benefits are not as clear as in young men. Depo-testosterone was administered to delayed pubertal boys in 3-month blocks alternating with placebo. Although there were modest increases in measures of sexuality, there were significant hormone effects on physical aggressive behaviors and aggressive impulses. A causal correlation is difficult to dispute because numerous studies have shown that withdrawal of exogenous TS to hypogonadal or castrated males is followed by a rapid and marked decrease in sexual interest and activity that is reinstated in a few weeks with TS replacement therapy (Meston and Frohlich 2000).

Nonetheless, there are data to jolt us back to the recognition that sexuality is dependent on factors other than normal androgens in circulation (OCarroll and Bancroft 1984). Hormonal supplementation that results in normal TS values does not always restore libido and erectile function in hypogonadal males. Moreover, many hypogonadal men are capable of sexual erections. Almost a third of men receiving effective anti-androgen therapy for prostate disease can develop erections when tested with erotic stimulation (Morales and Heaton 2003).

Previous findings with normal males may provide a clue to understanding at least some of the exceptions. In one experiment, we treated gonadally intact male rats to increase TS levels in one group by exogenous TS injections and decreased TS effectiveness by administering an antiandrogen to a second group. We found that decreased TS potency had minimal effects on sexual and aggressive behaviors despite profound suppressive effects on reproductive organs and glands (Taylor, *et al* 1985).

In an elegant experiment with healthy young men (Buena, *et al* 1993), two groups were treated with a GnRH agonist that suppresses endogenous TS production. Both groups also received TS replacement by a sustained release, long-acting microcapsule formulation to restore serum TS levels at low and high ends of the normal male range, respectively. There were no differences between the two groups on any measure of libido or copulatory performance. The most plausible explanation is that the threshold for sexual behavior is considerably below the circulating TS value of normal males (Bhasin, *et al* 2001). This may explain why some partially hypogonadal men continue to have normal sexual function and the absence of correlation between sexuality in males with serum T levels either in the high or low normal ranges.

III.2.6. Supplements that produce supraphysiological increases in testosterone do not change behaviors of healthy young males

Inspired by the upsurge in abuse of anabolic steroids there is now a substantial literature on the behavioral outcomes of supraphysiological increases in TS in gonadally intact young males. Here, we are defining supraphysiological as being in the highest values (circa 1000 ng/dl), or slightly above these levels, of TS found in untreated, healthy men.

There are various reasons to predict that additional TS to men with normal endocrine function, the so-called eugonadal condition, would not change sociosexual behaviors. One is that androgen receptors in most tissues are either saturated or downregulated at physiological TS concentrations (Antonio, *et al* 1999). Additional TS would have no more binding sites.

Also, as cited in the previous section, the evidence points to the level of TS required for sexual interest and activity in adult males is lower than normal males' circulating levels of TS. The suggestion is that most males already are at high functional levels of circulating TS. Finally, the threshold model discussed earlier certainly predicts that exogenously induced TS changes above the threshold level would not be expected to influence sexual interest or behavior (Schiavi and Segraves 1995).

The data from men serving as subjects in biomedical experiments provide considerable support for the prediction. A meta-analysis concluded that supplements of TS had no effect on erectile function in eugonadal men compared to placebo (Isidori, *et al* 2005). In a similar paradigm, healthy young men with normal levels of TS were administered supplemental hormone to boost levels to supraphysiological TS values. The men showed an increased self-reported interest in sex during TS treatment. These changes, however, were not reflected in any change in overt sexual behavior, which in eugonadal men may be more determined by sexual relationship factors (Anderson, *et al* 1992).

Their work with gonadally intact male rats provides additional support. Additional hormone does not uniformly increase copulation in sexually experienced males, although TS therapy increased sexual performance of virgin males (Taylor, *et al* 1985).

The conclusion is that supplementation that increases TS to physiological, albeit high physiological, levels is unlikely to increase sexual performance. However, the treatment can increase sexual interest. Supplements that increase TS levels to pharmacologic levels may be quite another story.

III.2.7. Steroid abuse raises testosterone to pharmacological levels with increases in aggressiveness and perhaps sexual motivation

An important feature of the supraphysiological research cited above is that the TS supplements to eugonadal men were of minimal to modest dosages and of short durations. This is dictated by the consideration of human researchers bound by ethical considerations to keep the TS dosages to the participants in ranges that are unlikely to endanger their health. Even many researchers using animal models attempt to maintain as near physiological titers of steroid as possible to provide data that can be generalized to natural populations.

There are people outside the usual biomedical research protocols, however, who experience chronic, and greatly exaggerated, pharmacologic levels of circulating TS. These are, of course, professional or amateur athletes and others who abuse anabolic steroids. These compounds are more accurately identified as androgenic anabolic steroids (AAS) to indicate they have the significant androgenic effects of TS and muscle building (anabolic) features. AAS are synthetic derivatives of TS. Indeed, many AAS were developed by pharmaceutical firms as possible TS therapies with different characteristics (Clark and Henderson 2003).

The most potent AAS are injected to avoid the dangers of first-pass metabolism, with the result that androgen titers are chronically high and pharmacological. It is not uncommon for these values to be 20x or more of the highest, physiological values. Because these individuals are engaged in criminal activity, they are off-limits to responsible researchers. Thus, there are only informal, non-systematic data available on people abusing steroids.

Adding to the uncertainty of information on anabolic steroid abuse is that results of the supraphysiological biomedical studies cited in the previous section may not accurately reflect the outcomes of the high pharmacological dosages common among abusers of steroids (Yates, *et al* 1999). Fortunately, there are systematic data available from animal models administered high doses to mimic the pharmacological levels of steroid abusers (Blanco, *et al* 1997).

The behavioral results from these animal experiments suggest that AAS are more likely to elevate aggression than sexuality. For example, injection of TS propionate over 10 weeks to intact adult male rats increased inter-male aggression significantly with less effect on copulation (Lumia, *et al* 1994). Aggression was also increased toward the source of a tail pinch in intact male rats treated with high doses of TS for 12 weeks (McGinnis, *et al* 2002). Finally, a study of a highly strain of mice administered TS observed no further increases in their intact adults. Females of the strain, however, showed more aggression to the same dosage of TS (Bronson 1996). A recent review (Clark and Henderson 2003) of the animal literature concluded that AAS has minimal effects on sexual behavior of intact rats, although there were a few exceptions for animals treated chronically with very high dosages.

The available human data suggests that very high doses of TS may, in fact, increase both some aspects of sociosexual behaviors (Lukas 1993). Sexual performance in the form of impotency may be a significant risk factor of pharmacological dosages (Eklof, *et al* 2003), but heightened aggressiveness and libido may be increased. A 2-week, double-blind placebo-controlled crossover study administered high doses of methyltestosterone to 20 young, healthy volunteers. Results were statistically significant increases in sexual arousal, energy and irritability (Su, *et al* 1993). Self-reports by AAS abusing athletes have suggestion a similar conclusion (Clark and Henderson 2003). These results point to AAS agents that induce long-term pharmacologic elevation of systemic TS almost surely increase aggressive behaviors and also may increase sexual motivation. Sexual performance, however, is likely to suffer declines.

Conclusion

To summarize, we offer the following general principles of testosterone – sociosexual behavior relations. 1) The evidence is overwhelming that testosterone is critical for the organization and activation of sexual responses of the male. 2) In males, and likely also in females, testosterone is responsible for sexual motivation. 3) Probably the testosterone metabolites, DHT and especially E2, are ultimately responsible for much of the activation of brain system underlying the sociosexual behaviors of males. 4) Resting testosterone levels are unlikely to be related to individual differences in behavior, but momentary and, especially, chronic changes in testosterone in circulation are directly associated with changes in sociosexual behaviors. 5) Steroid supplements that increase circulating testosterone to high physiological levels are likely to improve the sexual well-being of hypogonadal and aged men, but anabolic steroids that produce pharmacologic testosterone levels are unlikely to produce beneficial behavioral outcomes. 6) The distribution of steroid receptors in brain areas unrelated to reproduction, along with the non-genomic effects of neuroactive steroids and neurosteroids, point to the likelihood that we have only scratched the surface of the impact steroids have on brain morphology and function, and behavior. The neuroendocrinology of testosterone and the other steroids are likely to have a most interesting future.

References

Abbud, R. A., Ameduri, R. K., Rao, J. S., Nett, T. M. & Nilson, J. H. (1999). Chronic hypersecretion of luteinizing hormone in transgenic mice selectively alters responsiveness of the alpha-subunit gene to gonadotropin-releasing hormone and estrogens. *Molecular Endocrinology, 13,* 1449-1459.

Adkins-Regan, E. (1981). Hormone specificity, androgen metabolism, and social behavior. *American Zoologist, 21,* 257-271.

Akingbemi, B. T. (2005). Estrogen regulation of testicular function. *Reproductive Biology and Endocrinology, 3,* doi: 10. 1186/1477-7827-1183-1151.

Aluja, A. & Torrubia, R. (2004). Hostility-aggressiveness, sensation seeking, and sex hormones in men: Re-exploring their relationship. *Neuropsychobiology, 50,* 102-108.

Anderson, R. A., Bancroft, J. & Wu, F. C. (1992). The effects of exogenous testosterone on sexuality and mood of normal men. *Journal of Clinical Endocrinology & Metabolism, 75,* 1503-1507.

Antonio, J., Wilson, J. D. & George, F. W. (1999). Effects of castration and androgen treatment on androgen-receptor levels in rat skeletal muscles. *Journal of Applied Physiology, 87,* 2016–2019.

Archer, J. (1994). Testosterone and aggression. In: *The Psychobiology of Aggression* (ed. by M. Hillbrand & N. J. Pallone), 3-25. The Haworth Press, New York.

Arlt, W., Haas, J., Callies, F., Reincke, M., Hubler, D., Oettel, M., Ernst, M., Schulte, H. & Allolio, B. (1999). Biotransformation of oral dehydroepiandrosterone in elderly men: significant increase in circulating estrogens. *Journal of Clinical Endocrinology & Metabolism, 84,* 2170-2176.

Arnold, A. P. & Gorski, R. A. (1984). Gonadal steroid induction of structural sex differences in the central nervous system. *Annual Review of Neuroscience, 7,* 413-442.

Arver, S., Dobs, A. S., Meikle, A. W., Allen, R. P., Sanders, S. W. & Mazer, N. A. (1996). Improvement of sexual function in testosterone deficient men treated for 1 year with a permeation enhanced testosterone transdermal system. *Journal of Urology, 155,* 1604-1608.

Ashmed, S. F., Boucher, A., Manni, A., Santen, R., Bartholomew, M. & Demers, L. (1988). Transdermal testosterone therapy in the treatment of male hypogonadism. *Journal of Clinical Endocrinology & Metabolism, 66,* 546-551.

Bachmann, G. A. (2002). The hypoandrogenic woman; pathophysiologic overview. *Fertility and Sterility, 77,* S72-S76

Ball, G. F. & Balthazart, J. (2006). Androgen metabolism and the activation of male sexual behavior: It's more complicated than you think! *Hormones and Behavior, 49,* 1-3.

Balthazart, J. & Ball, G. F. (1998). New insights into the regulation and function of brain estrogen synthase (aromatase). *Trends in Neuroscience, 21,* 243-249.

Bancroft, J. (2005). The endocrinology of sexual arousal. *Journal of Endocrinology, 186,* 411-427.

Bartke, A. & Dalterio, S. (1975). Episodic secretion of testosterone in laboratory mice. *Science., 100,* 1-5.

Baulieu, E. E. (1997). Neurosteroids: of the nervous system, by the nervous system, for the nervous system. *Recent Progress in Hormone Research, 52,* 1-32.

Baulieu, E. E. (1998). Neurosteroids: a novel function of the brain. *Psychoneuroendocrinology, 23,* 963-987.

Baum, M., Melamed, E. & Globus, M. (1986). Dissociation of the effects of castration and testosterone replacement on sexual behavior and neural metabolism of dopamine in the male rat. *Brain Research Bulletin, 16,* 145-148.

Baum, M. J. (2002). Neuroendocrinology of sexual behavior in the male. In: *Behavioral Endocrinology, 2nd Edition* (ed. by J. Becker, M. Breedlove & D. Crews), 153-203. The M. I. T. Press, Cambridge, MA.

Beach, F. A. (1981). Historical origins of modern research on hormones and behavior. *Hormones & Behavior, 15,* 325-376.

Beck, S. G. & Handa, R. J. (2004). Dehydroepiandrosterone (DHEA): A misunderstood adrenal hormone and spine-tingling neurosteroid? *Endocrinology, 145,* 1039-1041.

Belelli, D. & Lamber, J. J. (2005). Neurosteroids: endogenous regulators of the GABA-A receptor. *Nature Reviews of Neuroscience 6,* 565-566.

Beyer, C., Larsson, K., Perez-Placios, G. & Morali, G. (1973). Androgen structure and male sexual behavior in the castrated rat. *Hormones & Behavior, 4,* 99-107.

Bhasin, S., Woodhouse, L., Dzekov, C. & Others, X. (2001). Testosterone dose-response relationships in healthy young men. *American Journal of Physiology: Endocrinology & Metabolism, 281,* E1172-E1181.

Bialek, M., Zaremba, P., Borowicz, K. K. & Czuczwar, S. J. (2004). Neuroprotective role of testosterone in the nervous system. *Polish Journal of Pharmacology, 56,* 509-518.

Birchard, K. (1999) Body-building supplement fails to strengthen muscle and may harm health. *Lancet, 353,* 1943-1944.

Birzniece, V., Backstrom, T., Johansson, M. A. & Others, X. (2006). Neuroactive steroid effects on cognitive functions with a focus on the serotonin and GABA systems. *Brain Research Reviews, 51,* 212-239.

Blanco, C. E., Popper, P. & Micevych, P. (1997). Anabolic-androgenic steroid induced alterations in choline acetyltransferase messenger RNA levels of spinal cord motoneurons in the male rat. *Neuroscience, 78,* 873-882.

Bonsall, R., Clancy, A. & Michael, R. (1992). Effects of the nonsteroidal aromatase inhibitor, fadrozole, on sexual behavior in male rats. *Hormones & Behavior, 26,* 240-254.

Bonsall, R. W., Rees, H. & Michael, R. (1985). The distribution, nuclear uptake and metabolism of (3H) dihydrotestosterone in the brain, pituitary gland and genital tract of the male rhesus monkey. *Journal of Steroid Biochemistry, 23,* 389-398.

Breedlove, S. M. & Hampson, E. (2002). Sexual differentiation of the brain and behavior. In: *Behavioral Endocrinology, Second Edition* (ed. by J. B. Becker, S. M. Breedlove, D. Crews & M. M. McCarthy), 75-116. The MIT Press, Cambridge, MA.

Breedlove, S. M. & Jordan, C. L. (2001). The increasingly plastic, hormone-responsive adult brain. *Proceedings of the National Academy of Sciences, 98,* 2956-2957.

Bronson, F. H. (1996). Effects of prolonged exposure to anabolic steroids on the behavior of male and female mice. *Pharmacology Biochemistry & Behavior, 53,* 329–334.

Bronwyn, A. L., Crawford, C., Liu, P. Y., Kean, M. T., Bleasel, J. F. & Handelsman, D. J. (2003). Randomized placebo-controlled trial of androgen effects on muscle and bone in men requiring long- term systemic glucocorticoid treatment. *Journal of Clinical Endocrinology and Metabolism, 88,* 3167-3176.

Brown, W. A., Monti, P. & Corriveau, D. (1978). Serum testosterone and sexual activity and interest in men. *Archives of Sexual Behavior, 7,* 97-103.

Buena, F., Swerdloff, R. S., Steiner, B. S., Lutchmansingh, P., Peterson, M. A., Pandian, M. R., Galmarini, M. & Bhasin, S. (1993). Sexual function does not change when serum testosterone levels are pharmacologically varied within the normal male range. *Fertility & Sterility, 59,* 1118-1123.

Burris, A. S., Banks, S. M., Carter, S., Davidson, J. M. & Sherins, R. J. (1992). A long-term, prospective study of the physiologic and behavioral effects of hormone replacement in untreated hypogonadal men. *Journal of Andrology, 13,* 297-304.

Butera, P. C. & Czaja, J. A. (1989). Activities of sexual behavior in male rats by combined subcutaneous and intracranial treatments of 5 alpha-dihydrotestosterone. *Hormones & Behavior, 23,* 92-105.

Carlson, A. A., Young, A. J., Russell, A. F., Bennett, N. C., McNeilly, A. S. & Clutton-Brock, T. (2004). Hormonal correlates of dominance in meerkats (Suricata suricatta). *Hormones & Behavior, 46,* 141-150.

Carreau, S., Lambard, S., Delalande, C. & Others, X. (2003). Aromatase expression and role of estrogens in male gonad: a review. *Reproductive Biology and Endocrinology, 1,* 211-223.

Chambers, K. C. & Phoenix, C. H. (1992). Sexual behavior and serum levels of prolactin, testosterone, and estradiol in young and old rhesus males. *Physiology & Behavior, 52,* 13-16.

Chambers, K. C., Thornton, J. & Roselli, C. (1991). Age-related deficits in brain androgen binding and metabolism, testosterone, and sexual behavior of male rats. *Neurobiology of Aging, 12,* 123-130.

Chen, F., K., K., E., B., J., F. & Others, X. (2005). Direct agonist/antagonist functions of dehydroepiandrosterone. *Endocrinology, 146,* 4568-4576.

Chen, T. & Tu, W. (1992). Sex differences in estrogen and androgen receptors in hamster brain. *Life Sciences, 50,* 1639-1647.

Chubb, C. & Desjardins, C. (1984). Testicular function and sexual activity in senescent mice. *American Journal of Physiology, 247,* 569-573.

Clark, A. S. & Henderson, L. P. (2003). Behavioral and physiological responses to anabolic-androgenic steroids. *Neuroscience and Biobehavioral Reviews, 27,* 413-436.

Cooke, B., Hegstrom, C. D., Villeneuve, L. S. & Breedlove, S. M. (1999a). Sexual differentiation of the vertebrate brain: principles and mechanisms. *Frontiers in Neuroendocrinology, 20,* 323-362.

Cooke, B. M., Breedlove, S. M. & Jordan, C. L. (2003). Both estrogen receptors and androgen receptors contribute to testosterone-induced changes in the morphology of the medial amygdala and sexual arousal in male rats. *Hormones & Behavior, 43,* 336-346.

Cooke, B. M., Tabibnia, G. & Breedlove, S. M. (1999b). A brain sexual dimorphism controlled by adult circulating androgens. *Proceedings of the National Academy of Sciences (U. S. A.), 96,* 7538-7540.

Cooke, P. S., Buchanan, D. L., Lubahn, D. B. & Cunha, G. R. (1998). Mechanism of estrogen action: Lessons from the estrogen receptor-alpha knockout mouse. *Biology of Reproduction, 59,* 470-475.

Corona, G., Mannucci, E., Mansani, R. & Others, X. (2004). Aging and pathogenesis of erectile dysfunction. *International Journal of Impotence Research, 16,* 395-402.

Corpechot, C., Robel, P., Axelson, M., Sjovall, J. & Baulieu, E. (1981). Characterization and measurement of dehydroepiandrosterone sulfate in the rat brain. *Proceedings of the National Academy of Science, 78,* 4704-4707.

Craigen, W. & Bronson, F. (1982). Deterioration of the capacity for sexual arousal in aged male mice. *Biology of Reproduction, 26,* 869-874.

Dabbs, J. & Hargrave, K. R. (1997). Age, testosterone, and behavior among female prison inmates. *Psychosomatic Medicine, 59,* 477-480.

Damassa, D. A., Smith, E. R., Tennent, B. & Davidson, J. M. (1977). The relationship between circulating testosterone levels and male sexual behavior in rats. *Hormones & Behavior, 8,* 275-286.

Davidson, J. M. (1966). Characteristics of sex behaviour in male rats following castration. *Animal Behaviour, 14,* 266-272.

Davidson, J. M., Kwan, M. & Greenleaf, W. J. (1982). Hormonal replacement and sexuality in men. *Journal of Clinical Endocrinology and Metabolism, 11,* 599-623.

Davis, S. R. (1999). The therapeutic use of androgens in women. *Journal of Steroid Biochemistry & Molecular Biology, 69,* 177-184.

Davis, S. R., Goldstat, R., Papalia, M. A., Shah, S., Kulkarni, J., Donath, S. & Bell, R. J. (2006). Effects of aromatase inhibition on sexual function and well-being in postmenopausal women treated with testosterone: a randomized, placebo-controlled trial. *Menopause, 13,* 37-45.

Davis, S. R., McCloud, P., Strauss, B. J. & Burger, H. (1995). Testosterone enhances estradiol's effects on postmenopausal bone density and sexuality. *Maturitas, 21,* 227-236.

Dennerstein, L. M. B., Randolph, J., Taffe, J., Dudley, E. & Burger, H. (2002). Hormones, mood, sexuality, and the menopausal transition. *Fertility and Sterility, 77,* S42-S48.

Dewsbury, D. A. (1981). Effects of novelty on copulatory behavior: The Coolidge effect and related phenomena. *Psychological Bulletin, 89,* 464-482.

Dhatariya, K. (2005). Self-reported sexual function in women and androgen levels. *JAMA, 294,* 2167-2168.

Dobs, A. S., Nguyen, T., Pace, C. & Roberts, C. P. (2002). Differential effects of oral estrogen versus oral estrogen-androgen replacement therapy on body composition in postmenopausal women. *Journal of Clinical Endocrinology & Metabolism, 87,* 1509-1516.

Dominguez, J. M. & Hull, E. M. (2005). Dopamine, the medial preoptic area, and male sexual behavior. *Physiology & Behavior, 86,* 356-368.

DonCarlos, L. L., Garcia-Ovejero, D., Sarkey, S., Garcia-Segura, L. M. & Azcoitia, I. (2003). Androgen receptor immunoreactivity in forebrain axons and dendrites in the rat. *Endocrinology, 144,* 3632-3638.

Dougherty, D. M., Bjork, J. M., Moeller, F. G. & Swann, A. C. (1997). The influence of menstrual-cycle phase on the relationship between testosterone and aggression. *Physiology & Behavior, 62,* 431-435.

Eklof, A. C., Thurelius, A. M., Garle, M., Rane, A. & Sjoqvist, F. (2003). The anti-doping hot-line, a means to capture the abuse of doping agents in the Swedish society and a new service function in clinical pharmacology. *European Journal of Clinical Pharmacology, 59,* 571-577.

Engel, S. R. & Grant, K. A. (2001). Neurosteroids and behavior. *International Review of Neurobiology, 46,* 321-348.

Everitt, B. J. (1990). Sexual motivation: A neural and behavioral analysis of the mechanisms underlying appetitive and copulatory responses in male rats. *Neuroscience and Biobehavioral Reviews, 14,* 217-232.

Ewing, L., Gorski, R., Sbordane, R., Tyler, J., Desjardins, C. & Robaire, B. (1979). Testosterone-estradiol filled polydimethylsiloxane subdermal implants: Effect on fertility and masculine sexual and aggressive behavior of male rats. *Biology of Reproduction, 21,* 765-772.

Federman, D. D. (2004). Three facets of sexual differentiation. *New England Journal of Medicine, 350,* 323-324.

Fernandez-Guasti, A., Kruijver, F. P., Fodor, M. & Swaab, D. F. (2000). Sex differences in the distribution of androgen receptors in the human hypothalamus. *Journal of Comparative Neurology, 425,* 422-435.

Frankel, E. (1984). Plasma testosterone levels are higher in old mating rats than in old non-mating rats. *Experimental Gerontology, 16,* 345-348.

Frye, C. A. (2001). The role of neurosteroids and non-genomic effects of progestins and androgens in mediating sexual receptivity of rodents. *Brain Research Reviews, 37,* 201-222.

Frye, C. A. & McCormick, C. M. (2000). Androgens are neuroprotective in the dentate gyrus of adrenalectomized female rats. *Stress, 3,* 185-194.

Fukada, S., Nagashima, H., Marioka, K. & Aoki, J. (1988). Fluctuation in peripheral serum testosterone levels within a day with age and by sexual stimulation in male beagle dogs bred indoors. *Experimental Animals, 37,* 381-386.

Goldstein, I., Traish, A., Kim, N. & Munarriz, R. (2004). The role of sex steroid hormones in female sexual function and dysfunction. *Clinical Obstetrics And Gynecology, 47,* 471-484.

Goldstein, J. S. & Sites, C. K. (2002). Selective modulation of sex steroids. *Ageing Research Reviews, 1,* 17-28.

Gordon, R. J., Breedlove, M. S., Bernstein, S. & Lichtman, J. W. (1990). Neuromuscular junctions shrink and expand as muscle fiber size is manipulated: in vivo observations in the androgen-sensitive bulbocavernosus muscle of mice. *Journal of Neuroscience, 10,* 2660-2671.

Gray, G. D., Smith, E., Dorsa, D. & Davidson, J. M. (1981). Sexual behavior and testosterone in middle-aged rats. *Endocrinology, 109,* 1597-1604.

Gray, P. B., Singh, A. B., Woodhouse, L. J. & Others, X. (2005). Dose-dependent effects of testosterone on sexual function, mood, and visuospatial cognition in older men. *Journal of Clinical Endocrinology & Metabolism, 90,* 3838-3846.

Greenstein, A., Plymate, S. R. & Katz, P. G. (1995). Visually stimulated erection in castrated men. *Journal of Urology, 153,* 650-652.

Gruber, C. J., Tschugguel, W., Schneeberger, C. & Huber, J. C. (2002). Production and actions of estrogens. *New England Journal of Medicine, 346,* 340-352.

Guay, A., Munarriz, R., Jacobson, J., Talakoub, L., Traish, A., Quirk, F., Goldstein, I. & Spark, R. (2004). Serum androgen levels in healthy premenopausal women with and without sexual dysfunction: Part A. Serum androgen levels in women aged 20-49 years with no complaints of sexual dysfunction. *International Journal of Impotence Research, 16,* 112-120.

Hall, C. M., Jones, J. A., Meyer-Bahlburg, H. F., Dolezal, C., Coleman, M., Foster, P., Price, D. A. & Clayton, P. E. (2004). Behavioral and physical masculinization are related to genotype in girls with congenital adrenal hyperplasia. *Journal of Clinical Endocrinology & Metabolism, 89,* 419-424.

Haller, J., Millar, S., van de Schraaf, J., de Kloet, R. E. & Kruk, M. R. (2000). The active phase-related increase in corticosterone and aggression are linked. *Journal of Neuroendocrinology, 12,* 431-436.

Hamann, S. (2005). Sex differences in the responses of the human amygdala. *Neuroscientist, 11,* 288-293.

Haren, M. T., Morley, J. E., Chapman, I. M., O'Loughlin, P. D. & Wittert, G. A. (2002). Defining 'relative' androgen deficiency in aging men: how should testosterone be measured and what are the relationships between androgen levels and physical, sexual and emotional health?. *Climacteric, 5,* 15-25.

Hayes, F. J. (2000). Testosterone - fountain of youth or drug of abuse? *Journal of Clinical Endocrinology & Metabolism, 85,* 3020-3023.

Hijazi, R. A. & Cunningham, G. R. (2005). Andropause: Is androgen replacement therapy indicated for the aging male? . *Annual Review of Medicine, 56,* 117-137.

Hodes, G. E. & Shors, T. J. (2005). Distinctive stress effects on learning during puberty. *Hormones and Behavior, 48,* 163-171.

Howell, S. & Shalet, S. (2001). Testosterone deficiency and replacement. *Hormone Research, 56 (Suppl. 1),* 86-92.

Huang, J., Chang, L., Ho, D. & Ho, L. (1989). The effect of sexual activity on androgen metabolism, androgen-receptor translocation and glandular weight of ventral prostates of rats. *Endocrinology, 120,* 505-510.

Huhtaniemi, I. (2000). Mutations of gonadotrophin and gonadotrophin receptor genes: what do they teach us about reproductive physiology? *Journal of Reproduction and Fertility, 119,* 173–186.

Hull, E. M., Lorrain, D. S., Du, J., Matuszewich, L., Lumley, L., Putnam, S. K. & Moses, J. (1999). Hormone-neurotransmitter interactions in the control of sexual behavior. *Behavioural Brain Research, 105,* 105-116.

Isidori, A. M., Giannetta, E., Gianfrilli, D. & Others, X. (2005). Effects of testosterone on sexual function in men: results of a meta-analysis. *Clinical Endocrinology, 63,* 381-394.

Johannsson, G., Burman, P., Wiren, L. & Others, X. (2002). Low dose dehydroepiandrosterone affects behavior in hypopituitary androgen-deficient women: a placebo- controlled trial. *Journal of Clinical Endocrinology & Metabolism, 87,* 2046–2052.

Johnston, P. & Davidson, J. M. (1972). Intracerebral androgens and sexual behavior in the male rat. *Hormones & Behavior, 3,* 345-357.

Jones, K. J., Coers, S., Storer, P. D., Tanzer, L. & Kinderman, N. B. (1999). Androgenic regulation of the central glia response following nerve damage. *Journal of Neurobiology, 40,* 560-573.

Kalantaridou, S. N. & Calis, K. A. (2006). Testosterone therapy in premenopausal women. *Seminars in Reproductive Medicine, 24,* 106-114.

Keast, J. R. (1999). The autonomic nerve supply of male sex organs--an important target of circulating androgens. *Behavioural Brain Research, 105,* 81-92.

Kelliher, K. R., Liu, Y. C., Baum, M. J. & Sachs, B. D. (1999). Neuronal Fos activation in olfactory bulb and forebrain of male rats having erections in the presence of inaccessible estrous females. *Neuroscience, 92,* 1025-1033.

King, D. S., Sharp, R. L., Vukovich, M. D., Brown, G. A., Reifenrath, T. A., Uhl, N. L. & Parsons, K. A. (1999). Effect of oral androstenedione on serum testosterone and adaptations to resistance training in young men: a randomized controlled trial. *The Journal of the American Medical Association (JAMA), 281,* 2020-2028.

Knussmann, R., Christiansen, K. & Couwenbergs, C. (1986). Relations between sex hormone levels and sexual behavior in men. *Archives of Sexual Behavior, 15,* 429-445.

Kohl, J. V., Atzmueller, M., Fink, B. & Grammer, K. (2001). Human pheromones: Integrating neuroendocrinology and ethology. *Neuroendocrinology Letters, 22,* 309-321.

Kruger, T. H., Haake, P., Chereath, D., Knapp, W., Janssen, O. E., Exton, M. S., Schedlowski, M. & Hartmann, U. (2003). Specificity of the neuroendocrine response to orgasm during sexual arousal in men. *Journal of Endocrinology, 177,* 57-64.

Labrie, F., Belanger, A., Luu-The, V., Labrie, C., Simard, J., Cusan, L., Gomez, J. & Candas, B. (1998). DHEA and the intracrine formation of androgens and estrogens in peripheral target tissues: Its role during aging. *Steroids, 63,* 322-328.

Labrie, F., Luu-The, V., Belanger, A., Lin, S. X., Simard, J., Pelletier, G. & Labrie, C. (2005). Is dehydroepiandrosterone a hormone? *Journal of Endocrinology, 187,* 169-196.

Leranth, C., Hajszan, T. & MacLusky, N. J. (2004a). Androgens increase spine synapse density in the CA1 hippocampal subfield of ovariectomized female rats. *Journal of Neuroscience, 24,* 495- 499.

Leranth, C., Prange-Kiel, J., Frick, K. M. & Horvath, T. L. (2004b). Low CA1 spine synapse density is further reduced by castration in male non-human primates. *Cerebral Cortex, 14,* 503-510.

Lieberman, S. & Prasad, V. (1990). Heterodox notions on pathways of steroidogenesis. *Endocrine Rev., 11,* 469-493.

Linkowski, P., Mendlewicz, J., Leclercq, R. & Others, X. (1985). The 24-hour profile of adrenocorticotropin and cortisol in major depressive illness. *Journal of Clinical Endocrinology & Metabolism, 61,* 429-438.

Lu, S. F., McKenna, S. E., Cologer-Clifford, A., Nau, E. A. & Simon, N. G. (1998). Androgen receptor in mouse brain: sex differences and similarities in autoregulation. *Endocrinology, 139,* 1594-1601.

Lukas, S. E. (1993). Current perspectives on anabolic-androgenic steroid abuse. *Trends in Pharmacological Science, 14,* 61-68.

Lumia, A. R., Thorner, K. M. & McGinnis, M. Y. (1994). Effects of chronically high doses of the anabolic androgenic steroid, testosterone, on intermale aggression and sexual behavior in male rats. *Physiology & Behavior, 55,* 331-335.

Lupo-DiPrisco, C. & Dessi-Fulgheri, F. (1980). Endocrine and behavioral modifications in aging male rats. *Hormone Research, 12,* 149-160.

Mantzoros, C., Georgiadis, E. & Trichopoulos, D. (1995). Contribution of dihydrotestosterone to male sexual behaviour. *British Medical Journal, 310,* 1289-1291.

Martini, L., Celotti, F., Lechuga, M., Melcangi, R., Motta, M., Negri-Cesi, P., Poletti, A. & Zoppi, S. (1990). Androgen metabolism in different target tissues. *Annals New York Academy of Sciences, 595,* 184-198.

Matthews, K. A., Berga, S. L., Owens, J. F. & Flory, J. D. (1998). Effects of short-term suppression of ovarian hormones on cardiovascular and neuroendocrine reactivity to stress in women. *Psychoneuroendocrinology, 23,* 307-322.

Mazur, A., Mueller, U., Krause, W. & Booth, A. (2002). Causes of sexual decline in aging married men: Germany and America. *International Journal of Impotence Research, 14,* 101-106.

McEwen, B. S. (2001). Estrogens effects on the brain: multiple sites and molecular mechanisms. *Journal of Applied Physiology, 91,* 2785-2801.

McEwen, B. S., Gould, E., Orchinik, M., Weiland, N. & Woolley, C. S. (1995). Oestrogens and the structural and functional plasticity of neurons: implications for memory, ageing and neurodegenerative processes. In: *Non-reproductive actions of sex steroids* (ed. by C. R. Brock & J. A. Goode), 52-73. John Wiley, New York.

McGinnis, M. Y., Lumia, A. R., Breuer, M. E. & Possidente, B. (2002). Physical provocation potentiates aggression in male rats receiving anabolic androgenic steroids. *Hormones & Behavior, 41,* 101-110.

McGivern, R. F., Handa, R. J. & Raum, W. J. (1998). Ethanol exposure during the last week of gestation in the rat: inhibition of the prenatal testosterone surge in males without long-term alterations in sex behavior. *Neurotoxicology & Teratology, 20,* 483-490.

Meisel, R. L. & Sachs, B. D. (1994). The physiology of male reproductive behavior. In: *The Physiology of Reproduction, Volume 2* (ed. by E. Knobil & J. Neill), 3-106. Raven Press, Inc., N. Y.

Mellon, S. H. (1994). Neurosteroids: Biochemistry, modes of action, and clinical relevance. *Journal of Clinical Endocrinology & Metabolism, 78,* 1003-1008.

Meston, C. M. & Frohlich, P. F. (2000). The neurobiology of sexual function. *Archives of General Psychiatry, 57,* 1012-1030.

Meston, C. M. & Heiman, J. R. (2002). Acute dehydroepiandrosterone effects on sexual arousal in premenopausal women. *Journal of Sex & Marital Therapy, 28,* 53-60.

Michael, R. P., Bonsall, R. W. & Zumpe, D. (1987). Testosterone and its metabolites in male cynomologus monkeys (Macaca fascicularis behavior and biochemistry. *Physiology & Behavior, 40,* 527-537.

Michael, R. P., Clancy, A. N. & Zumpe, D. (1995). Distribution of androgen receptor-like immunoreactivity in the brains of cynomolgus monkeys. *Journal of Neuroendocrinology, 7,* 713-719.

Michael, R. P., Zumpe, D. & Bonsall, R. W. (1984). Sexual behavior correlates with the diurnal plasma testosterone range in intact male rhesus monkeys. *Biology of Reproduction, 30,* 652-657.

Miller, K., Sesmilo, G., Schiller, A., Schoenfeld, D., Burton, S. & Klibanski, A. (2001). Androgen deficiency in women with hypopituitarism. *Journal of Clinical Endocrinology & Metabolism, 86,* 561-567.

Miller, K. K. (2002). The androgen deficiency syndrome in women. *Endocrinology Rounds, 1,* 1-8.

Moffat, S. D., Zonderman, A. B., Metter, E. J., Kawas, C., Blackman, M. R., Harman, S. M. & Resnick, S. M. (2004). Free testosterone and risk for Alzheimer disease in older men. *Neurology, 62,* 188-193.

Morales, A. & Heaton, J. P. (2003). Hypogonadism and erectile dysfunction: pathophysiological observations and therapeutic outcomes. *BJU International, 92,* 896-899.

Nakamura, N., Fujita, H. & Kawata, M. (2002). Effects of gonadectomy on immunoreactivity for choline acetyltransferase in the cortex, hippocampus, and basal forebrain of adult male rats. *Neuroscience, 109,* 473-485.

Nottebohm, F. & Arnold, A. P. (1976). Sexual dimorphism in vocal control areas of the songbird brain. *Science, 194,* 211–213.

Nyunt, A., Stephen, G., Gibbin, J., Durgan, L., Fielding, A. M., Wheeler, M. & Price, D. E. (2005). Androgen status in healthy premenopausal women with loss of libido. *Journal of Sex & Marital Therapy, 31,* 73-80.

O'Carroll, R. E. & Bancroft, J. (1984). Testosterone therapy for low sexual interest and erectile dysfunction in men: a controlled study. *British Journal of Psychiatry, 145,* 146-151.

O'Connor, D. B., Archer, J. & Wu, F. C. W. (2004). Effects of testosterone on mood, aggression, and sexual behavior in young men: a double-blind, placebo- controlled, cross-over study. *Journal of Clinical Endocrinology & Metabolism, 89*, 2837-2845.

Occhiato, E. G., Guarna, A., Danza, G. & Serio, M. (2004). Selective non-steroidal inhibitors of 5alpha-reductase type 1. *Journal of Steroid Biochemistry & Molecular Biology, 88,* 1-16.

Payne, A. H. & Hales, D. B. (2004). Overview of steroidogenic enzymes in the pathway from cholesterol to active steroid hormones. *Endocrine Reviews, 25,* 947-970.

Penny, R. (1985). Episodic secretion of melatonin in pre-and post-pubertal girls and boys. *Journal of Clinical Endocrinology & Metabolism, 60,* 751-756.

Pfaus, J. G. (1996). Homologies of animal and human sexual behaviors. *Hormones & Behavior, 30,* 187-200.

Phoenix, C. H. & Chambers, K. C. (1986). Threshold for behavioral response to testosterone in old castrated male rhesus macaques. *Biology of Reproduction. 35,* 918-926.

Phoenix, C. H., Dixson, A. F. & Resko, J. A. (1977). Effects of ejaculation on levels of testosterone, cortisol, and luteinizing hormone in peripheral plasma of rhesus monkeys. *Journal of Comparative & Physiological Psychology, 91,* 120-127.

Phoenix, C. H., Goy, R. W., Gerall, A. A. & Young, W. C. (1959). Organizing action of prenatally administered testosterone propionate on the tissues mediating mating behavior in the female guinea pig. *Endocrinology, 65,* 369-382.

Piroli, G. G., Pietranera, L., Grillo, C. A. & DeNicola, A. F. (2002). Dehydroepiandrosterone regulation of prolactin gene expression in the anterior pituitary does not depend on galanin induction. *Neuroendocrinology Letters, 23,* 321-324.

Resko, J. A. & Roselli, C. E. (1997). Prenatal hormones organize sex differences of the neuroendocrine reproductive system: observations on guinea pigs and nonhuman primates. *Cellular & Molecular Neurobiology, 17,* 627-648.

Roselli, C. E. & Resko, J. A. (1997). Sex differences in androgen-regulated expression of cytochrome P450 aromatase in the rat brain. *Journal of Steroid Biochemistry & Molecular Biology, 61,* 365-374.

Rosler, A. & Witztum, E. (1998). Treatment of men with paraphilia with a long-acting analogue of gonadotropin-releasing hormone. *New England Journal of Medicine, 338,* 416-422.

Rupprecht, R. & Holsboer, F. (1999). Neuropsychopharmacological properties of neuroactive steroids. *Steroids, 64,* 83-91.

Sachs, B. D. (1997). Erection evoked in male rats by airborne scent from estrous females. *Physiology & Behavior, 62,* 921-924.

Sachs, B. D., Glater, G. B. & O'Hanlon, J. K. (1984). Morphology of the erect penis in rats under various gonadal hormone conditions. *Anatomical Record, 210,* 45-52.

Saltzman, E. & Guay, A. (2006). Dehydroepiandrosterone therapy as female androgen replacement. *Seminars in Reproductive Medicine, 24,* 97-105.

Samuels, M., Veldhuis, J., Henry, P. & Ridgway, E. (1990). Pathophysiology of pulsatile and copulsatile release of thyroid-stimulating hormone, luteinizing hormone, follicle-stimulating hormone, and alpha-subunit. *Journal of Clinical Endocrinology & Metabolism, 71,* 425-432.

Sarkola, T., Makisalo, H., Fukunaga, T. & Eriksson, C. J. (1999). Acute effect of alcohol on estradiol, estrone, progesterone, prolactin, cortisol, and luteinizing hormone in premenopausal women. *Alcoholism: Clinical & Experimental Research, 23,* 976-982.

Sarrel, P., Dobay, B. & Wiita, B. (1998). Estrogen and estrogen-androgen replacement in postmenopausal women dissatisfied with estrogen-only therapy. Sexual behavior and neuroendocrine responses. *Journal of Reproductive Medicine, 43,* 847-856.

Schiavi, R. C., Schreiner, P., White, D. & Mandeli, J. (1991). The relationship between pituitary-gonadal function and sexual behavior in healthy aging men. *Psychosomatic Medicine, 53,* 363-374.

Schiavi, R. C. & Segraves, R. T. (1995). The biology of sexual function. *Psychiatric Clinics of North America, 18,* 7-23.

Schiavi , R. C. & White, D. (1976). Androgens and male sexual function: a review of human studies. *Journal of Sex & Marital Therapy, 2,* 214-228.

Schiavi, R. C., White, D., Mandeli, J. & Levine, A. C. (1997). Effect of testosterone administration on sexual behavior and mood in men with erectile dysfunction. *Archives of Sexual Behavior, 26,* 231-241.

Scott, C., Kuehl, D., Ferreira, S. & Jackson, G. (1997). Hypothalamic sites of action for testosterone, dihydrotestosterone, and estrogen in the regulation of luteinizing hormone secretion in male sheep. *Endocrinology, 138,* 3686-3694.

Scott, C. J., Tilbrook, A. J., Rawson, J. A. & Clarke, I. J. (2000). Gonadal steroid receptors in the regulation of GnRH secretion in farm animals. *Animal Reproduction Science, 60-61,* 313-326.

Seidman, S. N. (2003). Testosterone deficiency and mood in aging men: pathogenic and therapeutic interactions. *World Journal of Biological Psychiatry, 4,* 14-20.

Sharpe, R. M. (1998). The roles of oestrogen in the male. *Trends in Endocrinology & Metabolism, 9,* 371-377.

Sherwin, B. B., Gelfand, M. M. & Brender, W. (1985). Androgen enhances sexual motivation in females: a prospective, crossover study of sex steroid administration in the surgical menopause. *Psychosomatic Medicine, 47,* 339-351.

Shifren, J. L. (2004). The role of androgens in female sexual dysfunction. *Mayo Clinic Proceedings, 79 (Supplement),* S19-S24.

Shors, T. J., Chua, C. & Falduto, J. (2001). Sex differences and opposite effects of stress on dendritic spine density in the male versus female hippocampus. *Journal of Neuroscience, 21,* 6292-6297.

Shughrue, P. J., Scrimo, P. J. & Merchenthaler, I. (2000). Estrogen binding and estrogen receptor characterization (ERalpha and ERbeta). in the cholinergic neurons of the rat basal forebrain. *Neuroscience, 96,* 41-49.

Simerly, R. B. (2002). Wired for reproduction: organization and development of sexually dimorphic circuits in the mammalian forebrain. *Annual Review of Neuroscience, 25,* 507-536.

Sodersten, P., Enertoh, P. & Petersson, A. (1983). Episodic secretion of luteinizing hormone and androgen in male rats. *Journal of Endocrinology, 97,* 145-153.

Somboonporn, W., Davis, S., Seif, M. W. & Bell, R. (2005). Testosterone for peri- and postmenopausal women. *Cochrane Database of Systematic Reviews, 2005,* DOI: 10. 1002/14651858. CD14004509. pub14651852.

Southworth, M. B., Matsumoto, A., Gross, K., Soules, M. & Bremner, W. (1991). The importance of signal pattern in the transmission of endocrine information: Pituitary gonadotropin responses to continuous and pulsatile gonadotropin-releasing hormone. *Journal of Clinical Endocrinology and Metabolism, 72,* 1286-1289.

Stalenheim, E. G., Eriksson, E., von Knorring, L. & Wide, L. (1998). Testosterone as a biological marker in psychopathy and alcoholism. *Psychiatry Research, 77,* 79-88.

Sternbach, H. (1998). Age-associated testosterone decline in men: Clinical issues for psychiatry. *American Journal of Psychiatry, 155,* 1310-1318.

Stoffel-Wagner, B. (2001). Neurosteroid metabolism in the human brain. *European Journal of Endocrinology, 145,* 669-679.

Stone, T. H., Winslade, W. J. & Klugman, C. M. (2000). Sex offenders, sentencing laws and pharmaceutical treatment: a prescription for failure. *Behavioral Sciences & the Law, 18,* 83-110.

Su, T. P., Pagliaro, M., Schmidt, P. J., Pickar, D., Wolkowitz, O. & Rubinow, D. R. (1993). Neuropsychiatric effects of anabolic steroids in male normal volunteers. *JAMA The Journal of the American Medical Association, 269,* 2760-2764.

Swerdloff, R. S. & Wang, C. (2004). Androgens and the ageing male. *Best Practice & Research Clinical Endocrinology & Metabolism, 18,* 349-362.

Taylor, G., Bardgett, M., Farr, S., Humphrey, W., Womack, S. & Weiss, J. (1996). Aging of the brain-testicular axis: Reproductive systems of healthy old males with or without endocrine stimulation. *Proceedings of the Society of Experimental Biology & Medicine, 211,* 69-75.

Taylor, G. T. (1980a). Fighting in juvenile rats and the ontogeny of agonistic behavior. *Journal of Comparative & Physiological Psychology, 94,* 953-961.

Taylor, G. T. (1980b). Sex pheromones and aggressive behavior in male rats. *Animal Learning & Behavior, 8,* 485-490.

Taylor, G. T., Bardgett, M. E., Griffin, M. G. & Weiss, J. (1989). Reproductive behavior and physiology of nulliparous female rats after sexual experience. *Behavioural Processes, 19,* 31-46.

Taylor, G. T., Griffin, M. G. & Bardgett, M. E. (1991). Search for a male contraceptive: the effect of gossypol on sexual motivation and epididymal sperm. *Journal of Medicine, 22,* 29-44.

Taylor, G. T., Haller, J. & Regan, D. (1982). Female rats prefer an area vacated by a high testosterone male. *Physiology & Behavior, 28,* 953-958.

Taylor, G. T., Haller, J., Rupich, R. & Weiss, J. (1984). Testicular hormones and intermale aggressive behaviour in the presence of a female rat. *Journal of Endocrinology, 100,* 315-321.

Taylor, G. T. & Pitha, J. (1988). Hormone-cyclodextrin complexes in behavioral endocrinology: Simulating natural episodic release during therapy. *Biomaterials, Artificial Cells & Artificial Organs, 15,* 759-760.

Taylor, G. T., Scherrer, J., Weiss, J. & Pitha, J. (1994). Endocrine interactions: Adrenal steroids and precursors. *American Journal of Physiology, 266,* E676-E681.

Taylor, G. T. & Weiss, J. (1987). Behaviour and fecundity of female rats mated with preferred and non-preferred males. *Animal Behaviour, 35,* 115-121.

Taylor, G. T., Weiss, J. & Rupich, R. (1985). Suprathreshold manipulations of testosterone and reproductive functioning in gonadally intact sexually experienced and inexperienced male rats. *Physiology & Behavior, 35,* 735-739.

Timiras, P. & Cons, J. M. (1982). Hormones during prenatal and neonatal development. In: *Hormones in Development and Aging* (ed. by A. Vernadakis & P. Timiras), 25-79. Spectrum Publications: Medical & Scientific Books, New York.

Tuiten, A., Van Honk, J., Koppeschaar, H., Bernaards, C., Thijssen, J. & Verbaten, R. (2000). Time course of effects of testosterone administration on sexual arousal in women. *Archives of General Psychiatry, 57,* 149-153.

VandePoll, N. E., Taminiau, M. S., Endert, E. & Louwerse, A. L. (1988). Gonadal steroid influence upon sexual and aggressive behavior of female rats. *lnternational]ournal of Neuroscience, 47,* 271-286.

Vanderschueren, D. & Bouillon, R. (2000). Estrogen deficiency in men is a challenge for both the hypothalamus and pituitary. *Journal of Clinical Endocrinology & Metabolism, 85,* 3604-3606.

Wade, J. (2006). Relationships among hormones, brain and behavior: Exceptions in search of a rule? *Hormones and Behavior, 49,* 577-579.

Weiss, J., Taylor, G. T., Zimmermann, F. & Nebenahl, K. (2000). Collection and analyses of biological fluids. In: *Handbook of experimental laboratory animals* (ed. by F. Zimmermann), 485-510. Academic Press, New York.

Welt, C. K., Jimenez, Y., Sluss, P. M., Smith, P. C. & Hall, J. E. (2006). Control of estradiol secretion in reproductive ageing. *Human Reproduction, 21,* 2189-2193.

Wespes, E. & Schulman, C. C. (2002). Male andropause: myth, reality, and treatment. *International Journal of Impotence Research, 14,* S93-98.

Wickham, L. A., Gao, J., Toda, I., Rocha, E. M., Ono, M. & Sullivan, D. A. (2000). Identification of androgen, estrogen and progesterone receptor mRNAs in the eye. *Acta Ophthalmologica Scandinavica, 78,* 146-153.

Widstrom, R. L. & Dillon, J. S. (2004). Is there a receptor for dehydroepiandrosterone or dehydroepiandrosterone sulfate? *Seminars in Reproductive Medicine, 22,* 289-298.

Williams, J. R. (2000). The effects of dehydroepiandrosterone on carcinogenesis, obesity, the immune system, and aging. *Lipids, 35,* 325-331.

Wilson, J. D. (2000). Endocrinology: Survival as a discipline in the 21st century? *Annual Review of Physiology,* 947–950.

Wilson, J. D., Leihy, M. W., Shaw, G. & Renfree, M. B. (2002). Androgen physiology: unsolved problems at the millennium. *Molecular & Cellular Endocrinology, 198,* 1-5.

Woolley, C. S. (1998). Estrogen-mediated structural and functional synaptic plasticity in the female rat hippocampus. *Hormones & Behavior, 34,* 140-148.

Woolley, C. S., McEwen, B. S. & Beatty, W. W. (1993). Roles of estradiol and progesterone in regulation of hippocampal dendritic spine density during the estrous cycle in the rat. *Journal of Comparative Neurology, 336,* 293-306.

Xiao, L. & Jordan, C. L. (2002). Sex differences, laterality, and hormonal regulation of androgen receptor immunoreactivity in rat hippocampus. *Hormones & Behavior, 42,* 327-336.

Yates, W. R., Perry, P. J., MacIndoe, J., Holman, T. & Ellingrod, V. (1999). Psychosexual effects of three doses of testosterone cycling in normal men. *Biological Psychiatry, 45,* 254-260.

Young, E. A., Midgley, A. R., Carlson, N. E. & Brown, M. B. (2000). Alteration in the hypothalamic-pituitary-ovarian axis in depressed women. *Archives of General Psychiatry, 57,* 1157-1162.

Zhang, J. Q., Cai, W. Q., Zhou de, S. & Su, B. Y. (2002). Distribution and differences of estrogen receptor beta immunoreactivity in the brain of adult male and female rats. *Brain Research, 935,* 73-80.

Zitzmann, M. & Nieschlag, E. (2001). Testosterone levels in healthy men and the relation to behavioural and physical characteristics: facts and constructs. *European Journal of Endocrinology, 144,* 183-197.

In: Neuroendocrinology Research Developments
Editor: Nejc S. Penkava et al., pp. 193-238

ISBN: 978-1-60876-983-4
© 2009 Nova Science Publishers, Inc.

Chapter 11

EFFECT OF PSYCHOSOCIAL INTERVENTIONS ON PSYCHOENUROENDOCRINE OUTCOMES IN CANCER PATIENTS: WHERE DO WE GO FROM HERE?

Linda E. Carlson[1,2,3,*] and Sheila N. Garland[1,3]
[1]Department of Psychology, University of Calgary, Canada
[2]Department of Oncology, University of Calgary, Canada
[3]Department of Psychosocial Resources, Tom Baker Cancer Centre, Canada

ABSTRACT

A significant literature exists on the role of psychosocial factors in cancer initiation and progression, and effects of psychosocial interventions on eventual survival, but research investigating the effects of psychosocial interventions on psychoneuroendocrine and psychoneuroimmune outcomes in cancer patients is rare. There is some evidence that stress-reduction interventions may affect cortisol secretion profiles and aspects of cellular immunity, but the clinical significance of any observed effects is not known. Questions that require additional investigation concern: 1) the significance of various endocrine and immune outcome measures for predicting disease outcome in cancer patients (i.e. disease recurrence and/or survival); 2) the optimal timing of psychosocial interventions to affect biological outcomes (i.e. pre- or post-surgery, chemotherapy); 3) the type and stage of cancers that are potentially most responsive to psychosocial interventions (e.g. early vs. late stage, tumour type), and; 4) consideration of other factors that may be mediating any biological changes seen as a result of psychosocial interventions (i.e. health behaviours). The research in these areas will be reviewed and fruitful directions for future research outlined.

* Correspondence concerning this article should be addressed to Linda E. Carlson, Ph. D., C. Psych. Alberta Cancer Board - Holy Cross Site, Department of Psychosocial Resources, 2202 2nd St. S.W. Calgary, Alberta, Canada T2S 3C1. Phone: (403) 355-3209; Fax: (403) 355-3206; E-mail: l.carlson@ucalgary.ca.

Overview

The study of interactions between psychological and social factors and eventual disease initiation and progression in psychosocial oncology has been a hot-button issue for several decades. Controversy began with the introduction of the "Type C" personality style, purported to lead to higher incidence of cancer diseases [1,2]. The "Type C" personality was characterized by emotional repression, agreeableness, passivity and patience combined with a helpless/hopeless coping style that deferred to authority – the type of person often referred to as a "good patient" [1]. The theory holds that this type of person often unconsciously represses or purposively suppresses their emotions and turns them inward, resulting in pathophysiological internal changes that could contribute to the development of cancer. The psychoneuroimmunological (PNI) or psychoneuroendocrinological (PNE) routes by which this process was thought to occur were relatively unspecified. However, a good deal of research over the last two decades has explored these questions with increasing rigour. Another large body of literature exists detailing the associations between chronic stress and health outcomes as diverse as colds, heart disease, asthma, allergies, rheumatoid arthritis and wound healing [3-7] – the question now is - does the same apply to cancer?

The underlying rationale for this type of research is based on an understanding of the stress response and its physiological concomitants – the research on stress is also illustrative of how other psychosocial factors such as depression and social support may affect disease. Essentially, psychosocial processes which result in the perception of psychological or physical threat trigger a cascade of events in the central nervous system (CNS) and periphery that result in stress responses in the autonomic nervous system (ANS) and through the hypothalamic-pituitary-adrenal (HPA) axis. HPA responses are mediated by production of corticotrophin-releasing factor (CRF) and arginine vasopression in the hypothalamus. These releasing factors activate the pituitary gland to secrete hormones such as adrenocorticotrophic hormone (ACTH), enkephalins and endorphins. ACTH then triggers the release of glucocorticoids (cortisol in humans) from the adrenal glands, situated atop the kidneys. Glucocorticoids have a whole host of effects throughout the body, many of which are necessary for regulatory functions, but can also cause downregulation of immune function when exposure is prolonged or chronic [8]. Often in disease states such as cancer or depression, HPA feedback is dysregulated, which can result in chronic hyper-arousal of the HPA axis, or eventual collapse and exhaustion [9]. ANS responses to stress are mediated primarily through the sympathetic nervous system (SNS) through release of catecholamines (epinephrine (EP) and norepinepherine (NE)) both from sympathetic nerve endings and through the medulla of the adrenal glands. In short time frames under acute stressors, elevations in cortisol and catecholamines are adaptive, but if they become chronically elevated as a consequence of exposure to chronic stress, many physiological systems can be negatively affected, resulting in increased risk for viral infections such as common colds [4], increased risk for cardiac disease [6], and slower wound healing [7]. There is also a growing body of evidence, primarily from animal research, that chronic alterations in neuroendocrine feedback dynamics and balance can alter an array of physiological parameters related to cancer tumour development [10]. This research will be reviewed later in this chapter.

A general biopsychosocial or biobehavioral model of cancer development and progression can be helpful to tie together the different inputs and outcomes often measured in

PNI and PNE research. Such a model has been proposed by a number of researchers [11-13] – Figure 1 is their adaptation showing in simple terms their understanding of interactions among a number of key elements, many of which will be discussed in this chapter. It includes the influence of psychological, social and biological background variables such as temperament, social support, and heredity, as well as health behaviours such as diet, exercise and smoking, on health outcomes. These factors interact with the experience of life stress, which can in turn influence neuroendocrine, immune and central nervous system processes that effect disease course and recovery. Psychosocial interventions can act to affect psychological processes as indicated, and change health behaviours, both of which may impact biological processes. These in turn affect disease processes and subsequent morbidity and mortality. This model will be used as a guide to understand the areas in the field that have been relatively well researched, and highlight areas and associations where little empirical understanding exists.

Returning to the clinical study of these potential effects in humans, however, it is important to consider how such relationships can accurately be investigated. Several types of research methodologies have been applied to studying relationships between psychological and social factors and cancer initiation and progression. The question of disease etiology has been addressed primarily through long-term prospective (or retrospective) epidemiological cohort studies that have tracked large groups of initially healthy individuals over time to determine if social, personality or psychological variables predict later cancer incidence in the small proportion who do go on to develop cancers. Very rarely have biomarkers been collected in these studies that might also be associated with disease initiation, so little can be said about potential pathways to disease that any psychosocial factors may affect.

Other methodology has been applied to determine the effects of psychosocial factors on disease progression, recurrence and survival in people once they have been diagnosed with cancer. Because the time-frame is shorter and sample sizes are smaller, this research is substantially less expensive, time consuming and difficult to conduct than large-scale prospective cohort studies with initially healthy populations, and hence there is a much larger body of research in this area. Again, however, the pathways by which psychosocial factors may influence disease outcome are rarely investigated, and research methodology in general has not been of very good quality. However, these studies do provide some tantalizing findings that suggest psychosocial factors may be influencing relevant endocrine and immune markers that may be important in cancer progression [14-16].

Other researchers have begun to investigate the effects of manipulation of psychosocial factors, through different supportive and stress reductive interventions, on outcomes as diverse as quality of life, psychological well-being and symptomatology, endocrine and immune measures, and eventual survival. This work is well known and the survival literature has been extensively reviewed on numerous occasions, with equivocal results [17-21]. There have been a small number of reviews of studies looking at immune and endocrine changes as a result of psychosocial interventions in cancer [22,23], and much speculation about potential pathways [23,24]. Hence, the picture is far from complete.

This chapter will review studies of the above two types (predicting cancer incidence and progression from psychosocial factors, and effects of interventions on survival and psychological, immune and endocrine outcomes). This will not be an exhaustive review but carried out from the perspective of providing a general overview of the field. This chapter will then address several outstanding, relatively unresearched and unresolved areas of inquiry that may help to direct the thinking of the field regarding the larger questions. These include addressing the specific usefulness of various endocrine and immune measures for predicting disease outcome in cancer patients (i.e. disease recurrence and/or survival). This question in many cases can only be addressed indirectly through noting associations between psychosocial and immune or endocrine measures and linking this with any existing research documenting pathways between certain immune or endocrine measures and disease status.

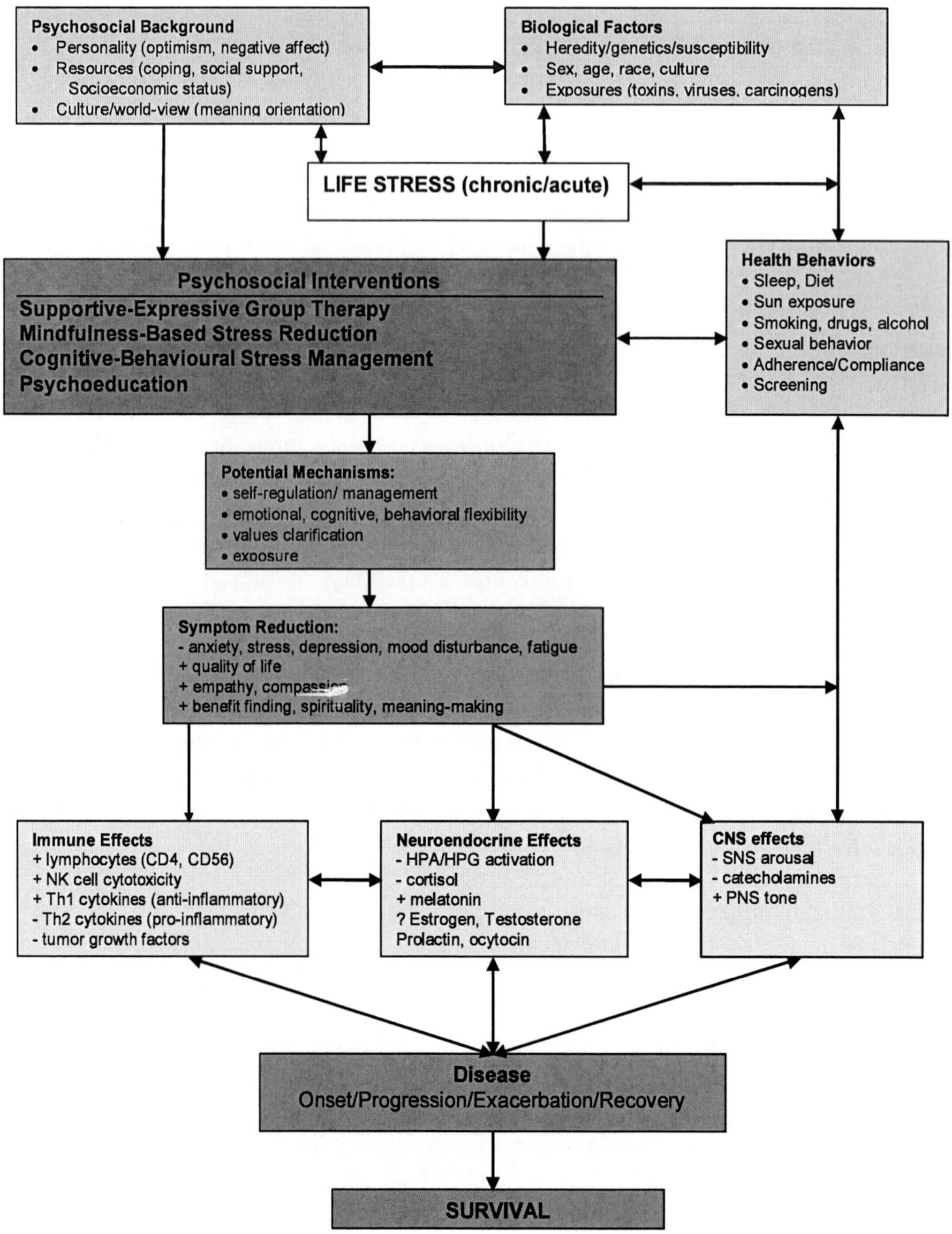

Figure 1. Biobehavioral Model of Cancer Progression.

Other more specific questions of interest for those considering the implementation of psychosocial interventions designed to alter immune/endocrine function or survival include the optimal timing of psychosocial interventions to affect biological outcomes (i.e. pre- or post-surgery, chemotherapy), the type and stage of cancers that are potentially most biologically responsive to psychosocial interventions (e.g. early vs. late stage, solid vs. hematological vs. virally-mediated tumours), and consideration of other factors that may be mediating any biological changes seen as a result of psychosocial interventions (i.e. health behaviours).

The quality and quantity of research available to be drawn upon to address each of these issues varies, and hence this review will also vary in terms of the level of detail and certainty of the conclusions that can be put forth.

Finally, before reviewing the area of psychosocial effects on cancer, the research should be put into perspective: although all the risk factors for different cancers are not definitively known, and because cancer is a term which encompasses over 200 different diseases, it is difficult to determine the relative weight associated with various risk factors. Information on specific risk factors for the major types of cancer is readily available, but it has proven more difficult to obtain actual percentage values in terms of the risk carried for the various factors. One estimate of this data suggests that 30-32% of the variability in incidence for all cancers is related to tobacco, 30-35% to diet, 10% to viruses and infection and so on (including alcohol, sexual factors, heredity, and occupational and environmental exposures), without the inclusion of any psychosocial factors and approximately 5% left unexplained [25]. Hence, the maximum amount of variance in the incidence of cancers that could be accounted for by psychosocial factors would be up to but not likely much beyond five percent. This is not insignificant, and about on par with the effects of alcohol consumption overall. Of course, these values are different for different forms of cancer; for example smoking accounts for approximately 85% of lung cancer cases but is not a risk factor for colon cancer or melanoma. Hence, it may be the case that psychosocial factors play a larger role in some cancers and are inconsequential in others. This possibility has only begun to be investigated.

Psychosocial Factors and Disease Initiation

The research in this area spans 30 years and has been reviewed on several occasions [9,26-33]. The most recent and rigorous review included only studies that used true prospective longitudinal designs, and excluded all those that were cross-sectional, comparisons between groups or semi-prospective, as these study designs do not allow conclusions about causality – 38 studies of this type were excluded [30]. Seventy studies were included in the review, but only 25 of these looked specifically at cancer initiation (while the others focussed on disease progression – reviewed below). Psychosocial factors were divided into several commonly-studied categories: stressful life events; bereavement and other losses; social relations (i.e social support); negative emotions (distress, psychiatric diagnoses); repression of emotions; and personality. Another critical review of studies looking only at disease initiation focussed on similar factors but assessed a broader base of studies, including retrospective cohort studies and case-controlled studies [28]. Several studies published after these most recent reviews also addressed issues of the association between perceived stress and breast cancer incidence, in particular [34-37].

In terms of major life events and bereavement, a meta-analytic review by Petticrew et al [38] of 15 studies looking at only breast cancer patients found that patients reported adverse life events more than twice as often as control subjects. However, they included studied of low quality including group comparisons and semi-prospective studies. Two more rigorous reviews conclude that large population-based studies using independently collected registry data failed to support the link between major life events and increased risk for cancer [28,30]. Garssen [30] did suggest, however, that negative life events in combination with other risk factors, such as social support or hopelessness, could interact to potentially effect cancer initiation. Bereavement too was concluded not to have a clear-cut effect on cancer incidence [28], but perhaps a stronger effect on death from cancer [30]. This conclusion is based on several large-scale studies which looked at the effects of death of a spouse in the UK [39], widowhood [40] and death of a child [41] in Norway, and loss of a son through war in Israel [42] – findings were suggestive of associations but effects were small or inconclusive in most cases. In the Levav study [42], there were no effects on incidence of all cancers together, but the odds of being diagnosed with lymphoma for bereaved parents compared to the rest of the population was 1.5 times higher, and for melanoma it was 1.7 times higher.

Methodologically, it is important to note that these studies use major life events as surrogate markers for the experience of stress, but none of the studies took into account how the individuals actually perceived these events and subsequently reacted to them. For example, widowhood may be perceived very differently by a young woman with small children and a happy marriage, compared to an older woman with an unsatisfactory relationship. Hence, the subjective stressfulness of these life events rather than their mere presence or absence may be more important in determining psychophysiological responses, but this was not measured in these studies. Newer studies not covered in the most recent review have looked at specific reports of subjective life stress, and found further conflicting results. In a report from the Nurses' Health Study of a subsample of 665 women, subjective stress associated with caregiving did not predict incidence of breast cancer, but women who spent a lot of time caregiving had lower circulating levels of estradiol, which may be significant as major risk factors for breast cancer are related to estrogen exposure – in fact lower estrogen levels may be a protective factor against the growth of breast neoplasms [35]. Hence, in this case, the stress of caregiving may have the opposite effect, of lowering estradiol levels and decreasing cancer risk. Another report from the Nurses' Health Study cohort found that job stress was not related to development of breast cancer in 37, 562 women followed for up to 8 years [43]. Hence, the role of major life events and even subjective stress is likely minor in terms of the development of cancers, but the research is not conclusive.

The research evidence for the role of social support is stronger for disease progression than for cancer incidence, with fewer studies in the area of social support and incidence – some reviews of cancer incidence don't even consider this factor (e.g. 28;33). Of those that were conducted and considered of high methodological quality, one failed to find associations [44] but one found that women with few friends who experienced feelings of social isolation were at higher risk for developing cancer [45]. Issues around how to measure social support and the differential effects of structural measures of support (i.e. number of people in the social network) and perceived emotional support (i.e. satisfaction with the network) continue to make interpretation of the data difficult [30].

Negative emotions associated with mood disturbance or more serious psychiatric illness such as major depressive disorder have also been investigated, and again the results are equivocal. Specifically looking at depression, Dalton [28] found of 10 major prospective studies and two retrospective studies that the support for a link between depression and cancer incidence was strongest for specific types of cancers (i.e. breast; lung) and that the duration of depression was also an important, yet not often assessed factor. In studies that did look at the duration of depression through repeated measurements over a period of years, those who suffered more chronic and stable depression were more likely to be diagnosed with cancer [28]. There was also a moderating effect of smoking, such that smokers who were also depressed were more likely to get cancer than similarly heavy smokers who were not depressed. Garsson [30] expressed the most support for the strength of the evidence associating depression with cancer initiation, but two earlier reviewers [32,33] were less convinced. McKenna [33] failed to find a convincing link between depression or anxiety and breast cancer initiation, and McGee [32] reported a small but marginally statistically significant association, which amounted to an almost negligible effect.

It is important to note, also, that the measures of depression were quite varied and not necessarily the most up-to-date instruments that are known to be valid and reliable in this context. Summarizing the evidence, Garssen [30] noted that of nine studies looking at formal psychiatric diagnosis and incidence of cancer, four studies found a relationship as predicted, whereas five did not. Similarly, of 14 studies on measures of depressive affect and disease initiation, six studies found no effect, seven found an association between depression and cancer incidence, and one study even found depression to be a protective factor against cancer incidence. An additional newer study adds to their knowledge in this area: in a large sample of 81,612 women from the Nurses' Health Study in the USA, depressive symptoms were associated with increased risk for colorectal cancer 4-8 years later, in that those women in the highest quartile of depressive symptoms were at higher risk than those with the lowest levels [46]. Hence, the research is mixed, but there are indicators that chronic levels of depression may be associated with higher risk for cancer initiation, particularly in the case of lung cancer.

Finally, returning to the initial question of the effect of certain personality characteristics on cancer initiation, the cancer-prone or "Type C" personality (described as cooperative, unassertive, patient, suppressing negative emotions and accepting external authority) was investigated as a causal factor in several studies. Because no one theory of personality is universally accepted, many different methods for measuring personality have been utilized in this research. Results in this area have again been varied, with two of four high-quality studies finding positive associations. However, the measures of this construct have varied considerably. The most well-designed study found that men classified as "acting out/emotional" were less likely to develop cancer than those classified as normal, healthy/sensitive, loners, or having a personality characteristic of interpersonal conflict [47]. There was little direct support for a role of the entire Type C personality cluster as defined previously in cancer initiation [28,30].

Emotional repression is a characteristic of the Type C personality described as a tendency to consciously suppress or unconsciously repress negative emotions, often accompanied with denial that difficult emotions even exist. It has been studied independently of other aspects of the personality style. Again, this is a difficult construct to measure, and has been operationally defined in some studies by combining a low score on a measure of anxiety with a high score on a measure of defensiveness. Hence, the typical highly repressive person would report low levels of anxiety and have a tendency to refuse to acknowledge any emotional difficulties. There are also specific measures for emotional repression that have been developed. In terms of the initiation of cancer, the role of repression is considered questionable, as only two high quality studies support the association, while three others refute it [28,30]. One study that did support an association found that "anti-emotionality" was associated with a 19% increase in breast cancer diagnoses in a group of over 9,000 women in the Netherlands [48].

In summary, it is clear from this overview that there are a tremendous number of conflicting results regarding the role of various psychosocial factors in cancer initiation. For each factor reviewed, there were both supporting and refuting studies published. None can be ruled out as important, and the degree of support for the different factors, from strongest to weakest, can be summarized as: chronic depression, social support, emotional repression, major life events and Type C personality. The issue of how these conditions or characteristics could lead to cancer development will be addressed in subsequent sections. First however, we will consider issues around psychosocial factors and disease progression and survival, in order to better understand the nuances of this research.

Psychosocial Factors and Disease Progression/Survival

Research in this area mirrors in some ways the results of studies on psychosocial factors and cancer initiation; however in some cases the effects are much stronger when looking at disease progression. This may have as much to do with research methodology as actual effects, but it does inspire greater confidence in the results. Reviews have also been conducted in this area [49,50] and some of the reviews of factors related to cancer incidence also studied progression and survival [9,30,31,51]. Factors considered include bereavement and stressful life events, perceived stress, social support, depression, hopelessness/ helplessness, emotional repression, and also the coping strategies one uses to deal with cancer and its treatments.

Considering the effect of stressful life events on disease outcome, only one study of major life events found a negative relationship between higher total number of life events and shorter disease-free interval and survival [52], where five other studies found no associations (reviewed in Garssen 2004 [30]). Specifically regarding bereavement studies, mixed results have been reported, with large population-based studies showing conflicting results. For example, in a study of 84,000 participants, no effect of losing a partner was found in women, but men were more likely to die from lung cancer and "other cancers", but not from stomach cancer – this effect was highest in younger men (aged 35-64 years) [53]. However, another study of 20,000 people found no increase in death from cancer in people who had lost a spouse [54]. Garssen concluded a weak effect exists for the impact of loss events on death from cancer, based on two studies of child-loss and one bereavement study, but the effect seems stronger for men than women [30].

Twelve studies reviewed by Garssen [30] investigated the relationships between social support and disease progression. In seven reports experiencing social support, having confidantes and a sufficient network of relatives and friends were related to a longer disease-free interval and longer survival. An example of a well-conducted study in this area is Maunsell et al (1995) [55] who identified the presence of different types confidantes in 224 newly diagnosed breast cancer patients. The larger number of categories in which women had close confidantes (i.e. spouse, children, friends, colleagues, etc), the higher the survival rate 7 years later. Fifty-six percent of women without a confidante had survived compared to 72% of those with one or more confidantes – a dose-response relationship was also seen, in that having more confidantes improved the survival rate.

There were also five negative reports reviewed that found no associations between measures of social support and cancer progression. Reasons for these discrepancies may include the specific ways that social support has been measured – structural versus functional. It may be the case that the quality of the support sytem is more important than its size, as indicated in one study which found no relationships between structural measures of support and survival, but did find associations between the subjective judgment of experienced social support and mortality [56]. A more recent report of 2,835 women who were diagnosed with breast cancer from the Nurses' Health Study in the USA found that women who were socially isolated before the diagnosis of cancer had a 66% increased risk of mortality from any cause, and twice the chance of dying from breast cancer [57]. Women without close relatives, friends or children also had elevated risks of death from breast cancer. Added to the data reviewed by Garssen in 2004 [30], this recent study suggests that women who feel less isolated and have a larger support network may have better outcomes.

The case of depression is yet another in which the evidence for a relationship with survival may be stronger than with incidence, with a good deal of research having been conducted in this area. Garssen [30] summarized that of 33 well-conducted studies in this area, six found that negative emotions predicted a more favorable disease outcome, 11 found a negative relationship, and 16 failed to find a relationship at all. When looking at studies that considered only psychiatric diagnoses, a similar pattern is seen, with two studies finding that having a psychiatric diagnosis was a favourable prognostic indicator, three studies finding the opposite, and no relationship in an additional two.

A well-conducted study published in 2003 and not included in earlier reviews followed similar methodology [58]. Measures were collected on a range of emotional and cognitive factors in the early postdiagnostic period and at 4-month intervals up to 15 months after diagnosis. These were used to predict survival time up to 10 years among 205 cancer patients heterogeneous in disease site, status, and progression. Depressive symptomology was the most consistent psychological predictor of shortened survival time using both baseline and repeated measures, after controlling for several known demographic and medical risk factors. Although controversy remains, most reviewers state that the evidence for an effect of depression on disease course is still inconclusive [23,30,50] although one major review concluded more strongly that depression likely plays a role in cancer survival [9]. These authours noted also that emotional overcontrol or repression of emotions likely adds to the deleterious effect of the depression itself.

Indeed, considering more specifically emotional repression and survival, five studies found that "repressors" had shorter disease-free intervals and shorter survival time. However, three others found no associations. Nonetheless, the role of emotional repression finds more support in terms of cancer progression than for initial cancer etiology and is described as one of the more "promising factors" for further investigation [30].

The final area that was evaluated as a factor in disease progression is coping style and adjustment to illness. Several hypothesized coping styles loosely related to the Type-C personality have been investigated. These include having a "fighting spirit", denial or minimization of the impact of the illness, stoic acceptance or fatalism, and a helpless/hopeless or pessimistic coping style. This latter type of response to cancer is also linked with depression, as some of the symptoms of depression are hopelessness and pessimism. The most support is found for a negative role of this factor in disease progression, with six of 10 studies finding patients with more hopelessness and pessimism had shorter survival times. For the other factors, little support was found for the importance of fighting spirit (1/6 studies), denial (0/5 studies), or fatalism (1/5 studies) [30].

Hence, overall a poor prognostic profile emerges of a person prone to feelings of helplessness, hopelessness and pessimism, with a tendency to repress emotions, and with the perception of little social support. The question then arises of what the physiological consequences of having a predominance of these psychological characteristics may be, and how this profile might promote cancer development. The question also arises of whether psychosocial interventions can, though altering these psychological characteristics, change this internal state and arrest cancer promoting processes already set in motion. The latter question regarding survival will be addressed next.

Psychosocial Interventions and Survival

This type of research investigates more specifically whether it is possible to manipulate some of the factors identified in the research reviewed previously that seem important for disease outcome, and subsequently change the course of the illness. This is an ambitious undertaking that many researchers would consider the final test for the role of psychosocial factors in disease processes. Again, this work has been reviewed on numerous occasions [17-21].

A recent review used the technique of meta-analysis to quantify the relative effect of psychosocial interventions on survival across all studies in the area that met criteria for good methodological quality [21]. There were 14 studies included in the review; interventions included components such as supportive therapy, emotional expression, cognitive behavioural therapy, psychoeducation, coping skills training, stress management, mental imagery, psychotherapy and hypnotherapy. Most were in formats of weekly group meetings from 6 weeks to one year in duration with follow-up periods ranging from 9-months to 20 years. When hazard ratios (HR) were calculated for each study and aggregated, the average HR was 0.85 (with a confidence interval (CI) of 0.65-1.11). In meta-analytic terminology, a HR of 1.0 means there is no advantage of the intervention over the control condition on survival – both the control patients and those who got the intervention lived about the same length of time. Values below 1.0 favour the interventions, over 1.0 favour the control group. Only if the value is below 1.0 and the confidence interval is entirely above or below 1.0 can the results be considered statistically significant. Hence, even though the HR is below one, the range of the CI includes 1.0, so one cannot conclude with certainty that the interventions prolonged survival. When interventions were analyzed separately by group vs. individual delivery, there was no effect of group programs on survival (HR=0.97, CI=0.73-1.27). However, individually-delivered interventions did have a positive effect on survival time (HR=0.55, CI=0.43-0.70). What this value means is that the odds of dying first were 35% greater for patients in no-treatment groups compared to those receiving the individual interventions.

As a well-known example of research in this area, consider the case of the Spiegel at al Supportive Expressive Group Therapy (SEGT) study [59,60]. SEGT is a form of professionally-led group psychosocial intervention that evolved specifically to address the support needs of seriously ill medical patients. Two key interrelated goals of SEGT are to build social bonds and to facilitate the expression of emotion. Thus, the group creates a context for the expression, containment, and processing of current distress. This enables patients and their families to proactively address foreseeable challenges, to marshal appropriate resources and to make the most of whatever life remains [59]. Given that lack of social support and emotional repression were two of the strongest predictive factors for poor disease outcomes, this type of approach makes intuitive sense.

The Spiegel study of SEGT, published in 1989, reported on 10-year follow-up of women with metastatic breast cancer randomly assigned to weekly SEGT meetings over the course of an entire year, or care-as-usual, which in the late 1970s included no formal psychosocial support. They found that after 10 years, the women in the treatment group lived an average of 18-months longer than those assigned to the control condition [60]. This caused a great deal of interest internationally and a large replication study was carried out in Canada, known as the Breast Expressive-Supportive Therapy pan-Canadian trial (BEST; [61]). However, that study failed to find any survival advantage for the SEGT group, although it was successful in alleviating pain and suffering, as well as enriching the lives of patients diagnosed with metastatic cancer.

Another long-awaited replication by the original group at Stanford released the results in an abstract format in 2006 [62]: 125 women with metastatic (n = 122) or locally recurrent (n = 3) breast cancer were randomly assigned to the SEGT condition (n = 64), or to the control condition (n = 61) receiving only educational materials for a minimum of 1 year. No overall statistically significant effect of treatment on survival was found for treatment compared to control patients, but there was a statistically significant site by treatment interaction such that estrogen receptor (ER) negative participants randomized to treatment survived longer (median = 29.8 months) than ER negative controls (median = 9.3 months), while the ER positive participants showed no treatment effect (this was a secondary post-hoc unplanned analysis and hence the results must be considered cautiously).. Hence there was no overall effect of the intervention on survival, except perhaps for those whose cancers were *not* responsive to estrogens These cancers also typically have a poorer prognosis than ER positive cancers. If this result were bourne out, it can be speculated that because ER positive cancers respond well to hormonal therapies which may also have effects on HPA functioning, that any putative effect of psychosocial support on survival among ER positive women has been superseded. However, outcome among ER negative women is less affected by hormonal treatments, perhaps leaving room for the impact of other treatments including psychosocial interventions. This study illustrates well the ongoing controversy about the possible life-extending properties of psychosocial interventions and hints at some of the potential neuroendocrine moderators of potential survival effects of psychosocial interventions.

Psychosocial Interventions and Immune and Endocrine Outcomes

There is surprisingly little known about the effects of psychosocial interventions on immune and endocrine outcomes in cancer patients. A small number of narrative reviews speculated on these associations in the 1990s [22,23], but little of a conclusive nature has been discussed. Given the dearth of information, we conducted a systematic review of studies in this area by searching every combination of the following search terms in Medline, Pubmed and PsychInfo: cancer, neoplasm, psychosocial, intervention, treatment, outcomes, immune, endocrine, psychoneuroimmunology, psychoneuroendocrinology, PNI, PNE, biological, cortisol, natural killer, lymphocyte as well as searching the reference lists of selected articles in a snowball technique. Details of the sample, methods, interventions, and outcomes of each study are presented in Table 1. Papers were not vetted or rated on their methodological quality, as relatively few (17 studies) were identified, so all are included in the review. Hence the list includes study designs ranging from pre-post observational studies to larger randomized controlled trials (RCTs). Sample sizes vary from a low of 13 [63] to a high of 227 participants [64]. Of the 17 studies, 11 were RCTs with one or more comparison groups [63,65-67] [64,68-72], another 2 had nonrandomized assignment to one or more comparison groups [73,74], and 4 were pre-post assessments of one intervention only without a control group [75-78]. This distribution is not optimal, as the only study design that allows inferences of causality between participation in interventions and outcome measures is the RCT, but almost two-thirds of the studies did utilize this design. The other study designs can provide provocative preliminary evidence for promising avenues of future research.

Intervention types also varied considerably across studies, as did outcome measures. Interventions ranged from existential psychotherapy [67] to cognitive-behavioural stress management [70], mindfulness-based stress reduction [77,78] (an intervention involving intensive training in meditation and yoga), support groups [66], music therapy [76] and biofeedback [63]. Outcomes, as well, included a range of measures, mostly cortisol (measured both in saliva and blood), and indices of immune functioning (white blood cells, lymphocytes, NK cells, proliferative responses, immunogloblulins, cytokines). A broad range of psychological outcome measures were also used to assess an array of constructs, including stress, depression, anxiety, quality of life, mood, coping strategies, personality, loneliness, optimism and benefit finding. Studies primarily looked at women with breast cancer (13/17) with 2 studies investigating prostate cancer [63-71,73,77-79], 2 with mixed participants [75,76] and one each in malignant melanoma [72] and ovarian cancer [74]. In addition, the stage of cancer also was varied, as was the timing of the intervention. Most participants were diagnosed with non-metastatic disease (stages I=III) in 12/17 studies [63,64,66-68,70-73,77-79], two studies investigated metastatic cancer patients only [65,75], and three included patients with any stage of cancer [69,74,76]. Finally, in terms of timing, the majority of studies were conducted after the completion of surgery and adjuvant treatment (8/17) [63,66,67,71,75-78], followed by during the post-surgical phase (5) [72] [64,70,73,79], during treatment (3) [65] [68,74] and one was conducted pre-surgery [69].

Table 1.

	Year	Reference	Sample and Methods	Intervention	Biological Outcomes	Psychological Outcomes
1.	1989	Length of survival and lymphocyte percentage in women with mammary cancer as a function of psychotherapy [65]	100 women with metastatic breast cancer were randomly assigned to concurrent psychotherapy and chemotherapy (25 in each group: chemo, no chemo, therapy, no therapy). The groups were matched on age, social background, cancer stage, and medical treatments received.	Patients in the therapy group were randomly assigned to 1 of 3 therapies (creative novation therapy, depth psychotherapy, and relaxation therapy with desensitization). Total psychotherapy time was 30 hours. The chemotherapy group received Doxorubicin and 1 of 3 other combination of agents (cyclophosphamide, fluoruracil and vincristine, cyclophosphamide and prednisolone). Chemotherapy was given in 3-4 week cycles and was repeated 4-9 times	Leucocyte concentration and lymphocyte percentage was measured in the women in the chemotherapy group. Measurements were taken prior to chemo, two weeks after treatment initiation, and one month after for all consecutive cycles resulting in 7 samples. *Patients with no psychotherapy showed a steady decrease in lymphocyte production. Patients in therapy showed an initial decrease but then demonstrated an increase past levels at treatment initiation.*	Psychological outcomes not included
2.	1990	A structured psychiatric intervention for cancer patients: II. Changes over time in immunological measures [72]	61 patients (28 mean and 33 women, mean age = 42) with stage I or II malignant melanoma were randomly assigned to a standard care (n=35) or intervention (n=26) group. Immunological and psychological assessments were taken at baseline, 6 weeks, and 6 months. All patients had completed surgery	A short term structured psychiatric group, 9 hours in duration was provided for the treatment group. The intervention was delivered to groups of 7-10 patients for 11/2 hours for 6 weeks. The intervention consisted of health education, enhancement of problem solving skills, stress management and relaxation, and psychological support	Immune outcomes included NK cells, LGLs, major T-cell subsets, CD8 and CD4 T-cells. Groups did not differ at baseline on immunological variables. *At 6 weeks, the treatment group had higher levels of LGLs. At 6 months, the treatment group remained higher in LGLs but also had higher levels of NK cells. The majority of patients in the treatment group had increases in the percent of LDLs, NK cell and NK function and decreased in CD4 t-cells compared to the control group*	The POMS and the Dealing with Illness-Coping Inventory were used to assess affective state and coping. Coping and affective state were improved after the intervention but no significant correlations were found between affective state and immune changes when groups were analyzed independently.

Table 1. (Continued)

	Year	Reference	Sample and Methods	Intervention	Biological Outcomes	Psychological Outcomes
3.	1993	Immunological responses of breast cancer patients to behavioral interventions [63]	13 stage I breast cancer patients were enrolled in the study, mean age of 45 years. 7 patients were randomly assigned to immediate treatment and 6 patients to delayed treatment (6 months into the study). All patients had undergone surgery and completed adjuvant treatment.	The intervention was a 9 week sequence of relaxation training, guided imagery and biofeedback training in group format. The first 3 weeks were focused on relaxation and guided imagery with biofeedback being introduced in week 4. Participants were given relaxation tapes and were asked to practice twice daily. After completion of the 9 week intervention, monthly brush up sessions were held.	Blood samples were provided at baseline, throughout treatment and during 3 month follow up for both groups. Immune assays performed included NK cell activity, Con-A, MLR, IL-2, plasma IgA, IgG and IgM, total WBC and PBL. Baseline measures of psychophysiological stress response was taken to evaluate biofeedback training effects. *Between group comparisons demonstrated significant differences in PBL, WBC, Con-A, and MLR. Within group comparisons demonstrated significant effects for PBL, Con-A, MLR, and IgM.*	Psychological tests were administered at baseline and following training. Measurements includ-ed the MMPI, Millon Behavioral Health Inventory, Sarason Social Support Scale, Rotter Locus of control, the Affects Balance Scale, and the MAC Scale. *There were no significant changes demonstrated on the psychological measures from pre- to post-training.*
4.	1994	Effects of behavioral interventions on plasma cortisol and lymphocytes in breast cancer patients: An exploratory study [73]	24 women with stage I and II breast cancer. All patients had surgery and were not undergoing additional treatment. 14 patients volunteered to participate in the treatment and 10 chose to wait and serve as controls (non-randomized)	The intervention consisted of 2 hour session, once a week for 10 weeks. The intervention consisted of relaxation techniques based on autogentic principles and guided imagery, health education, development of stress and illness coping skills	Blood samples were obtained to determine plasma concentration of cortisol and WBC before and after the 2nd and 10th sessions. *There was a significant reduction in cortisol after the 2nd session and were further decreased after the 10th session, totaling a 23% decrease in cortisol levels. No significant differences were seen in numbers of leukocytes and monocytes. Lymphocyte numbers increased overall and specifically after the second session, but not after the 10th session.* There were no correlations between biological outcomes.	A German questionnaire assessed coping with severe bodily disease. Personality factors were controlled for using the Freiburger Personality Inventory. *There were no significant differences in personality factors or coping strategies*

Table 1. (Continued)

	Year	Reference	Sample and Methods	Intervention	Biological Outcomes	Psychological Outcomes
5.	1997	Coping, life attitudes, and immune responses to imagery and group support after breast cancer treatment [66]	47 women who completed treatment for stage 1-3 breast cancer with a mean age of 46. Patients were randomly assigned to a standard care control group (n=15), standard care plus six weekly 1 hour support session (n=16), or imagery/relaxation sessions (n=16).	Themes for both groups were of giving and receiving support and preparing for the future. The support group focused on the exploration of feelings, returning to normal, the impact of relationships, fears of recurrence, loss and saying goodbye. The imagery group focused on relaxation, setting goals and finding purpose, the impact of beliefs on health, coping with fears, giving and receiving support and concluding.	NK cytotoxicity, cytokines (IL-1α, IL-1β, IL-2 and IFN-γ), and beta endorphins were assessed. *Quality of imagery and frequency of practice was associated with increased NK activity and improved psychical quality of life. No significant differences were found between the groups on any of the immune measures. Neopterin decreased and IFN-γ increased for all the women.*	Assessment instruments included the FACT-B, POMS-Brief, Ways of Coping with Cancer, and the Duke-UNC Functional Social Support Questionnaire. *Coping skills improved for the support and imagery groups. The treatment groups also sought more support from others.* No significant differences were found between treatment groups
6.	1997	Effectiveness of a short-term group psychotherapy program on endocrine and immune function in breast cancer patients: An exploratory study [67]	The sample consisted of women with early stage breast cancer and distant or lymph metastases (mean age = 59). Patients were randomly assigned to an intervention group (11 patients) or a control group (12 patients). A healthy age matched control group of 15 women (mean age = 56) was included for comparison	Patients were randomly assigned to either the existential-experiential group psychotherapy or a wait list control group. The group was semi-structured and focused on fears of death, limitations of freedom, existential isolation, relationships with family, relatives and the medical professions, autonomy, helplessness and dependence and the meaning of life. Sessions were held once a week for 2.5 hours.	*Patients provided 2 blood samples before and after the intervention or at concurrent time periods for the control group. Biological measures included cortisol, ACTH, peripheral blood cells, NK cell activity and proliferative responses. Women with breast cancer had significantly higher cortisol levels than healthy matched women and lower levels of CD3 and CD4 cells. When baseline levels were adjusted, women in the treatment group had lower levels of prolactin and cortisol and lower levels of NK cells, CD4 and CD8 cells.*	*Measures were com-pleted before and after program participation and included the BDI, the STAI, and the POMS. No correlations were found for psychological and endocrine outcomes. Trait anxiety was positively related to changes in CD4 levels. BDI scores were posi-ively related to percent-age of NK cells. Mood disturbance was related to proliferative responses*

Table 1. (Continued)

	Year	Reference	Sample and Methods	Intervention	Biological Outcomes	Psychological Outcomes
7.	1997	Immune effects of relaxation during chemotherapy for ovarian cancer [74]	22 patients (Mean age= 57) receiving 4 cycles postoperative chemotherapy for stage 1-4 ovarian cancer. 12 patients were in the relaxation group, 10 patients were in the control group. Allocation was based on hospital ward and non-random.	Intervention was designed to train patients how to use cue controlled progressive relaxation skills rapidly and apply them when needed. Audiotapes were provided for practice and patients were asked to practice twice a day. Patients received 3 relaxation training sessions with a clinical psychologist. The relaxation sessions were delivered prior to initiation of treatment, during treatment and prior to the second course of treatment	Venous blood sampling was performed 2 days before chemotherapy and on the morning of their 3rd or 4th cycle. Routine hematological date was assessed (white blood cells, lymphocytes, granulocytes, monocytes, Con-A and NK). Groups were not different at baseline. *After intervention, the relaxation group had higher white blood cell counts and more lymphocytes.* Nonsignificant trends were observed for monocyte levels and proliferative responses to Con-A. NK levels were similar between groups.	The STAI was completed immediately before each blood sampling. No results were reported for psychological outcomes.
8.	1997	Phase II study of psychotherapeutic intervention in advanced cancer [75]	35 patients (16 males, 19 females) enrolled in the study with a mean age of 55 years. The group was heterogeneous but the primary tumor site was colorectal. No control group.	Patients were offered 12, 1.5-2 hour sessions once a week of individual counselling. They also attended twice monthly group meetings lasting 2.5 hours. Psychotherapy was experiential-existentially based and focused on feelings, needs, aims and potential of the individual.	NK cell cytotoxicity and activity was measured prior to the intervention, at 6 weeks and 12 weeks of the intervention and at 6 and 12 months following intake. *5 patients experienced an arrest in tumour growth. No effect of treatment on NK cell activity was observed. No significant relationships were found between NK and psychological outcomes.*	*Patients completed the Purpose in Life Test, Zung's Depression Scale, the Loneliness Inventory and the Cancer Locus of Control scale at the same time as blood sampling. No changes were observed on measures of loneliness, depression or locus of control. Purpose in life increased significantly.*

Table 1. (Continued)

	Year	Reference	Sample and Methods	Intervention	Biological Outcomes	Psychological Outcomes
9.	2000	Cognitive-behavioral stress management reduces serum cortisol by enhancing benefit finding among women being treated for early stage breast cancer [70]	34 women (mean age = 46) with stage I or II breast cancer recruited within 8 weeks post surgery. 24 women were randomized to the intervention group and 10 to a waitlist control group.	Cognitive behavioral stress management was delivered in 2 hour classes over the course of 10 weeks. Class material consisted of progressive muscle relaxation, meditation, abdominal breathing, guided imagery, cognitive restructuring and techniques to improve coping, assertiveness, anger management and the use of social support.	Blood samples were provided pre and post intervention or control period to assess cortisol levels. There were no significant differences between groups at baseline. *Significant decreases in cortisol were produced for the intervention group compared to the control. Cortisol reductions were significantly associated with improvements in benefit finding.*	Perceived positive contribution for women experiencing breast cancer were measured by the Benefit Finding Scale. Distress was measured by the POMS. *Significant improvements were observed in benefit finding but not in distress levels after program participation.*
10.	2000	A presurgical psychosocial intervention for breast cancer patients: psychological distress and the immune response [69]	41 women (mean age=56). All women were awaiting either surgery or surgery plus adjuvant therapy at enrolment. Patients were randomly assigned to standard care or standard care plus a 2 session psychosocial intervention. Assessments and blood draws were performed before surgery and prior to intervention, before surgery and following intervention, and 1 week following surgery.	The intervention was delivered by two clinical psychologists to individuals or small groups of 2-3. Duration was 90 minutes. The intervention had 3 objectives: psychoeducation about somatic and emotional responses to stress, problems solving skills for use in crisis, relaxation techniques and psychosocial support	NK cell activity and IFN-γ were measured. No significant time or interaction effects were observed in NK cell activity. *A significant interaction was seen for IFN-γ levels, whereby the levels of IFN-γ in the control group decreased steadily and the levels in the therapy group remained constant.* This was no longer significant when baseline measures were included as a covariate	Patients completed the CES-D scale; the Differential Emotions Scale-IV, the IES and the Life Orientation Test. *The therapy group experienced an increase on measures of overall interest and enjoyment and a decrease in sadness compared to the control group.* Optimism increased regardless of group

Table 1. (Continued)

	Year	Reference	Sample and Methods	Intervention	Biological Outcomes	Psychological Outcomes
11.	2001	Effects of stress management on testosterone levels in women with early stage breast cancer [79]	34 women (mean age = 46) with stage I or II breast cancer recruited within 8 weeks post surgery. 24 women were randomized to the intervention group and 10 to a waitlist control group.	Cognitive behavioral stress management was delivered in 2 hour classes over the course of 10 weeks. Class material consisted of progressive muscle relaxation, meditation, abdominal breathing, guided imagery, cognitive restructuring and techniques to improve coping, assertiveness, anger management and the use of social support.	Blood samples were provided pre and post intervention or control period to assess total testosterone levels. There were no significant differences between groups at baseline. *Post intervention, there were significant reductions in free testosterone and total testosterone. Reduction in testosterone were positively correlated to increases in benefit finding.*	Perceived positive contribution for women experiencing breast cancer were measured by the Benefit Finding Scale
12.	2001	A pilot study into the therapeutic effects of music therapy at a cancer help center [76]	29 patients (21 women and 8 men) participated in a residential 1 week course at the care center with an average age of 49 years (no control group). Cancer type and stage was mixed but breast cancer was predominant. All were in the process or had completed treatment Physiological and psychological assessments were conducted before and after each session.	The intervention was completed over 3 days. Day 1 included listening to 1 hour of music in a relaxed state. Day 2 included active playing of instruments for 1.5 hours in a group format. Day 3 included a 1 hour focus group meeting to discuss, compare and contract their experiences in both the listening and playing sessions.	Two salivary measures were examined: Salivary cortisol and sIgA. *Listening to music resulted in increased levels of sIgA compared to levels before music listening session. Cortisol levels decreased significantly from Day 1 to Day 2, but were not significantly affected by either music treatment.* No significant correlations were found between the physiological and psychological measures	The University of Wales Institute of Science and Technology (UWIST) Mood Adjective Checklist provided information on hedonic tone (well-being), tense arousal and energetic arousal. *Listening to music produced significant decreases in tense arousal and increases in hedonic tone. Active playing of music produced a significant increase in energetic arousal.*

Table 1. (Continued)

	Year	Reference	Sample and Methods	Intervention	Biological Outcomes	Psychological Outcomes
13.	2003	Mindfulness-based stress reduction in relation to quality of life, mood, symptoms of stress, and immune parameters in breast and prostate cancer outpatients [77]	49 women with breast and 10 men with prostate cancer. The sample had a mean age of 55 years and were diagnosed with early stage cancer a median of 1.1 years prior. Treatment was completed a median of 6 months prior (excluding hormonal). The sample was mostly comprised of patients with stage II cancer. No control group.	Mindfulness-based Stress Reduction was delivered over 8 weeks with weekly 90 minute group sessions and 1 3 hour silent retreat. Primary components of the program are: mindfulness meditation and yoga practice, psychoeducation regading stress and the stress response and group support.	Biological measurements included all leukocyte subclasses and intracellular cytokines. *Increases in eosinophils and IL-4 production in T-cells were observed as well as decreases in monocytes, T-cell production of IFN-γ, and NK cell production of IL-10.* There were no significant relationships between psychological and immunological measures	Psychological outcomes were measured with the EORTC-QLQ-30, POMS, and the SOSI. *Improvements were observed in quality of life, mood disturbance (13% reduction) and symptoms of stress (19.3% reduction).*
14.	2004	Psychological, behavioral, and immune changes after a psychological intervention: A clinical trial [64]	227 women (mean age = 51) with stage II or III breast cancer who can completed surgery but were awaiting adjuvant therapy were accrued. 113 were randomly assigned to the assessment only group and 114 were assigned to the intervention group. At 4 month assessment, the sample sizes were 91 in the assessment group and 107 in the intervention group.	The intervention was provided to small groups of 8-12 patients and led by 2 clinical psychologists. Groups met for 1.5 hours for 18 sessions. Therapy content included stress management, emotional distress and social adjustment, health behaviors and adherence to treatment.	Immune assays investigated were T lymphocytes, T-cell subsets and NK cells, NK cell cytotoxicity and blastogetnic response to PHA and Con-A. No significant group effects were found for T-lymphocyte counts. *A significant effects was reported for Con-A and PHA induced T-cell blastogenesis in the intervention group.* NK cell count and cell lysis were not significant	Psychological measures were the IES, the POMS, the Social Network Index, the Perceived Social Support Scale, the Food Habits Questionnaire and the Seven Day exercise Recall. *Patients in the intervention group showed a reduction in anxiety and for patients with higher cancer stress, the group produced reduction in mood disturbance and fatigue.* The intervention group also perceived more support

Table 1. (Continued)

	Year	Reference	Sample and Methods	Intervention	Biological Outcomes	Psychological Outcomes
						whereas the assessment only group reported a reduction in support. Health behaviors (diet and smoking) improved for the intervention group only
15.	2004	A pilot randomiz-ed trial assessing the effects of auto-genic training in early stage cancer patients in relation to psychological status and immune system responses [71]	31 women with early stage breast cancer post surgery and radiotherapy, not undergoing further treatment were randomized to autogentic relaxation training or a wait list control	Autogenic relaxation training was taught in groups and focused on heaviness of limbs, warmth of limbs, calm regular heart beat, easy breathing, abdominal warmth and cooling of the forehead. Measurements were taken before and after the intervention.	CD4, CD8, B cells, NK cells, neutrophils and monocytes were examined. *There was a statistically significant difference in CD8 and NK cells after the intervention.* Caution in interpretation is warranted due to small sample size.	Anxiety and depression were measured using the HADS. *Intervention and control groups were significantly different on measures of anxiety and depression after the intervention*
16.	2004	Mindfulness-based stress reduction in relation to quality of life, mood, symptoms of stress and levels of cortisol, dehydroepiandrost erone sulphate (DHEAS) and melatonin in breast and prostate cancer outpatients [78]	49 women with breast and 10 men with pros-tate cancer. The sample had a mean age of 55 years and were diagnosed with early stage cancer a median of 1.1 years prior. Treatment was completed a median of 6 months prior (excluding hormonal). The sample was mostly comprised of patients with stage II cancer. No control group.	Mindfulness-based Stress Reduction was delivered over 8 weeks with weekly 90 minute group sessions and 1 3 hour silent retreat. Primary components of the program are: mindfulness meditation and yoga practice, psychoeducation regading stress and the stress response and group support.	A blood sample was taken for DHEAS testing and saliva samples for melatonin and cortisol. Cortisol samples were provided at 8am, 2pm, and 8pm. Melatonin samples were provided at 2pm. Patients with abnormal cortisol profiles at baseline also had higher stress scores. *No changes were observed in mean cortisol levels, but patients with higher initial cortisol levels decreased over time on mean cortisol levels as well as morning, afternoon and evening levels.* No significant changes were seen in DHEAS or melatonin levels	Psychological outcomes were measured with the EORTC-QLQ-30, POMS, and the SOSI. Psychological data is presented in the paper by Carlson, Speca, Patel and Goodey (2003) [77]

Table 1. (Continued)

	Year	Reference	Sample and Methods	Intervention	Biological Outcomes	Psychological Outcomes
17.	2006	A randomized controlled trial of psychological interventions using the psychophysiological framework for Chinese breast cancer patients [68]	76 participants (mean age = 49) were randomly assigned to a body-mind-spirit (BMS; n=27), supportive-expressive (SE; n=16), social support self help group (SS; n=16), or a no intervention group (n=17). Psychological and physiological measurements were administered at baseline, 4 months and 8 months post intervention.	The BMS group and integrated western psychotherapeutic elements with eastern philosophy and Chinese health practices. It focused on the normalization of traumatic experiences, letting go of attachments, forgiveness and self love and social support and commitment to others (15 total hours). The SE group was designed to build social support, deal with concerns of death, dying and body image, reorder life priorities, improve relationships, communication and symptom control (16 total hours). The SS group was unstructured and members decided topics (15 total hours).	The physiological outcome measure was salivary cortisol. Samples were taken at 5 times thoughout the day (waking, 45 min after waking, 12pm, 5pm, and 9pm). *Only the BMS group showed a significant reduction in total salivary cortisol level after 8 months. Mean cortisol concentration was significantly related to positive social support in that higher support was associated with lower cortisol at 8 months.*	psychological outcome measures included the General Health Questionnaire, the PSS, the Mini MAC Scale, the Courtauld Emotional Control Scale, and the Yale Social Support Index. *After 4 months, a significant reduction in health concerns, emotionality, negative emotion, and positive support was reported for the BMS group. The SS group showed and increase in negative emotion after 8 months. The control group showed a reduction in positive support after 4 months*

What can be concluded from this broad array of study designs, samples, interventions and outcome measures? Overall, 6 studies found some effect of the intervention on measures of cortisol [67,68,70,73,76,78], 14 reported positive effects on immune function [63-67,69,71-74,76-79], and one study reported no effect on immune function [75]. It might not be expected that biological changes would occur in the absence of psychological changes; hence it's important to note that 13 studies found positive effects of the intervention on psychological outcomes [64,66-72,75-78] but 2 studies did not [63,73]. The numbers don't always add up to 17 as some studies included both cortisol and immune measures, and other did not report psychological outcomes at all. It is also important to take into account publication bias, as most papers with negative results either aren't submitted for publication or are rejected at peer review. Also, most studies conducted multiple comparisons and had multiple outcome measures – hence, the finding of one of two positive outcomes inflates the error rate and perhaps exaggerates the effects of these interventions. If the percent positive outcomes were to be assessed on the basis of how many comparisons of all those conducted were statistically significant, the number would be far lower. However, this data does serve as "proof of principle" that it is possible to affect changes, particularly in measures of immune function and cortisol levels, through psychosocial intervention.

As mentioned previously, the quality of the studies varied considerably, with some of quite low quality, so perhaps it is useful to review one or two of the best studies in detail, to illustrate the potential effects. The largest study, conducted by Andersen et al (2004) [64] randomly assigned 227 women with stage II or III breast cancer who had completed surgery to either usual care or group therapy consisting of techniques for stress management, social support, emotional and social adjustment to cancer, enhancing health behaviours and adherence to treatment. After four months during which participants received chemotherapy, retention was good (80-93%) and the intervention group demonstrated greater t-cell proliferative responses to the mitogens ConA and PHA. Patients in the intervention also had greater reductions in anxiety, improvements in social support, and better health behaviors such as sleep and diet.

Similarly, a recent study reported a sample of 76 patients who were randomly assigned to a body-mind-spirit group, supportive-expressive therapy or a social support self-help group [68]. This type of study pitting various psychosocial interventions against one another creates a very hard test of specificity, as it is quite difficult to demonstrate the superiority of one group over another. Nonetheless, the authours found that only the body-mind-spirit group showed reductions in total salivary cortisol after 8-months, and higher social support was related to lower cortisol concentrations. Participants in the body-mind-spirit group also had decreases in health concerns, fewer negative emotions and felt more positive support than the other two groups.

To summarize, then, this body of work has demonstrated the potential for psychosocial interventions to affect a wide array of outcomes such as increasing NK cell cytotoxicity and decreasing salivary cortisol levels. Research in this area has focused mostly on immune and cortisol outcomes, and mostly on women with breast cancer. The potential significance of these changes will be addressed in the following section.

Endocrine/Immune Measures and Disease Progression/Survival

Much of the motivation behind investigating the neuroendocrine and immune impacts of psychosocial interventions in the previous section is based on the assumption that the intermediary outcome measures used are meaningful. Hence, the studies reviewed document associations between manipulating psychosocial factors and consequent changes in immune and endocrine measures. However, whether or not these outcomes have much or anything to do with disease processes has not been well explored. This question can be addressed by looking at both the animal and human research into the psychobiology of cancer, which has been reviewed by a number of investigators [9,10,13,14,22-24,80,81].

Researchers have looked at several potential pathways between immune and endocrine function, some of which can be altered by psychosocial factors, and disease progression in both humans and animals. Simply speaking, at least five interacting systems are involved in these relationships: 1) psychological factors (i.e. stress; depression); 2) CNS factors including HPA and SNS reactivity and regulation; 3) endocrine factors, including HPG reactivity of estrogens and testosterone and circadian rhythms of melatonin; 4) immune factors including immunosurveillance; and 5) tumour-related factors in the tumour microenvironment itself, including processes such as angiogenesis and programmed cell death (apoptosis). These systems clearly interact, so breaking them down into separate categories is an artificial heuristic that may help with understanding, but it is quickly obvious that they interact with one another in a myriad of ways. The first factor, psychological processes, has been addressed in earlier sections; the remainder of this section will selectively look at interactions between the other systems and disease progression.

HPA Axis

A growing body of research has investigated the stress-related concept of allostatic load, and a large body of evidence has associated excessive release of cortisol with suppression of the immune system (for reviews see [11,82,83]). Cortisol is largely responsible for the downregulation of immune function as a result of stress. Its hypersecretion also results in depressed mood [84,85]. Cortisol levels are typically highest in the morning, and decrease during the day, resulting in the downward sloping profile characteristic of most healthy individuals. However, cortisol levels have been reported to be elevated and overall diurnal profiles flatter in breast cancer patients compared to control women [86-88]. This supportive data stems primarily from women with metastatic, rather than earlier stage, cancers. For example, abnormal patterns of cortisol secretion have been reported in up to 75% of a sample of metastatic breast and ovarian cancer patients [89]. Further, the slope of the rate of change of cortisol levels measured four times a day for three consecutive days was associated with survival time in a group of 104 women with metastatic breast cancer. Those women who displayed less variation in salivary cortisol levels, expressed as a flatter slope and indicating a lack of normal diurnal cortisol variation, experienced earlier mortality over a 7-year follow-up period [15].

When these patients were split at the median cortisol slope for descriptive purposes, 77% of those with flat rhythms had died after surviving an average of 3.2 years. In contrast, 60% of the patients with relatively steep rhythms had died, with an average survival of 4.5 years. Hence, the women with steeper slopes survived more than 1 year longer on average. This relationship held even when other prognostic medical variables were taken into account, such as markers of disease status (e.g. location of metastases, estrogen receptor status), medical treatment (e.g. chemotherapy drugs) and psychosocial variables (e.g. stress levels and marital satisfaction) [15]. The authors speculate that these abnormal circadian rhythms of cortisol secretion represent compromised HPA axis functioning, which may be responsible for earlier mortality. Indeed other studies have reported circadian abnormalities in the secretion of 12 hormones in women at high risk for developing occurrences of breast cancer [90], as well as associations with later stages of cancer development and other prognostic indicators such as poorer performance status and more metastatic involvement [89,91]. In addition to affecting hormones, potentially through cell receptors and cell signalling pathways, excess cortisol may directly facilitate tumour growth through metabolic pathways, such that normal cells in which cortisol inhibits glucose uptake may become resistant to this effect when they mutate into cancer cells. Hence, glucocorticoids may suppress energy uptake in healthy cells but facilitate the ability of cancer cells to preferentially utilize energy, providing a metabolic advantage [92].

HPA axis dysregulation also has direct effects on immune function, both in terms of cellular and innate immunity. Immune defences against tumours are very complicated and include specific mechanisms such as tumour cell targeting by cytotoxic and helper T-cells and B-cell mediated cell lysis, and also natural immunity channels including cell death through NK cells, macrophages and ganulocytes. Abnormal cortisol rhythms were associated with reduced NK cell number and cytotoxicity in women with metastatic breast cancer [15], and decreased NK activity has been associated with tumour progression in animals [81] and humans [93]. Hence, excess cortisol in the blood stream of cancer patients due to allostatic load and HPA axis dysregulation can affect both numbers and activity levels of lymphocytes, macrophages and granulocytes [10].

SNS Factors

There is preliminary evidence suggesting that autonomic control may sometimes be impaired among BC patients [94]. Women at high familiar risk for breast cancer showed a greater catecholamine response to laboratory stressors than healthy women with normal risk levels [95], and they also had higher urinary levels of epinephrine (EP) during the work day [96]. During sleep there is usually a reduction of sympathetic nervous system (SNS) activity and an increase in parasympathetic (PNS) function, but the quality of sleep contributes to these autonomic changes. Deep-wave sleep is characterized by markedly reduced SNS activity, in that both norepinephrine (NE) and EP levels decline [97]. Hence, sleep quality can impact production of SNS catecholamines, or vice versa (higher SNS arousal can negatively impact sleep quality). If SNS activity is not reduced sufficiently during sleep, other systems may also suffer dysregulation. Hence, sleep is an important variable in maintaining SNS regulation and potentially contributing to cancer outcomes as well.

Influences of stress-related SNS products on *in vivo* tumour growth is illustrated by a wealth of studies demonstrating the negative effects of various types of stressors on tumour growth and metastasis in animal models. Typically animals may be injected with tumour cell lines, subjected to stress, and tumour growth quantified. For example, immobilization stress led to increased incidence of tumours and more growth in rats injected with the carcinogen diethylnitrosamine [98]. Other physical, social and psychological stressors including swimming stress, surgical stress, social confrontation and hypothermia all lead to increased lung metastasis from injected breast cancer cell lines [81,99,100]. In a chemical model simulating stressor effects, animals were subjected to elevated levels of injected β-adrageneric agonists, which simulate the effect of SNS activation, on tumour growth. Several animal studies have found β-adrageneric agonists cause increases in lung and mammary tumour metastases [101]. Conversely, pre-treatment of animals with β-adrageneric antagonists to block SNS activity also blocked effects of behavioural stress on lung tumour metastases previously observed [102]. There is also evidence that stress in animals may compromise mechanisms of DNA repair [10], thought to be important for recovery of cells from DNA damage due environmental or therapeutic exposure to radiation. Hence, products of the SNS elevated during the stress response or when circadian systems are dysregulated have direct facilitative effects on tumour growth and metastasis. The molecular basis for this effect is not fully understood but being actively researched.

Hormonal Factors

Estrogen (E)

Endocrine factors altered through stress and other psychological processes are extremely important for cancer development and progression, particularly in the case of cancers such as breast and prostate. Researchers have reported circadian abnormalities in the secretion of 12 hormones in women at high risk for developing occurrences of breast cancer [103] , as well as associations with later stages of cancer development and other prognostic indicators such as poorer performance status and more metastatic involvement [89,91]. Although estrogen is essential for normal mammary development and ductal growth, it also plays a role in the development and progression of breast cancer, and increased exposure to estrogens and increases in estrogen receptor expression in mammary epithelial cells increases risk. Primary risk factors for breast cancer include measures of lifelong E exposure, such as early menarche, fewer or no children, later age of parity, later menopause and obesity (for a review see Velie, 2005) [104]. Typically, women are tested at the time of diagnosis for E receptors and tumours with a high concentration of E receptors are referred to as positive (ER-positive) whereas those with a low or non-existent concentration of receptors are negative (ER-negative). Generally, ER-positive tumours respond best to hormonal treatments like Tamoxifen, which preferentially bind to ERs on breast cancer cells, taking the place of the naturally occurring estrogen and inhibiting the expression of estrogen-regulated genes that would normally induce cell proliferation [105].

Estrogen biosynthesis is catalyzed by the aromatase enzyme (aromatase cytochrome P450), which converts androgens to estrogens through the process of aromatization. Aromatase levels increase with age and BMI. The increase with rising BMI is thought to be due to tumour-adipocyte interactions [106]. Adipocytes are endocrine cells making up the bulk of the human breast (epithelial cells account for only 10% of the volume), and their numbers increase with increasing body weight and fat concentrations. They secrete various cytokines, polypeptide and hormone-like molecules, such as TNF-alpha and IL-6, which stimulate the production of aromatase [106]. Hence, more aromatase available for conversion of T to E may account for higher levels of E in obese women, as aromatase (and not T) is usually the rate-limiting factor.

Recall also that psychosocial interventions have been observed to alter levels of these aromatase-producing cytokines [78] which may result in less aromatase and subsequent less conversion of T to E in women with breast cancer participating in these interventions. No studies to their awareness have directly measured E level changes as a result of participation in psychosocial interventions. However it is well known that IL-6, TNF-alpha and other proinflammatory cytokines are elevated during periods of stress, and also in depression [107]. The cytokine pattern of depression is in fact very similar to that of cancer, leading researchers to suggest a high degree of similarity between the pathobiochemistry and immunology of cancer, cancer pain and depression [108]. Cancer treatment incorporating immune therapy with IL-2 and/or IFN-alpha is associated with depressive symptoms in a large proportion of patients [109,110]. This effect seems to be mediated by the activation of the cytokine network, including IL-6 [111], which is also elevated in depressed patients [112-114]. It makes sense, then, that if levels of pro-inflammatory cytokines can be decreased through the treatment of stress and depression, this may also affect levels of bioavailable E, especially in obese women, which is important for the development and progression of many breast cancers.

Testosterone

There is an interesting controversy around the role of testosterone in the development and progression of prostate cancer. Although the common assumption is that testosterone (T) plays a role in prostate cancer development due to the observation that castration (either surgical or biochemical) is an effective treatment for prostate cancer disease [115,116], a review of 34 studies investigating T levels in individuals newly diagnosed with prostate cancer compared to those without is inconclusive. That is, there is no clear-cut evidence that men who get prostate cancer have higher circulating levels of testosterone than those free of the disease [116]. This non-association between T levels and prostate cancer incidence has been shown in clinical trials of T supplementation, in longitudinal population-based studies, and in men who receive exogenous T treatment for hypogonadism. These findings have lead researchers to propose an indirect link between T and prostate cancer, perhaps through the acquisition of multiple non-specific sexually-transmitted diseases (STDs) caused by higher levels of sexual activity in men with higher T in their youth. This may promote transformation of prostate cells and damage to Leydig cells in the testis, which may contribute to the pathogenesis of prostate cancer, but not be observed as higher T levels around the time of diagnosis [116].

Not all researchers agree, as another meta-analysis found a 2.34 fold increase in the risk of prostate cancer in men in the highest quartile of T production, but they also found the same level of risk associated with higher serum IGF-1, and conversely, higher levels of sex hormone-binding globulin were associated with lower risk. Estrogens and DHT did not seem to play a role in prostate cancer risk [117]. The question of whether T levels can be altered through stress or psychosocial interventions is open. It is well known that T can affect mood states, and in aging there is a moderate decline of total T and a more significant decline of bioavailable T [118]. Elderly men who are most depressed also have the lowest T values, and T replacement in men with low T levels often results in improved mood. Indeed, even in hypogonadal men with clinical depression, T administration in some cases alleviated the depression [118]. Whether treatment of depression through psychosocial interventions may influence T production (and potentially prostate cancer progression) is not known, but one study did find that a combination treatment of diet, stress reduction, meditation and yoga resulted in arrest or regression, in some cases, of prostate-specific antigen (PSA) levels, the primary marker of disease activity in prostate cancer [119]. The mechanism for any such action is currently unknown.

Melatonin

The pineal hormone melatonin has been implicated in the treatment of many types of cancers and other diseases [120,121]. Proposed mechanisms of action include its effects as a free radical scavenger, an antioxidant, as well as an immunomodulatory agent and through the promotion of apoptosis of cancer cells in animal and human models [122]. In both *in vitro* and *in vivo* investigations, melatonin protected healthy cells from radiation-induced and chemotherapeutic drug-induced toxicity [123,124]. In humans, a series of clinical trials using melatonin in conjunction with standard treatment found superior survival response in patients with advanced cancer receiving adjuvant melatonin therapy [125], and higher tolerance of standard chemotherapy regimes [125,126]. A review of the animal and human literature concluded that converging evidence supports large transnational research-based clinical trials of melatonin therapy for a wide variety of cancers [122]. For years reports have indicated that women with breast cancer have suppressed or absent nocturnal melatonin peaks [127]. Epidemiological studies have also shown increased risk of breast cancer in women who work night shifts [128,129]. One biologically plausible explanation for this association is that these women have blunted melatonin secretion rhythms, and lack the nocturnal melatonin peak that is associated with normal sleep cycles.

We have evaluated the associations between sleep, stress, urinary melatonin and catecholamines in women recovering from breast cancer and matched healthy controls, and found higher levels of depressive symptoms, anxiety, fatigue, confusion, cardiopulmonary symptoms of stress and sleep disturbance in breast cancer patients than the comparison women; however, despite these disturbances there were no group differences on any of the biomarkers, including salivary cortisol, urinary catecholamines and melatonin, with the exception of higher dopamine levels in the control participants [130]. The women with breast cancer in their group were diagnosed with stages I-III breast cancer, primarily stage II, with no metastatic spread. This may account for the failure to find differences in any of the endocrine measures. However, the issue of the potential role of melatonin in disease development, circadian rhythm dysregulations and mood and stress remains a promising area of research [91,122].

Immune Factors

Cell-mediated immunity is the most studied outcome area in the intervention studies reviewed above, but the question arises as to the importance of the measures shown to be responsive to psychosocial interventions – most commonly increases in the number of lymphocytes, including NK cells, [64,67,72,73] NK cell cytotoxicity [72] and cytokine production [69,77].

Even though NK cells have been the target outcome measure in a number of psychosocial intervention trials and some changes have been observed, they have rarely been correlated with disease outcome (i.e. Fawzy et al, 1991 [72]). Many authours are skeptical of a role for immune factors in cancer progression (e.g. [23], including mainstream cancer biologists). Points raised by Garssen and Goodkin [23] against an important role of immune factors in cancer development include observations that: 1) spontaneously arising cancers in mice (in contrast to those induced by experimental methods) provoke little or no immune response; 2) tumour cells can easily mutate and avoid being targeted by cytotoxic T cells by constantly changing their antigens; 3) tumour cells can directly suppress the efficacy of various immune cells; and 4) due to the fast proliferation of some tumour cells the immune response is not capable of limiting their growth.

However, decreased NK activity has been associated with tumour progression in some studies of animals [81] and humans [93] and abnormal cortisol rhythms were associated with reduced NK cell number and cytotoxicity in women with metastatic breast cancer [15]. A persuasive argument has been made by Ben-Eliyahu for a role of cell-mediated immunity in the promotion of metastatic spread [81]. He speculates that the postoperative period when immunosupression occurs as a result of the surgical assault is a vulnerable period, in that dislodged tumour cells are most likely to travel through the bloodstream and metastasize to other parts of the body, if not controlled through immunomodulatory mechanisms. Mechanisms thought to be important for this process include cell-mediated immunity (CMI) though cytotoxic T lymphocytes, NK cells, NKT cells, tissue macrophages, dendritic cells and helper T cells. Research has shown that cell-mediated immunosuppression following surgery or stress coincides with periods of compromised resistance to metastasis of a cancer cell line known to be NK-sensitive [131]

Hence Ben-Eliyahu (2003) [81] makes an argument for the role of surgery in promoting metastatic spread through suppression of CMI based on the following points: 1) In human models, general anaesthesia has been shown to suppress aspects of human CMI, such as NK activity and helper T-cell ratios, but local or regional anaesthesia is not immunosuppressive. When given in conjunction, local anaesthesia blunts the SNS and HPA reactivity to surgery and attenuates the degree of immunosuppression. In animals local anaesthesia when added to general, results in less suppression of CMI and less metastatic spread; 2) Blood transfusions suppress CMI (decreased NKCC and T-cell blastogenesis) and are also associated with poorer prognosis, independent of other complications and risk factors; 3) In the past, colorectal cancer was treated with two successive surgeries; when these were reduced to one, lower rates of metastatic spread and better survival was seen, in both humans and animal models; 4) minimally invasive surgeries are less immunosuppressive and also reduce the promotion of metastatic spread, in both animals and humans. Hence, an argument can be made for an important role of CMI in preventing metastatic spread after surgery, but little is known about what specific level of various immune cells or function is required to prevent such spread. It may also be the case that beyond the post-surgical period immune factors are relatively *unimportant* in the progression of tumour growth, which is supported by angiogenesis and the failure of apoptosis.

Growth Factors and Angiogenesis

Effects of stress on the tumour microenvironment including effects on the growth of a blood supply to tumours have been investigated quite extensively in recent years. Associations between elevated stress, lower social support and elevated levels of IL-6, a proinflammatory cytokine, and vascular endothelial growth factor (VEG-F), both promoters of angiogenesis in the tumour site, have been documented in ovarian cancer patients as well as *in vitro* cell cultures [13,132-134]. Immobilization stress increased tumour burden and enhanced angiogenesis and production of VEG-F within the tumour cell – angiogenesis is critical for tumour mass to increase beyond a certain size as the tumour cannot nourish itself without this development of its own blood supply. VEG-F also stimulates endothelial cell migration and proliferation and interferes with the development of T cells and the functional maturation of dendritic cells, which suggests additional negative effects on anti-tumour immune responses [10].

There are also effects of stress on viral oncogenesis, with many studies demonstrating accelerated growth of virally-induced tumours in animals who have been subjected to stressors [10]. Antoni et al [10] reviewed the neuroendocrine influences on various virally-related tumours and drew associations between HPA dysregulations and liver as well as cervical and head and neck cancers caused in part by Hepatitis B and C and human papilomavirus (HPV) viral exposure. They also drew associations between ANS reactivity and leukemia/lymphoma and Kaposi sarcomas cased in part by T-cell lymphotropic virus and Kaposi sarcoma-associated herpes virus, respectively [10], based on a review of primarily *in vitro* studies.

In summary, there are many potential avenues that stress and other psychological factors can "get in the body" and affect a whole host of processes important in cancer development and progression. Although the role of immunosurveillance is not a promising area of study for many cancer biologists, it may play an important role in prevention of metastatic spread of cancer cells following surgery. Other substances such as elevated epinephrine and cortisol may be cancer-promoting through several different mechanisms such as suppression of CMI. Elevated estrogens as a result of stress may also play a role in the pathogenesis of breast cancer, and testosterone may be important indirectly for its ability to aromatize to estrogens which can feed breast cancer cells, or by directly impacting prostate cancer development.

Other Issues for Intervention Research

Timing of Interventions

Little research has been done to investigate the importance of the timing of psychosocial intervention delivery, but there is reason to believe that the impact may be different depending on where in the process of diagnosis, treatment and recovery interventions are applied. Keeping in mind the research on the effects of surgery on CMI, it seems that post-surgery might be an opportune time to apply psychosocial interventions likely to enhance cellular immunity. Levels of distress are also high at this time, as evidenced not only by large surveys of distress levels [78,125], but also by studies of anxiety around the time of biopsy [136,137]. Women assessed at that time, both pre- and post-biopsy also showed changes in immune function. Lymphocytes at pre biopsy showed a lower expression of NFkB and Ap-1, transcription factors that regulate lymphocyte function, compared to post-biopsy. At post biopsy NFkB activity increased threefold and AP-1 activity nearly doubled. Post biopsy, the transcription factors were similar to those of the healthy controls [137]. In another similar study, women undergoing breast biopsy (later confirmed either malignant or benign) and a control group were assessed on levels of T-lymphocytes, NK cells, helper lymphocytes, cytotoxic lymphocytes, circulating monocytes and cytokines [136]. NK cell activity was reduced pre-biopsy and remained so for 3 months after results for the benign group of women. NK cell activity remained reduced for the women in the malignant group. IFN-γ was reduced in the malignant and nonmalignant groups pre and post biopsy but returned to normal levels for both groups at 3 months. This data illustrates that the time around biopsy and initial surgery is not only stressful, but also may be a time of biological vulnerability.

Only one study we are aware of investigated the effects of delayed versus early psychosocial interventions for women with early stage breast cancer [138], but they did not assess any immune or endocrine markers. All participants had received surgery no longer than 4 months prior to study participation. Participants were randomized to 1 of 4 conditions: early or late start and experiential existential group psychotherapy or a support group. Groups were closed and limited to 6-10 women. Thirty-three women were assigned to the early start: 19 in psychotherapy and 14 in social support, and 34 women were assigned to the delayed start condition: 16 in psychotherapy and18 in social support. In both interventions, women met for 2.5 hours for 12 weeks and included follow up groups at 1 and 2 months post-completion. Women who were assigned to the late intervention appeared more distressed at follow up than did the early starters, after controlling for baseline differences. Overall there were improvements in distress, body image, social interaction, and recreational activities.

Hence it may be possible, through carefully choosing the timing of interventions, to maximize the effects of psychosocial treatments to have the most beneficial effects on both reduction of psychological symptoms, and biological processes potentially important for disease course. Whether concomitant changes occurred in important parameters related to CMI as a result of these interventions, either soon after surgery or later, remains to be investigated in further research.

Type and Stage of Cancer

The issue of the importance of the specific type of cancer for determining psychological and biological responses to interventions has been addressed only infrequently in the psychosocial literature, but it is likely quite a critical point, as the pathophysiology of cancers varies greatly. Unfortunately, most of the research in these areas has been conducted on breast cancer populations, and most in early stage women after treatment. Hence it is difficult to directly compare effects of interventions on different types of cancer patients at a variety of stages of disease progression.

However, in one review on the etiology and progression of cancer in relation to psychosocial characteristics, effects were compared among different types and stages of cancers. The proportion of studies that found a link between psychosocial factors and disease progression was 73% in breast cancer, 75% in malignant melanoma, 67% in haematological malignancies, and an astounding 100% in lung cancers [30]. This is interesting as some researchers have suggested that psychosocial factors are more likely to be important in diseases with more favourable prognoses, where the tumour burden is perhaps less and more amenable to respond to changes in immune and endocrine function caused by psychosocial interventions [50]. The result that all studies included in this review found an association between lung cancer incidence and psychosocial factors can partly be explained by the behaviour of smoking, as not all studies controlled for the correlation between depression and smoking. Looking just at those that did statistically control for smoking, two-thirds failed to find a relationship between depression and lung cancer initiation, but one-third still upheld the relationship. However, if smoking is controlled for, there appears to be no stronger association between psychosocial factors and disease initiation in lung cancer than other commonly studied types. The authors of this review conclude that there is little convincing evidence that psychosocial factors are more important in the initiation of some types of cancers more than others.

Another perspective on this issue is put forth by Antoni et al [24], who suggest that virally-mediated tumours are likely to be more responsive to psychosocial influences than solid epithelial tumours. This is based on their work in HIV and AIDS-related conditions where they have shown significant effects of cognitive-behavioral stress management on numbers and function of important T-cell subtypes and NK cells. They speculate that cervical cancer, a causal factor of which is HPV infection, may be more responsive to psychosocial interventions than solid tumours with different pathogenesis such as breast cancers. This possibility has not yet been tested empirically.

The impact of the stage of tumour development on the effect that psychosocial interventions can have on disease progression has also been considered in the literature, but not extensively evaluated. The literature in the area of breast cancer is the only area extensive enough within which to directly address this question. In one review, 64% of 14 studies looking at nonmetastatic breast cancer found relationships between psychosocial factors and disease initiation or progression, and this was even higher in metastatic breast cancer at 83% [30]. However, some reviewers have concluded that interventions for treating cancer patients might best be applied to earlier-stage diseases, in the hopes of intervening earlier in the disease process before the tumour burden becomes overwhelming [50]. This issue awaits resolution with further research.

Health Behaviours

Included in the biopsychosocial model of disease etiology and progression are other factors with potential to influence disease outcomes, including health behaviours such as sleep, exercise, and diet. There is evidence linking each of these to cancer initiation and progression. In terms of sleep, in the general North American population 1/3 of adults experience intermittent insomnia, and 10% suffer chronic insomnia [139,140]. The prevalence of chronic insomnia is much higher in cancer, with anywhere from 30-50% of patients reporting sleep difficulties [141,142] that often persist well into the post-treatment period. In metastatic breast cancer patients, 63% reported serious sleeping problems [143]. Individuals with insomnia have been characterized by increases SNS activity, increased 24-hour metabolic rate, and elevated cortisol and NE. A general state of physiological hyperarousal is considered to be symptomatic of these poor sleepers, and insufficient sleep duration has recently been shown to be associated with all-cause mortality [144]. Hence, it is very important to consider the effects of sleep quality on disease outcome, and the impact improving sleep during psychosocial interventions such as stress reduction could have on overall outcomes.

Exercise has emerged in the literature of late as a risk factor for both cancer incidence and progression [145,146]. Recent epidemiological research analyzed the relation between physical activity and breast cancer incidence between 1990 and 2002 among 90,509 French women between 40 and 65 years of age [147]. A linear decrease in risk of breast cancer was observed with increasing amounts of moderate and vigorous recreational activities. Compared with women who reported no recreational activities, those with more than five weekly hours of vigorous exercise had a relative risk of 0.62 (CI=0.49-0.78). This decrease was still observed among women who were overweight, had no children, had a family history of breast cancer, or used hormone replacement therapy [147]. After diagnosis, exercise rehabilitation programs have been successful in improving quality of life and reducing all-cause mortality [148,149], and recent observational evidence suggests that moderate levels of physical activity may reduce the risk of death from breast cancer after diagnosis [150]. This study was based on responses from 2987 nurses in the Nurses' Health Study who were diagnosed with stage I, II, or III breast cancer. Women who engaged in higher levels of physical activity (the equivalent of walking at average pace of 2 to 2.9 mph for 1 hour, 3 times/week, at minimum) were less likely to die from breast cancer than those who exercised less. The benefit of physical activity was particularly apparent among women with hormone-responsive tumours (ER positive). This is the opposite of the recent study of supportive-expressive therapy which found effects only for women who were ER negative [62]. The potential interactions between ER status and psychosocial interventions have yet to be investigated in great detail.

Another study examined colorectal cancer death rates and exercise, and found similar results: Increasing levels of exercise after diagnosis of nonmetastatic colorectal cancer reduced cancer-specific mortality ($p = .008$) and overall mortality ($p = .003$) [151]. In this case, prediagnosis physical activity was not predictive of mortality. Women who increased their activity (when comparing prediagnosis to postdiagnosis values) had a hazard ratio of 0.48 for colorectal cancer deaths and a hazard ratio of 0.51 for any-cause death, compared with those with no change in activity. Hence, there is little question that physical activity can be an important factor in improving disease outcomes, and changes in this variable associated with decreased depression and stress should be addressed in future research.

Finally, diet is known as one of the most important risk factors for the development of a host of cancers, and thought to account for about 30-35% of overall risk [25]. In general, plant-based diets high in fruits and vegetables and low in red meat and saturated fats are considered to be the healthiest in terms of avoiding or recovering from cancer. Specifically, according to Key et al., (2004) [152] fruits and vegetables probably reduce the risk for cancers of the oral cavity, oesophagus, stomach and colorectum; preserved meat and red meat probably increase the risk for colorectal cancer; salt preserved foods and high salt intake probably increase the risk for stomach cancer; and very hot drinks and foods probably increase the risk for cancers of the oral cavity, pharynx and oesophagus.

Recommendations regarding diet in several other reviews are similar, but focussing more on the role of obesity and alcohol consumption. Indeed, as reviewed previously, obesity increases breast cancer risk in postmenopausal women by around 30%, probably by increasing serum concentrations of estradiol. Moderate alcohol intake increases breast cancer risk by about 7% per alcoholic drink per day, perhaps also by increasing estrogen levels. Populations with high fat intake generally have higher rates of breast cancer, but studies of individual women have not confirmed an association of high fat diets with breast cancer risk. Speculation is that nutrition might affect breast cancer risk by altering levels of growth factors such as insulin-like growth factor (IGF)-I [153].

In colorectal and other gastric cancers, consumption of fruits and vegetables appeared to have a modest role in prevention [154]. In contrast, the roles of alcohol consumption and overweight on risk of gastrointestinal cancer are more clear and similar to breast cancer: overweight and obesity are important risk factors for adenocarcinoma (but not squamous carcinoma) of the esophagus and colorectal cancer (particularly in men). Alcohol consumption is a risk factor for squamous carcinoma (but not adenocarcinoma) of the esophagus, gastric cancer and colorectal cancer [154].

One research group wished to investigate the interactions among diet, exercise and markers of prostate cancer risk including measures of insulin, free T, E, and IGF as well as sex hormone-binding globulin (SHBG), a positive prognostic marker [155]. They found that in men who undertook a low-fat diet and/or exercise program all these factors changed in the predicted directions, and these changes impacted prostate cancer cell lines in vitro to reduce cell growth and induce apoptosis (programmed cell death), primarily through increasing tumour cell p53 proteins [155]. This is a compelling example of the potential for dietary factors to directly affect processes known to be important for cancer development and progression.

In summary, it is possible that psychosocial interventions that often include discussion of health behaviours and extol the virtues of taking control of lifestyle factors may also result in changes in these important behaviours, not to mention stopping smoking, which accounts for about 30% of the risk for all cancers combined. Stress reduction interventions often report better sleep in participants [156], which may be a pathway though which changes in immune and endocrine function are mediated. Some interventions explicitly recommend or include exercise, and the literature on specific exercise effects in cancer patients is growing, although it was not reviewed in this paper [145,146].

Conclusion

In conclusion, this chapter has addressed associations between psychosocial variables and both disease initiation and progression, showing that the evidence is strongest for a role of social support, emotional repression, hopelessness and depression as potentially important factors in disease progression. As well, the evidence that psychosocial interventions can effect survival was reviewed, with the conclusion that there may be effects, but if so they are quite weak. The literature on the effects of psychosocial interventions on immune and endocrine outcomes was reviewed in greater detail, with the conclusion that a wide variety of psychosocial programs may effect aspects of cell-mediated immunity and stress hormone production. Potential mechanisms of action between immune and endocrine variables and cancer progression were summarized, including HPA and SNS mechanisms, the role of various hormones, immunosuppression and other mechanisms such as HPA promotion of angiogenesis and virally-induced tumour growth. All pathways show some promise but perhaps the most hope for future research finding links between psychosocial interventions and important factors in disease pathogenesis lies with the effect of stress on the regulation of circadian rhythms, growth factors such as VEG-F, and hormones such as melatonin, although very little research has been conducted in these areas to date. Finally, specific factors such as the timing of interventions, the types of cancers targeted and the stage of disease progression are important to consider, as are other factors that may affect outcomes such as sleep, exercise, diet and smoking. Application of a comprehensive biopsychosocial model of disease progression will help to guide future research efforts.

Abbreviations

ACTH	adrenocorticotropic hormone
ANS	autonomic nervous system
AP-1	activator protein 1
BDI	Beck Depression Inventory
BEST	breast expressive-supportive therapy
BMI	body mass index
CD3, CD4, CD8	specific t-cell cluster of differentiation
CES-D	Center for Epidemiological Studies-Depression
CI	confidence interval
CMI	cell mediated immunity
CNS	central nervous system
Con-A	canavalin A
CRF	corticotrophin-releasing factor
DHEAS	dehydroepiandosterone sulphate
EORTC-QLQ-30	European Organization for the Treatment of Cancer-Quality of Life Questionnaire-30
E	estrogen
EP	epinephrine
ER	estrogen receptor

FACT-B	Functional Assessment of Cancer Therapy-Breast
HADS	Hospital Anxiety and Depression Scale
HA	hazard ratio
HPA	hypothalamic-pituitary-adrenal
HPG	hypothalamic-pituitary-gonadal
HPV	human papillomavirus
HRT	hormone replacement therapy
IES	Impact of Events Scale
IFN-γ	Interferon-gamma
IgA	immunoglobulin-A
IGF	insulin-like growth factor
IgG	immunoglobulin-G
LGL	large granular lymphocyte
IgM	immunoglobulin-M
IL-1α	interluekin-1 alpha
IL-1β	interleukin-1 beta
IL-2	interleukin 2
IL-4	interleukin 4
IL-10	interleukin 10
MAC	Mental Adjustment to Cancer
MLR	mixed lymphocyte responsiveness
MMPI	Minnesota Multiphasic Personality Inventory
NK cells	natural killer cells
NE	norepinephrine
NFkB	Nuclear Factor kappa B
PBL	peripheral blood lymphocytes
PHA	phytohemagglutinin
PNE	psychoneuroendocrine
PNI	psychoneuroimmune
PNS	parasympathetic nervous system
POMS	Profile of Mood States
PSA	prostate-specific antigen
PSS	Perceived Stress Scale
RCT	randomized controlled trial
SEGT	supportive expressive group therapy
SHBG	sex hormone-binding growth factor
SIgA	salivary immunoglobulin A
SNS	sympathetic nervous system
SOSI	Symptoms of Stress Inventory
STAI	State-Trait Anxiety Inventory
STD	sexually transmitted disease
T	testosterone
VEG-F	vascular endothelial growth factor
WBC	white blood cell

Acknowledgments

Dr. Linda E. Carlson is supported by a New Investigator Award from the Canadian Institutes of Health Research and holds the Enbridge Endowed Research Chair in Psychosocial Oncology . Sheila Garland is funded by the University of Calgary and the Social Sciences and Humanities Research Council of Canada. Thanks to Jennifer Lowden for help with managing references.

References

[1] Temoshok, L. Personality, coping style, emotion and cancer: towards an integrative model. *Cancer Surv*, 1987, 6(3), 545-567.

[2] Greer, S; Watson, M. Towards a psychobiological model of cancer: psychological considerations. *Soc Sci Med*, 1985, 20(8), 773-777.

[3] Chen, E; Hanson, MD; Paterson, LQ; Griffin, MJ; Walker, HA; Miller, GE. Socioeconomic status and inflammatory processes in childhood asthma: the role of psychological stress. *J Allergy Clin Immunol*, 2006, 117(5), 1014-1020.

[4] Cohen S, Doyle WJ, Skoner DP. Psychological stress, cytokine production, and severity of upper respiratory illness. *Psychosom Med*, 1999, 61(2), 175-180.

[5] Daruna, JD. *Introduction to psychoneuroimmonology*. London, UK, Elsevier Academic Press, 2004.

[6] Miller, GE; Cohen, S; Ritchey, AK. Chronic psychological stress and the regulation of pro-inflammatory cytokines: A glucocorticoid-resistance model. *Health Psychol*, 2002, 21(6), 531-541.

[7] Rozlog, LA; Kiecolt-Glaser, JK; Marucha, PT; Sheridan, JF; Glaser, R. Stress and immunity: implications for viral disease and wound healing. *J Periodontol*, 1999, 70(7), 786-792.

[8] Segerstrom, SC; Miller, GE. Psychological stress and the human immune system: a meta-analytic study of 30 years of inquiry. *Psychol Bull*, 2004, 130(4), 601-630.

[9] Spiegel, D; Giese-Davis, J. Depression and cancer: mechanisms and disease progression. *Biol Psychiatry*, 2003, 54(3), 269-282.

[10] Antoni, MH; Lutgendorf, SK; Cole, SW; Dhabhar, FS; Sephton, SE; McDonald, PG; Stefanek, M; Sood, AK. The influence of bio-behavioural factors on tumour biology: pathways and mechanisms. *Nat Rev Cancer*, 2006, 6(3), 240-248.

[11] Andersen, BL; Kiecolt-Glaser, JK; Glaser, R. A biobehavioral model of cancer stress and disease course. *Am Psychol*, 1994, 49(5), 389-404.

[12] Cameron, LD; Leventhal, H. *The self-regulation of health and behavior*. New York, Routledge, 2003.

[13] Lutgendorf, SK; Costanzo, ES. Psychoneuroimmunology and health psychology: an integrative model. *Brain Behav Immun*, 2003, 17(4), 225-232.

[14] Sephton, S; Spiegel, D. Circadian disruption in cancer: A neuroendocrine-immune pathway from stress to disease? *Brain, Behavior, & Immunity*, 2003, 17(5), 321-328.

[15] Sephton, SE; Sapolsky, RM; Kraemer, HC; Spiegel, D. Diurnal cortisol rhythm as a predictor of breast cancer survival. *Journal of the National Cancer Institute*, 2000, 92(12), 944-1000.

[16] Spiegel, D; Sephton, SE. Psychoneuroimmune and endocrine pathways in cancer. effects of stress and support. [Review] [184 refs]. *Seminars in Clinical Neuropsychiatry*, 6(4), 252-65, 2001.

[17] Classen, C; Koopman, C; Hales, R; Spiegel, D. Acute stress disorder as a predictor of posttraumatic stress symptoms. *Am J Psychiatry*, 1998, 155(5), 620-624.

[18] Newell, SA; Sanson-Fisher, RW; Savolainen, NJ. Systematic review of psychological therapies for cancer patients: overview and recommendations for future research. *J Natl Cancer Inst*, 2002, 94(8), 558-584.

[19] Ross, L; Boesen, EH; Dalton, SO; Johansen, C. Mind and cancer: does psychosocial intervention improve survival and psychological well-being? [Review] [69 refs]. *European Journal of Cancer*, 38(11), 1447-57, 2002.

[20] Meyer, TJ; Mark, MM. Effects of psychosocial interventions with adult cancer patients: a meta-analysis of randomized experiments. *Health Psychol*, 1995, 14(2), 101-108.

[21] Smedslund, G; Ringdal, GI. Meta-analysis of the effects of psychosocial interventions on survival time in cancer patients. *J Psychosom Res*, 2004, 57(2), 123-131.

[22] van der Pompe, G; Antoni, M; Visser, A; Garssen, B. Adjustment to breast cancer: the psychobiological effects of psychosocial interventions. [Review] [77 refs]. *Patient Education & Counseling*, 28(2), 209-19, 1996.

[23] Garssen, B; Goodkin, K. On the role of immunological factors as mediators between psychosocial factors and cancer progression. *Psychiatry Res*, 1999, 85(1), 51-61.

[24] Antoni, MH. Psychoneuroendocrinology and psychoneuroimmunology of cancer: Plausible mechanisms worth pursuing? *Brain Behav Immun* 2003, 17 Suppl 1:S84-S91.

[25] Dollinger, M; Resenbaum, EH; Cable, G. *Everyone's Guide to Cancer Therapy: How Cancer is Diagnosed*, Treated, and Managed Day to Day. ed 3, Kansas City, Andrews McMeel Publishing, 1997.

[26] Butow, PN; Hiller, JE; Price, MA; Thackway, SV; Kricker, A; Tennant, CC. Epidemiological evidence for a relationship between life events, coping style, and personality factors in the development of breast cancer. *J Psychosom Res*, 2000, 49(3), 169-181.

[27] Price, MA; Tennant, CC; Butow, PN; Smith, RC; Kennedy, SJ; Kossoff, MB; Dunn, SM. The role of psychosocial factors in the development of breast carcinoma: Part II. Life event stressors, social support, defense style, and emotional control and their interactions. *Cancer*, 91(4), 686-97, 2001.

[28] Dalton, SO; Boesen, EH; Ross, L; Schapiro, IR; Johansen, C. Mind and cancer. Do psychological factors cause cancer? *Eur J Cancer,* 2002, 38(10), 1313-1323.

[29] Edelman, S; Kidman, A. Mind and cancer: Is there a relationship? A review of evidence. *Australian Psycologist*, 1997, 32(2), 79-85.

[30] Garssen, B. Psychological factors and cancer development: evidence after 30 years of research. [Review] [81 refs]. *Clinical Psychology Review*, 24(3), 315-38, 2004.

[31] Geyer, S. The role of social and psychosocial factors in the development and course of cancer. *Wien Klin Wochenschr*, 2000, 112(23), 986-994.

[32] McGee, R; Williams, S; Elwood, M. Are life events related to the onset of breast cancer. *Psychol Med*, 1996, 26(3), 441-447.

[33] McKenna, MC; Zevon, MA; Corn, B; Rounds, J. Psychosocial factors and the development of breast cancer: a meta-analysis. *Health Psychol*, 1999, 18(5), 520-531.

[34] Duijts, SF; Zeegers, MP; Borne, BV. The association between stressful life events and breast cancer risk: a meta-analysis. *Int J Cancer*, 2003, 107(6), 1023-1029.

[35] Kroenke, CH; Hankinson, SE; Schernhammer, ES; Colditz, GA; Kawachi, I; Holmes, MD. Caregiving stress, endogenous sex steroid hormone levels, and breast cancer incidence. *Am J Epidemiol*, 2004, 159(11), 1019-1027.

[36] Helgesson, O; Cabrera, C; Lapidus, L; Bengtsson, C; Lissner, L. Self-reported stress levels predict subsequent breast cancer in a cohort of Swedish women. *Eur J Cancer Prev*, 2003, 12(5), 377-381.

[37] Nielsen, NR; Zhang, ZF; Kristensen, TS; Netterstrom, B; Schnohr, P; Gronbaek, M. Self reported stress and risk of breast cancer: prospective cohort study. *BMJ*, 2005, 331(7516), 548.

[38] Petticrew, M; Fraser, J; Regan, MF. Adverse life-events and risk of breast caner: A meta-analysis. *British Journal of Health Psychology*, 1999, 4, 1-17.

[39] Jones, DR; Goldblatt, PO; Leon, DA. Bereavement and cancer: some data on deaths of spouses from the longitudinal study of Office of Population Censuses and Surveys. *Br Med J (Clin Res Ed)* 1984, 289(6443), 461-464.

[40] Kvikstad, A; Vatten, LJ; Tretli, S; Kvinnsland, S. Death of a husband or marital divorce related to risk of breast cancer in middle-aged women. A nested case-control study among Norwegian women born 1935-1954. *Eur J Cancer*, 1994, 30A(4), 473-477.

[41] Kvikstad, A; Vatten, LJ. Risk and prognosis of cancer in middle-aged women who have experienced the death of a child. *Int J Cancer*, 1996, 67(2), 165-169.

[42] Levav, I; Kohn, R; Iscovich, J; Abramson, JH; Tsai, WY; Vigdorovich, D. Cancer incidence and survival following bereavement. *Am J Public Health*, 2000, 90(10), 1601-1607.

[43] Schernhammer, ES; Hankinson, SE; Rosner, B; Kroenke, CH; Willett, WC; Colditz, GA; Kawachi, I. Job stress and breast cancer risk: the nurses' health study. *Am J Epidemiol*, 2004, 160(11), 1079-1086.

[44] Bleiker, EM; van der Ploeg, HM. Psychosocial factors in the etiology of breast cancer: review of a popular link. *Patient Educ Couns*, 1999, 37(3), 201-214.

[45] Reynolds, P; Kaplan, GA. Social connections and risk for cancer: prospective evidence from the Alameda County Study. *Behav Med*, 1990, 16(3), 101-110.

[46] Kroenke, CH; Bennett, GG; Fuchs, C; Giovannucci, E; Kawachi, I; Schernhammer, E; Holmes, MD; Kubzansky, LD. Depressive symptoms and prospective incidence of colorectal cancer in women. *Am J Epidemiol*, 2005, 162(9), 839-848.

[47] Shaffer, JW; Graves, PL; Swank, RT; Pearson, TA. Clustering of personality traits in youth and the subsequent development of cancer among physicians. *J Behav Med*, 1987, 10(5), 441-447.

[48] Bleiker, EM; van der Ploeg, HM; Hendriks, JH; Ader, HJ. Personality factors and breast cancer development: a prospective longitudinal study. *J Natl Cancer Inst*, 1996, 88(20), 1478-1482.

[49] Petticrew, M; Bell, R; Hunter, D. Influence of psychological coping on survival and recurrence in people with cancer: systematic review. *BMJ*, 2002, 325(7372), 1066.
[50] Cwikel, JG; Behar, LC; Zabora, JR. Psychosocial factors that affect the survival of adult cancer patients: A review of research. *Journal of Psychosocial Oncology*, 1997, 15(3/4), 1-34.
[51] Fox, BH. The role of psychological factors in cancer incidence and prognosis. *Oncology (Williston Park)*, 1995, 9(3), 245-253.
[52] Forsen, A. Psychosocial stress as a risk for breast cancer. *Psychother Psychosom* 1991, 55(2-4), 176-185.
[53] Martikainen, P; Valkonen, T. Mortality after the death of a spouse: rates and causes of death in a large Finnish cohort. *Am J Public Health*, 1996, 86(8), 1087-1093.
[54] Jones, DR; Goldblatt, PO. Cancer mortality following widow(er)hood: Some further results from the office of population censuses and surveys longitudinal study. *Stress Medicine*, 1986, 2, 129-229.
[55] Maunsell E, Brisson J, Deschenes L. Social support and survival among women with breast cancer. *Cancer* 1995, 76(4), 631-637.
[56] Reynolds, P; Boyd, PT; Blacklow, RS; Jackson, JS; Greenberg, RS; Austin, DF; Chen, VW; Edwards, BK. The relationship between social ties and survival among black and white breast cancer patients. National Cancer Institute Black/White Cancer Survival Study Group. *Cancer Epidemiol Biomarkers Prev*, 1994, 3(3), 253-259.
[57] Kroenke, CH; Kubzansky, LD; Schernhammer, ES; Holmes, MD; Kawachi, I. Social networks, social support, and survival after breast cancer diagnosis. *J Clin Oncol*, 2006, 24(7), 1105-1111.
[58] Brown, KW; Levy, AR; Rosberger, Z; Edgar, L. Psychological distress and cancer survival: a follow-up 10 years after diagnosis. *Psychosom Med*, 2003, 65(4), 636-643.
[59] Spiegel, D; Classen, C. *Group psychotherapy for cancer patients: A research-based handbook of psycosocial care*. New York, Basic Books, 2000.
[60] Spiegel, D; Bloom, JR; Kraemer, HC; Gottheil, E. Effect of psychosocial treatment on survival of patients with metastatic breast cancer. *Lancet*, 1989, 2(8668), 888-891.
[61] Goodwin, PJ; Leszcz, M; Ennis, M; Koopmans, J; Vincent, L; Guther, H; Drysdale, E; Hundleby, M; Chochinov, HM; Navarro, M; Speca, M; Hunter, J. The effect of group psychosocial support on survival in metastatic breast cancer. *N Engl J Med*, 2001, 345(24), 1719-1726.
[62] Spiegel, D; Butler, LD; Giese-Davis, J; Koopman, C; Miller, E; DiMiceli, S; Classen, C; Fobair, P; Carlson, RW; Kraemer, H. Effects of Supportive-Expressive Group Therapy on Survival of Patients with Metastatic Breast Cancer: A Randomized Clinical Intervention Trial. *Breast Cancer Res Treat*, 2006, 100(Supplement 1), S240.
[63] Gruber, BL; Hersh, SP; Hall, NR; Waletzky, LR; Kunz, JF; Carpenter, JK; Kverno, KS; Weiss, SM. Immunological responses of breast cancer patients to behavioral interventions. *Biofeedback Self Regul*, 1993, 18(1), 1-22.
[64] Andersen, BL; Farrar, WB; Golden-Kreutz, DM; Glaser, R; Emery, CF; Crespin, TR; Shapiro, CL; Carson, WE, III. Psychological, behavioral, and immune changes after a psychological intervention: a clinical trial. *J Clin Oncol*, 2004, 22(17), 3570-3580.

[65] Grossarth-Maticek, R; Eysenck, HJ. Length of survival and lymphocyte percentage in women with mammary cancer as a function of psychotherapy. *Psychol Rep*, 1989, 65(1), 315-321.

[66] Richardson, MA; Post-White, J; Grimm, EA; Moye, LA; Singletary, SE; Justice, B. Coping, life attitudes, and immune responses to imagery and group support after breast cancer treatment. *Altern Ther Health Med*, 1997, 3(5), 62-70.

[67] van der Pompe, G; Duivenvoorden, HJ; Antoni, MH; Visser, A; Heijnen, CJ. Effectiveness of a short-term group psychotherapy program on endocrine and immune function in breast cancer patients: An exploratory study. *J Psychosom Res*, 1997, 42(5), 453-466.

[68] Chan, CL; Ho, RT; Lee, PW; Cheng, JY; Leung, PP; Foo, W; Chow, LW; Sham, JS; Spiegel, D. A randomized controlled trial of psychosocial interventions using the psychophysiological framework for Chinese breast cancer patients. *J Psychosoc Oncol*, 2006, 24(1), 3-26.

[69] Larson, MR; Duberstein, PR; Talbot, NL; Caldwell, C; Moynihan, JA. A presurgical psychosocial intervention for breast cancer patients. psychological distress and the immune response. *J Psychosom Res*, 2000, 48(2), 187-194.

[70] Cruess, DG; Antoni, MH; McGregor, BA; Kilbourn, KM; Boyers, AE; Alferi, SM; Carver, CS; Kumar, M. Cognitive-behavioral stress management reduces serum cortisol by enhancing benefit finding among women being treated for early stage breast cancer. *Psychosom Med*, 2000, 62(3), 304-308.

[71] Hidderley, M; Holt, M. A pilot randomized trial assessing the effects of autogenic training in early stage cancer patients in relation to psychological status and immune system responses. *European Journal of Oncology Nursing*, 2004, 8(1), 61-65.

[72] Fawzy, FI; Kemeny, ME; Fawzy, NW; Elashoff, R; Morton, D; Cousins, N; Fahey, JL. A structured psychiatric intervention for cancer patients. II. Changes over time in immunological measures. *Arch Gen Psychiatry*, 1990, 47(8), 729-735.

[73] Schedlowski, M; Jung, C; Schimanski, G; Tewes, U; Schmoll, H. Effects of behavioral interventions on plasma cortisol and lymphocytes in breast cancer patients: An exploratory study. *Psychooncology*, 1994, 3, 181-187.

[74] Lekander, M; Furst, CJ; Rotstein, S; Hursti, TJ; Fredrikson, M. Immune effects of relaxation during chemotherapy for ovarian cancer. *Psychother Psychosom*, 1997, 66(4), 185-191.

[75] de Vries, MJ; Schilder, JN; Mulder, CL; Vrancken, AM; Remie, M; Garssen, B. Phase II study of psychotherapeutic intervention in advanced cancer. *Psychooncology*, 1997, 6(2), 129-137.

[76] Burns, SJ; Harbuz, MS; Hucklebridge, F; Bunt, L. A pilot study into the therapeutic effects of music therapy at a cancer help center. *Altern Ther Health Med*, 2001, 7(1), 48-56.

[77] Carlson, LE; Speca, M; Patel, KD; Goodey, E. Mindfulness-based stress reduction in relation to quality of life, mood, symptoms of stress, and immune parameters in breast and prostate cancer outpatients. *Psychosom Med*, 2003, 65(4), 571-581.

[78] Carlson, LE; Speca, M; Patel, KD; Goodey, E. Mindfulness-based stress reduction in relation to quality of life, mood, symptoms of stress and levels of cortisol,

dehydroepiandrosterone sulfate (DHEAS) and melatonin in breast and prostate cancer outpatients. *Psychoneuroendocrinology*, 2004, 29(4), 448-474.

[79] Cruess, DG; Antoni, M; Kumar, M; McGregor, BA; Alferi, SM; Boyers, AE; Carver, CS; Kilshourn, L. Effects of stress management on testosterone levels in women with early stage breast cancer. *International Journal of Behavioral Medicine*, 2001, 8, 194-207.

[80] Bovbjerg, DH. Conditioning, cancer, and immune regulation. *Brain Behav Immun*, 2003, 17 Suppl 1, S58-S61.

[81] Ben-Eliyahu, S. The promotion of tumor metastasis by surgery and stress: immunological basis and implications for psychoneuroimmunology. *Brain Behav Immun*, 2003, 17 Suppl 1:S27-S36.

[82] Spiegel, D; Sephton, SE; Terr, AI; Stites, DP. Effects of psychosocial treatment in prolonging cancer survival may be mediated by neuroimmune pathways. *Ann N Y Acad Sci*, 1998, 840(674), 683.

[83] Cohen, S; Williamson, GM. Stress and infectious disease in humans. *Psychol Bull*, 1991, 109(1), 5-24.

[84] Sikes, CRA; Lasley, BJ. Cognitive sequelae of hypothalamic-pituitary-adrenal (HPA) dysregulation in depression. *Biological Psychiatry*, 1989, 25, 148A-149A.

[85] Wolkowitz, OM. Prospective controlled studies of the behavioral and biological effects of exogenous corticosteroids. *Psychoneuroendocrinology*, 1994, 3(19), 233-255.

[86] Abercrombie, HC; Giese-Davis, J; Sephton, S; Epel, ES; Turner-Cobb, JM; Spiegel, D. Flattened cortisol rhythms in metastatic breast cancer patients. P*sychoneuroendocrinology*, 2004, 29(8), 1082-1092.

[87] van der Pompe, G; Antoni, MH; Heijnen, CJ. Elevated basal cortisol levels and attenuated ACTH and cortisol responses to a behavioral challenge in women with metastatic breast cancer. *Psychoneuroendocrinology*, 1996, 21(4), 361-374.

[88] Porter, LS; Mishel, M; Neelon, V; Belyea, M; Pisano, E; Soo, MS. Cortisol levels and responses to mammography screening in breast cancer survivors: a pilot study. *Psychosom Med*, 2003, 65(5), 842-848.

[89] Touitou, Y; Bogdan, A; Levi, F; Benavides, M; Auzeby, A. Disruption of the circadian patterns of serum cortisol in breast and ovarian cancer patients: relationships with tumour marker antigens. *British Journal of Cancer*, 74(8), 1248-52, 1996.

[90] Ticher, A; Haus, E; Ron, IG; Sackett-Lundeen, L; Ashkenazi, IE. The pattern of hormonal circadian time structure (acrophase) as an assessor of breast-cancer risk. *International Journal of Cancer*, 1996, 65(5), 591-593.

[91] Mormont, MC; Levi, F. Circadian-system alterations during cancer processes: a review. *Int J Cancer*, 1997, 70(2), 241-247.

[92] Turner-Cobb, J; Sephton, SE; Spiegel, D. Psychosocial effects on immune function and disease progression in cancer:human studies., in: Ader R, Pelten D, Cohen N, (eds), *Psychoneuroimmunology*. San Diego, Academin Press, 2001, pp 565-582.

[93] Levy, SM; Herberman, RB; Lippman, M; D'Angelo, T; Lee, J. Immunological and psychosocial predictors of disease recurrence in patients with early-stage breast cancer. *Behav Med*, 1991, 17(2), 67-75.

[94] Bettermann, H; Kroz, M; Girke, M; Heckmann, C. Heart rate dynamics and cardiorespiratory coordination in diabetic and breast cancer patients. *Clin Physiol*, 2001, 21(4), 411-420.

[95] Gold, SM; Zakowski, SG; Valdimarsdottir, HB; Bovbjerg, DH. Stronger endocrine responses after brief psychological stress in women at familial risk of breast cancer. *Psychoneuroendocrinology*, 2003, 28(4), 584-593.

[96] James, GD; Berge-Landry, HH; Valdimarsdottir, HB; Montgomery, GH; Bovbjerg, DH. Urinary catecholamine levels in daily life are elevated in women at familial risk of breast cancer. *Psychoneuroendocrinology*, 2004, 29(7), 831-838.

[97] Linsell, CR; Lightman, SL; Mullen, PE; Brown, MJ; Causon, RC. Circadian rhythms of epinephrine and norepinephrine in man. *J Clin Endocrinol Metab*, 1985, 60(6), 1210-1215.

[98] Laconi, E; Tomasi, C; Curreli, F; Diana, S; Laconi, S; Serra, G; Collu, M; Pani, P. Early exposure to restraint stress enhances chemical carcinogenesis in rat liver. *Cancer Lett*, 2000, 161(2), 215-220.

[99] Ben-Eliyahu, S; Shakhar, G; Page, GG; Stefanski, V; Shakhar, K. Suppression of NK cell activity and of resistance to metastasis by stress: a role for adrenal catecholamines and beta-adrenoceptors. *Neuroimmunomodulation*, 2000, 8(3), 154-164.

[100] Page, GG; Ben-Eliyahu, S. A role for NK cells in greater susceptibility of young rats to metastatic formation. *Dev Comp Immunol*, 1999, 23(1), 87-96.

[101] Ben-Eliyahu, S; Yirmiya, R; Liebeskind, JC; Taylor, AN; Gale, RP. Stress increases metastatic spread of a mammary tumor in rats: evidence for mediation by the immune system. *Brain, Behavior, & Immunity*, 1991, 5(2), 193-205.

[102] Melamed, R; Rosenne, E; Shakhar, K; Schwartz, Y; Abudarham, N; Ben-Eliyahu, S. Marginating pulmonary-NK activity and resistance to experimental tumor metastasis: suppression by surgery and the prophylactic use of a beta-adrenergic antagonist and a prostaglandin synthesis inhibitor. *Brain Behav Immun*, 2005, 19(2), 114-126.

[103] Ticher, A; Haus, E; Ron, IG; Sackett-Lundeen, L; Ashkenazi, IE. The pattern of hormonal circadian time structure (acrophase) as an assessor of breast-cancer risk. *International Journal of Cancer*, 1996, 65(5), 591-593.

[104] Velie, EM; Nechuta, S; Osuch, JR. Lifetime reproductive and anthropometric risk factors for breast cancer in postmenopausal women. *Breast Dis*, 2005, 24:17-35.

[105] Jaiyesimi, IA; Buzdar, AU; Decker, DA; Hortobagyi, GN. Use of tamoxifen for breast cancer: twenty-eight years later. *J Clin Oncol*, 1995, 13(2), 513-529.

[106] Lorincz, AM; Sukumar, S. Molecular links between obesity and breast cancer. *Endocr Relat Cancer*, 2006, 13(2), 279-292.

[107] Reiche, EM; Morimoto, HK; Nunes, SM. Stress and depression-induced immune dysfunction: implications for the development and progression of cancer. *Int Rev Psychiatry*, 2005, 17(6), 515-527.

[108] Holden, RJ; Pakula, IS; Mooney, PA. An immunological model connecting the pathogenesis of stress, depression and carcinoma. *Med Hypotheses*, 1998, 51(4), 309-314.

[109] Hauser, P; Soler, R; Reed, S; Kane, R; Gulati, M; Khosla, J; Kling, MA; Valentine, AD; Meyers, CA. Prophylactic treatment of depression induced by interferon-alpha. *Psychosomatics*, 2000, 41(5), 439-441.

[110] Capuron, L; Ravaud, A; Dantzer, R. Early depressive symptoms in cancer patients receiving interleukin 2 and/or interferon alfa-2b therapy. *J Clin Oncol*, 2000, 18(10), 2143-2151.

[111] Tilg, H; Atkins, MB; Dinarello, CA; Mier, JW. Induction of circulating interleukin 10 by interleukin 1 and interleukin 2, but not interleukin 6 immunotherapy. *Cytokine*, 1995, 7(7), 734-739.

[112] Maes, M; Bosmans, E; De, JR; Kenis, G; Vandoolaeghe, E; Neels, H. Increased serum IL-6 and IL-1 receptor antagonist concentrations in major depression and treatment resistant depression. *Cytokine*, 1997, 9(11), 853-858.

[113] Seidel, A; Arolt, V; Hunstiger, M; Rink, L; Behnisch, A; Kirchner, H. Cytokine production and serum proteins in depression. *Scand J Immunol*, 1995, 41(6), 534-538.

[114] Sluzewska, A; Rybakowski, J; Bosmans, E; Sobieska, M; Berghmans, R; Maes, M; Wiktorowicz, K. Indicators of immune activation in major depression. *Psychiatry Res*, 1996, 64(3), 161-167.

[115] Morgentaler, A. Testosterone replacement therapy and prostate risks: where's the beef? *Can J Urol*, 2006, 13 Suppl 1:40-43.

[116] Slater, S; Oliver, RT. Testosterone: its role in development of prostate cancer and potential risk from use as hormone replacement therapy. *Drugs Aging*, 2000, 17(6), 431-439.

[117] Shaneyfelt, T; Husein, R; Bubley, G; Mantzoros, CS. Hormonal predictors of prostate cancer: a meta-analysis. *J Clin Oncol*, 2000, 18(4), 847-853.

[118] Margolese, HC. The male menopause and mood: testosterone decline and depression in the aging male--is there a link? *J Geriatr Psychiatry Neurol*, 2000, 13(2), 93-101.

[119] Saxe, GA; Hebert, JR; Carmody, JF; Kabat-Zinn, J; Rosenzweig, PH; Jarzobski, D; Reed, GW; Blute, RD. Can diet in conjunction with stress reduction affect the rate of increase in prostate specific antigen after biochemical recurrence of prostate cancer? *J Urol*, 2001, 166(6), 2202-2207.

[120] Saez, MC; Barriga, C; Garcia, JJ; Rodriguez, AB; Masot, J; Duran, E; Ortega, E. Melatonin increases the survival time of animals with untreated mammary tumours: neuroendocrine stabilization. *Mol Cell Biochem*, 2005, 278(1-2), 15-20.

[121] Bubenik, GA; Blask, DE; Brown, GM; Maestroni, GJ; Pang, SF; Reiter, RJ; Viswanathan, M; Zisapel, N. Prospects of the clinical utilization of melatonin. *Biol Signals Recept*, 1998, 7(4), 195-219.

[122] Vijayalaxmi, Thomas CR, Jr., Reiter, RJ; Herman, TS. Melatonin: from basic research to cancer treatment clinics. *J Clin Oncol*, 2002, 20(10), 2575-2601.

[123] Vijayalaxmi, Meltz ML; Reiter, RJ; Herman, TS. Melatonin and protection from genetic damage in blood and bone marrow: whole-body irradiation studies in mice. *Journal of Pineal Research*, 1999, 27(4), 221-225.

[124] Vijayalaxmi, Reiter RJ; Meltz, ML; Herman, TS. Melatonin: possible mechanisms involved in its 'radioprotective' effect. *Mutation Research*, 1998, 404(1-2), 187-189.

[125] Lissoni, P; Barni, S; Mandala, M; Ardizzoia, A; Paolorossi, F; Vaghi, M; Longarini, R; Malugani, F; Tancini, G. Decreased toxicity and increased efficacy of cancer chemotherapy using the pineal hormone melatonin in metastatic solid tumour patients with poor clinical status. *Eur J Cancer*, 1999, 35(12), 1688-1692.

[126] Lissoni, P; Cazzaniga, M; Tancini, G; Scardino, E; Musci, R; Barni, S; Maffezzini, M; Meroni, T; Rocco, F; Conti, A; Maestroni, G. Reversal of clinical resistance to LHRH analogue in metastatic prostate cancer by the pineal hormone melatonin: efficacy of LHRH analogue plus melatonin in patients progressing on LHRH analogue alone. *Eur Urol*, 1997, 31(2), 178-181.

[127] Tamarkin, L; Danforth, D; Lichter, A; DeMoss, E; Cohen, M; Chabner, B; Lippman, M. Decreased nocturnal plasma melatonin peak in patients with estrogen receptor positive breast cancer. *Science*, 1982, 216(4549), 1003-1005.

[128] Schernhammer, ES; Laden, F; Speizer, FE; Willett, WC; Hunter, DJ; Kawachi, I; Colditz, GA. Rotating night shifts and risk of breast cancer in women participating in the nurses' health study. *J Natl Cancer Inst*, 2001, 93(20), 1563-1568.

[129] Davis, S; Mirick, DK; Stevens, RG. Night shift work, light at night, and risk of breast cancer. *J Natl Cancer Inst*, 2001, 93(20), 1557-1562.

[130] Carlson, LE; Campbell, TS; Garland, SG; Grossman, P. Associations among salivary cortisol, melatonin, catecholamines, sleep quality and stress in women with breast cancer and healthy controls. *J Behav Med.*, In press.

[131] Ben-Eliyahu, S; Page, GG; Yirmiya, R; Shakhar, G. Evidence that stress and surgical interventions promote tumor development by suppressing natural killer cell activity. *Int J Cancer*, 1999, 80(6), 880-888.

[132] Costanzo, ES; Lutgendorf, SK; Sood, AK; Anderson, B; Sorosky, J; Lubaroff, DM. Psychosocial factors and interleukin-6 among women with advanced ovarian cancer. *Cancer*, 2005, 104(2), 305-313.

[133] Thaker, PH; Han, LY; Kamat, AA; Arevalo, JM; Takahashi, R; Lu, C; Jennings, NB; rmaiz-Pena, G; Bankson, JA; Ravoori, M; Merritt, WM; Lin, YG; Mangala, LS; Kim, TJ; Coleman, RL; Landen, CN; Li, Y; Felix, E; Sanguino, AM; Newman, RA; Lloyd, M; Gershenson, DM; Kundra, V; Lopez-Berestein, G; Lutgendorf, SK; Cole, SW; Sood, AK. Chronic stress promotes tumor growth and angiogenesis in a mouse model of ovarian carcinoma. *Nat Med* 2006, 12(8), 939-944.

[134] Lutgendorf, SK; Logan, H; Costanzo, E; Lubaroff, D. Effects of acute stress, relaxation, and a neurogenic inflammatory stimulus on interleukin-6 in humans. *Brain Behav Immun*, 2004, 18(1), 55-64.

[135] Zabora, J; BrintzenhofeSzoc, K; Curbow, B; Hooker, C; Piantadosi, S. The prevalence of psychological distress by cancer site. *Psycho-Oncology*, 10(1), 19-28, 2001, -Feb.

[136] Witek-Janusek, L; Gabram, S; Mathews, HL. Psychologic stress, reduced NK cell activity, and cytokine dysregulation in women experiencing diagnostic breast biopsy. *Psychoneuroendocrinology*, 2006.

[137] Nagabhushan, M; Mathews, HL; Witek-Janusek, L. Aberrant nuclear expression of AP-1 and NFkappaB in lymphocytes of women stressed by the experience of breast biopsy. *Brain Behav Immun*, 2001, 15(1), 78-84.

[138] Vos, PJ; Visser, AP; Garssen, B; Duivenvoorden, HJ, de Haes HC. Effects of delayed psychosocial interventions versus early psychosocial interventions for women with early stage breast cancer. *Patient Educ Couns*, 2006, 60(2), 212-219.

[139] Hossain, JL; Shapiro, CM. The prevalence, cost implications, and management of sleep disorders: an overview. *Sleep Breath*, 2002, 6(2), 85-102.

[140] Kushida, CA; Nichols, DA; Simon, RD; Young, T; Grauke, JH; Britzmann, JB; Hyde, PR; Dement, WC. Symptom-Based Prevalence of Sleep Disorders in an Adult Primary Care Population. *Sleep Breath*, 2000, 4(1), 9-14.

[141] Savard, J; Simard, S; Blanchet, J; Ivers, H; Morin, CM. Prevalence, clinical characteristics, and risk factors for insomnia in the context of breast cancer. *Sleep* 2001, 24(5), 583-590.

[142] Savard J, Morin CM. Insomnia in the context of cancer: a review of a neglected problem. *J Clin Oncol* 2001, 19(3), 895-908.

[143] Koopman C, Butler LD, Classen C, Giese-Davis J, Morrow GR, Westendorf J, Banerjee T, Spiegel D. Traumatic stress symptoms among women with recently diagnosed primary breast cancer. *J Trauma Stress* 2002, 15(4), 277-287.

[144] Kripke, DF; Garfinkel, L; Wingard, DL; Klauber, MR; Marler, MR. Mortality associated with sleep duration and insomnia. *Arch Gen Psychiatry*, 2002, 59(2), 131-136.

[145] Courneya, KS. Exercise in cancer survivors: an overview of research. *Med Sci Sports Exerc*, 2006, 35, 1846-1852.

[146] Courneya, KS. Exercise interventions during cancer treatment: biopsychosocial outcomes. *Exerc Sport Sci Rev*, 2001, 29(2), 60-64.

[147] Tehard, B; Friedenreich, CM; Oppert, JM; Clavel-Chapelon, F. Effect of physical activity on women at increased risk of breast cancer: results from the E3N cohort study. *Cancer Epidemiol Biomarkers Prev*, 2006, 15(1), 57-64.

[148] Farrell, SW; Braun, L; Barlow, CE; Cheng, YJ; Blair, SN. The relation of body mass index, cardiorespiratory fitness, and all-cause mortality in women. *Obes Res*, 2002, 10(6), 417-423.

[149] McNeely, ML; Campbell, KL; Rowe, BH; Klassen, TP; Mackey, JR; Courneya, KS. Effects of exercise on breast cancer patients and survivors. a systematic review and meta-analysis. *CMAJ*, 2006, 175(1), 34-41.

[150] Holmes, MD; Chen, WY; Feskanich, D; Kroenke, CH; Colditz, GA. Physical activity and survival after breast cancer diagnosis. *JAMA*, 2005, 293(20), 2479-2486.

[151] Meyerhardt, JA; Giovannucci, EL; Holmes, MD; Chan, AT; Chan, JA; Colditz, GA; Fuchs, CS. Physical activity and survival after colorectal cancer diagnosis. *J Clin Oncol*, 2006, 24(22), 3527-3534.

[152] Key, TJ; Schatzkin, A; Willett, WC; Allen, NE; Spencer, EA; Travis, RC. Diet, nutrition and the prevention of cancer. *Public Health Nutr*, 2004, 7(1A), 187-200.

[153] Key, TJ; Allen, NE; Spencer, EA; Travis, RC. Nutrition and breast cancer. *Breast*, 2003, 12(6), 412-416.

[154] van den Brandt, PA; Goldbohm, RA. Nutrition in the prevention of gastrointestinal cancer. *Best Pract Res Clin Gastroenterol*, 2006, 20(3), 589-603.

[155] Barnard, RJ; Aronson, WJ. Preclinical models relevant to diet, exercise, and cancer risk. *Recent Results Cancer Res*, 2005, 166, 47-61.

[156] Carlson, LE; Garland, SN. Impact of mindfulness-based stress reduction (MBSR) on sleep, mood, stress and fatigue symptoms in cancer outpatients. *International Journal of Behavioral Medicine*, 2005, 12(4), 278-285.

INDEX

A

B

C

D

E

F

G

H

I

J

K

L

M

N

O

P

Q

R

S

T

U

V

W

Y